A History of Epidemiologic Methods and Concepts

Edited by Alfredo Morabia

Birkhäuser Verlag
Basel · Boston · Berlin

Editor:

Alfredo Morabia
Division of Clinical Epidemiology
University Hospital
24 rue Micheli-du-Crest
1211 Geneva 14
Switzerland

Library of Congress Cataloging-in-Publication Data

A history of epidemiologic methods and concepts / edited by Alfredo Morabia.
   p. cm.
  Includes bibliographical references and index.
  ISBN 3-7643-6818-7 (alk. paper)
   1. Epidemiology--History. I. Morabia, Alfredo.

RA649.H55 2004
614.4--dc22

2004052802

Bibliographic information published by Die Deutsche Bibliothek
Die Deutsche Bibliothek lists this publication in the Deutsche Nationalbibliografie;
detailed bibliographic data is available in the Internet at <http://dnb.ddb.de>.

ISBN 978-3-7643-6818-0 Birkhäuser Verlag, Basel - Boston - Berlin

The publisher and editor can give no guarantee for the information on drug dosage and administration contained in this publication. The respective user must check its accuracy by consulting other sources of reference in each individual case.
The use of registered names, trademarks etc. in this publication, even if not identified as such, does not imply that they are exempt from the relevant protective laws and regulations or free for general use.
This work is subject to copyright. All rights are reserved, whether the whole or part of the material is concerned, specifically the rights of translation, reprinting, re-use of illustrations, recitation, broadcasting, reproduction on microfilms or in other ways, and storage in data banks. For any kind of use, permission of the copyright owner must be obtained.

© 2004 Birkhäuser Verlag, P.O. Box 133, CH-4010 Basel, Switzerland
Part of Springer Science+Business Media
Printed on acid-free paper produced from chlorine-free pulp. TCF ∞
Cover design: Micha Lotrovsky, CH-4106 Therwil, Switzerland
Printed in Germany
ISBN-10: 3-7643-6818-7
ISBN-13: 978-3-7643-6818-0

9 8 7 6 5 4 3

www.birkhauser.ch

Contents

List of contributors	xi
Preface	xiii
The Annecy workshop	xiii
What this book is and what it is not	xiii
Epidemiology teaching	xv
An antidote to dogmatism	xvi
How to use this book?	xvi
Acknowledgements	xvii

Alfredo Morabia
Part I: Epidemiology: An epistemological perspective 1

1.	Introduction	3
1.1.	A contextual name	3
1.2.	Historical contribution of epidemiology	4
1.3.	Theme of this essay	5
2.	Population thinking	7
2.1.	Definitions	7
2.1.1.	Ratios, risks, rates and odds	8
2.1.2.	Prevalence, incidence, mortality, case fatality	9
2.2.	Origin of population thinking	9
2.3.	Early ratios, proportions and rates	11
2.3.1.	Eighteenth century	11
	a) Proportions	12
	b) Ratios	12
	c) Rates	13
2.3.2.	Nineteenth century	14
	a) Ratios	14
	b) Proportions	15
2.4.	Risks and rates	16
2.4.1.	Burden of life destruction and force of mortality	16
2.4.2.	The fallacy resulting from neglect of the period of exposure to risk	19
2.4.3.	Incidence density and cumulative Incidence	21

2.5.	Prevalence and incidence	23
2.5.1.	Disease prevalence divided by incidence	23
2.5.2.	Exposure prevalence multiplied by (excess) incidence	25
2.6.	Risk and strength of association	28
2.7.	Evolution of population thinking in epidemiology	30
3.	Group comparisons	32
3.1.	Definition	32
3.2.	Eighteenth century	33
3.3.	Nineteenth century	37
3.3.1.	The bloodletting controversy	37
3.3.2.	The London 1854 natural experiment	39
3.4.	Evolution of confounding	42
3.4.1.	The paradoxical fate of a fallacy	43
3.4.2.	Early analyses of confounding	48
3.4.3.	Cohort analysis	53
3.4.4.	Alternate allocation of treatment	56
3.4.5.	Logic of confounding	58
3.5.	Case-control studies	59
3.6.	Cohort studies	62
3.7.	Selection bias	65
3.8.	Interaction	68
3.9.	Causal inference	72
3.10.	The rare disease assumption	75
3.11.	Refinements of the theory of case-control studies	78
3.11.1.	Sampling schemes of controls	79
3.11.2.	Sampling controls independent of exposure	82
3.12.	Evolution of group comparisons in epidemiology	83
3.12.1.	Comparing like with like	84
3.12.2.	Fallacies resulting from group incomparability	85
3.12.3.	Treatment allocation	85
3.12.4.	The name of the game	86
3.12.5.	Case-control and cohort studies	87
4.	Epistemology	89
4.1.	Tribute to Piaget	89
4.2.	Evolution of physics	91
4.3.	Was Hippocrates an epidemiologist?	92
4.4.	Traces of epidemiology in the Bible?	95
4.5.	The impossible comparison	96
4.6.	Why did epidemiology appear so late in human history?	97
4.7.	Emergence of probability	99

4.8.	A theory of group comparison	100
4.9.	Causal inference	102
4.10.	Principles of knowledge acquisition in epidemiology	105
5.	Phases of epidemiology	106
5.1.	Preformal epidemiology	107
5.1.1.	Preformal epidemiologists	107
5.1.2.	Population thinking and group comparisons	107
5.1.3.	More examples	110
5.1.4.	Definition of epidemiology	112
5.2.	Early epidemiology	112
5.2.1.	Early epidemiologists	112
5.2.2.	Population thinking	113
5.2.3.	Group comparisons	114
5.2.4.	Concepts	115
5.2.5.	Definitions of epidemiology	116
5.3.	Classic epidemiology	117
5.3.1.	Classic epidemiologists	117
5.3.2.	Population thinking	117
5.3.3.	Study designs	119
5.3.4.	Concepts	120
5.3.5.	Definition of epidemiology	120
5.4.	Modern epidemiology	121
5.4.1.	Modern epidemiologists	121
5.4.2.	Population thinking	122
5.4.3.	Study designs	122
5.4.4.	Concepts	123
5.4.5.	Definition of epidemiology	123
5.5.	What will come next?	124
6.	Conclusion	124

Part II: Collection of papers on the history of epidemiological methods and concepts 127

John M. Eyler
The changing assessments of John Snow's and William Farr's cholera studies .. 129

Jan P. Vandenbroucke
Changing images of John Snow in the history of epidemiology 141

John M. Eyler
Constructing vital statistics: Thomas Rowe Edmonds and William Farr,
1835–1845 149

William Farr
"On Prognosis" (British Medical Almanack 1838;
Supplement 199–216) 159

Gerry Bernhard Hill
Comments on the paper "On prognosis" by William Farr: a forgotten
masterpiece 179

B. Burt Gerstman
Comments regarding "On prognosis" by William Farr (1838), with reconstruction of his longitudinal analysis of smallpox recovery and death rates 183

Jan P. Vandenbroucke
Continuing controversies over "risks and rates" – more than a century
after William Farr's "On prognosis" 191

John M. Eyler
Understanding William Farr's 1838 article "On prognosis": comment 195

Anne Hardy
Methods of outbreak investigation in the "Era of Bacteriology" 1880–1920 .. 199

Anne Hardy, M. Eileen Magnello
Statistical methods in epidemiology: Karl Pearson, Ronald Ross,
Major Greenwood and Austin Bradford Hill, 1900–1945 207

George W. Comstock
Cohort analysis: W.H. Frost's contributions to the epidemiology of tuberculosis
and chronic disease 223

Benedetto Terracini, Roberto Zanetti
A short history of pathology registries, with emphasis on cancer registries 231

Sir Richard Doll
Cohort studies: history of the method 243

Steven D. Stellmann
Issues of causality in the history of occupational epidemiology 275

Nigel Paneth, Ezra Susser, Mervyn Susser
Origins and early development of the case-control study 291

Jan P. Vandenbroucke
The history of confounding 313

Paolo Vineis
History of bias 327

Paolo Vineis
Causality in epidemiology 337

Fang F. Zhang, Desireé C. Michaels, Barun Mathema, Shuaib Kauchali, Anjan Chatterjee, David C. Ferris, Tamarra M. James, Jennifer Knight, Matthew Dounel, Hebatullah O. Tawfik, Janet A. Frohlich, Li Kuang, Elena K. Hoskin, Frederick J. Veldman, Giulia Baldi, Koleka P. Mlisana, Lerole D. Mametja, Angela Diaz, Nealia L. Khan, Pamela Sternfels, Jeffery J. Sevigny, Asher Shamam, Alfredo Morbia
Evolution of epidemiologic methods and concepts in selected textbooks
of the 20th century 351

Kenneth J. Rothman
Commentary on the paper by Zhang et al. – Interaction and evolution
in epidemiology 363

Olli S. Miettinen
Commentary on the paper by Zhang et al. – Lack of evolution
of epidemiologic "methods and concepts" 365

References 367

Index of persons 397

Subject index 401

List of Contributors

George W. Comstock, The Johns Hopkins University, School of Hygiene and Public Health, Washington County Health Department, Box 2967, Hagerstown, MD 21742-2067, USA; e-mail: gcomstoc@jhsph.edu

Sir Richard Doll, CTSU, Harkness Building, Radcliffe Infirmary, Oxford OX2 6HE; UK

John M. Eyler, University of Minnesota, Program in the History of Medicine, 511 Diehl Hall, Minneapolis, MN 55455, USA; e-mail: eyler001@umn.edu

B. Burt Gerstman, Dept. of Health Science, San Jose State University, San Jose, California 95192-0052, USA; e-mail: gerstman@email.sjsu.edu

Anne Hardy, Wellcome Trust Centre for the History of Medicine at UCL, Euston House, 24 Eversholt Street, London NW1 1AD, UK; e-mail: a.hardy@ucl.ac.uk

Gerry B. Hill, 263 Chelsea Road, Kingston, Ontario K7M 3Z3, Canada; e-mail: hill1930@hotmail.com

M. Eileen Magnello, Wellcome Trust Centre for the History of Medicine at UCL, Euston House, 24 Eversholt Street, London NW1 1AD, UK

Olli S. Miettinen, Joint Departments of Epidemiology & Biostatistics and Occupational Health, McGill University, 1020 Pine Avenue West, Montreal, Quebec H3A 1A2, Canada; e-mail: olli.miettinen@mcgill.ca

Alfredo Morabia, Division of Clinical Epidemiology, University Hospital, 24 rue Micheli-du-Crest, 1211 Geneva 14, Switzerland; and Department of Epidemiology, Colombia University, Mailman School of Public Health, 722 West 168th Street, New York, NY 10032, USA, e-mail: Alfredo.Morabia@hcuge.ch

Nigel Paneth, Department of Epidemiology, 4660 S. Hagadorn, Ste. 600, Michigan State University, East Lansing, MI 48824, USA; e-mail: paneth@msu.edu

List of Contributors

Kenneth J. Rothman, Department of Epidemiology and Division of Preventive Medicine, Department of Medicine, Boston University School of Medicine, 715 Albany Street, Boston, MA 02118, USA; e-mail: KRothman@bu.edu

Steven D. Stellman, Department of Epidemiology, Columbia University, Mailman School of Public Health, 722 West 168th Street, New York, NY 10032; USA; e-mail: sds91@columbia.edu

Ezra Susser, Department of Epidemiology, Columbia University, Mailman School of Public Health, 722 West 168th Street, New York, NY 10032; and New York State Psychiatric Institute, USA; e-mail: ess8@columbia.edu

Mervyn Susser, School of Public Health, Sergievsky Center, 630 W. 168 St., New York, NY 10032, USA; e-mail: mws2@columbia.edu

Benedetto Terracini, University of Torino and Regional Center for Cancer Prevention of Piedmont, Via Santena 7, 10126 Torino, Italy; e-mail: terracini@etabeta.it

Jan P. Vandenbroucke, Clinical Epidemiology, Leiden University Medical Center, PO Box 9600, NL-2300 RC Leiden, The Netherlands; e-mail: j.p.vandenbroucke@lumc.nl; vdbroucke@mail.medfac.leidenuniv.nl

Paolo Vineis, Unit of Clinical Epidemiology, Ospedale S. Giovanni Battista, University of Torino, Via Santena 7, 10126 Torino, Italy; e-mail: paolo.vineis@unito.it

Roberto Zanetti, Cancer Registry of Torino and Regional Centre for Cancer Prevention of Piedmont, Via Santena 7, 10126 Torino, Italy; e-mail: zanetti-r@asl1.to.it

Fang F. Zhang, Department of Epidemiology, Mailman School of Public Health, Columbia University, 722 West 168th Street, New York, NY 10032, USA; e-mail: fz2004@columbia.edu

Preface

Alfredo Morabia

The Annecy workshop

This book has two parts. The first part presents the evolution of epidemiologic methods and concepts. It serves as introduction and synthesis to the second part which is a collection of papers originally published in *Social and Preventive Medicine (International Journal of Public Health)*. Most of these papers had been presented at a Workshop on the history of epidemiology entitled "Measuring our scourges", held in Annecy, France, on July 1–10 1996 and organized by the Wellcome Foundation and the Louis Jeantet Institute for the History of Medicine. The workshop focused on the historical emergence of the corpus of epidemiologic methods and concepts used today. A stimulating aspect of the workshop was the interaction between professional historians (William Bynum, John Eyler, Bernardino Fantini, Anne Hardy), who are world experts on Victorian and early 20th century epidemiology, and epidemiologists vested into the history of their discipline (Richard Doll, David Morens, Steven Stellman, Milton Terris, Jan Vandenbroucke, Paolo Vineis, Ernst L. Wynder and myself). Richard Doll, Ernst Wynder, Steven Stellman and Milton Terris have been prominent actors of the historical events we discussed. The other speakers were Luc Raymond, André Rougemont, Italo Scardovi and Jeanne Stellman. Four papers (on the history of cohort analysis, case-control studies, cancer registries and evolution of concepts and methods in textbooks) were written after the conference. The re-publication of the article of William Farr "On Prognosis" and its discussion by several scholars is also posterior to the Annecy workshop and was suggested by Gerry B. Hill. All papers have been available after publication on the website *www.epidemiology.ch*, choose history.

My introductory essay tries to synthesize the content of all these papers. I refer to the papers whenever possible, but this synthesis only reflects my personal view, just as each paper in part 2 expresses the views of its authors and not necessarily beyond.

What this book is and what it is not

This book retrieves the work of past scientists who in retrospect can be defined as epidemiologists and describe its evolution. This does not suffice to produce a historical analysis. Historians of science are able to integrate this analysis into its wider social, economical and political contexts, the general movement of science and of its ideas. But the history of epidemiology, and especially the history of its methods and concepts, is still in its infancy. We cannot rule out that historians who will dig more deeply into certain parts of this history will gather a mass of new facts that will substantially modify our vision of the whole. A striking example of such possibility is related to the use of quantified group comparisons in clinical research. We used to consider the work of Pierre Louis, in France, who promoted the comparison of groups of patients to evaluate the efficacy of treatment, as an exception in a medical world dominated by individual thinking and case series (Morabia, 1996). But when Ulrich Troehler, Professor of History of Medicine at the University of Freiburg im Breisgau, searched into the practice of medicine in 18th century England, he found that there had been dozens of examples, analogous to that of Louis, of group comparisons in clinical settings. Moreover, the physicians who conducted these analyses resembled Louis in that they usually were marginal to the medical establishment, but used quantitative analyses to distinguish themselves from ordinary physicians (Troehler, 2000, p. 119–120).

The challenging objective of writing a history of epidemiologic methods and concepts requires strong interdisciplinary collaborations between epidemiologists, because of their deep understanding of the matter, and historians, because of the breadth of their perspective. The present book is a step in that direction. In the future, the collaboration will hopefully go beyond the mere exchange of experiences, papers and visions that we did at the Annecy Workshop.

This book is not historical in another aspect. The work of past epidemiologists is revisited with a modern perspective. Data are sometimes re-analyzed and their results interpreted using concepts that may not have formally existed then. These "presentisms" are a form of bias, which is not acceptable for historians but which is almost inescapable when one tries to describe the evolution of methods and concepts.

This book is *not* about issues such as: a) the achievements of epidemiology in the control of plagues (e.g., cholera, tuberculosis, malaria, typhoid fever or lung cancer), or in describing the link between poverty and health; b) theories of disease causation (e.g., miasmatic, bacteriological, environmental, unilevel or multivevel), their evolution across time and their influence on the work of epidemiologists; c) biographies of epidemiologists even though some papers do retrace the lives and contributions of scientists like John Snow (Vandenbroucke, Part IIa; Eyler, Part IIa), William Farr (Eyler, Part IIa; Eyler, Part IIb; Eyler, Part IIc), Thomas Rowe Edmonds (Eyler, Part IIb), Wade Hampton Frost (Comstock, Part II), Major Greenwood, Ronald Ross and A. B. Hill (Hardy and Magnello, Part II). These are three very important and fascinating aspects of the history of epidemiology, but they were not our main subjects. This book focuses on the *work* of people who contributed to the *development* of epidemiologic methods or concepts.

Epidemiology teaching

I trust that this book has a place in the curriculum of students of epidemiology, because students may reach a better understanding of the methods and concepts when these are presented in their evolutionary context. Methods and concepts get refined when we are facing challenges that cannot be met using state-of-the-art approaches. These are situations of crisis that cry for innovative ideas. They provide great didactic examples.

Consider for example the distinction between the concepts of risks and incidence rates. Today students in epidemiology understand that a risk is a probability expressed over a specific period of time (e.g., the lifetime risk of breast cancer for a Western woman is 7%), and an incidence rate is a risk change by unit of time (e.g., the incidence rate of breast cancer in Geneva is 150 per 100,000 per year). But they have more difficulty catching the conceptual difference between risks and rates. Why and when should we use one or the other?

The separation of the concepts of risks and rates took place around 1838, when William Farr was responsible for the collection of vital statistics in England. Placing the students in the context, which led Farr to formally distinguish risks from rates, can illuminate the purpose of these two different measures of disease occurrence. Major killers of Farr's times were acute infections that killed quickly and whose behavior was well described by risks. Tuberculosis (then called phthisis) was not a disease of that type. It was a major threat for the public health but people perceived this menace as paradoxically less dangerous than that of less lethal diseases, such as cholera:

> *"Phthisis is more dangerous than cholera; but cholera, probably, excites the greatest terror."* (Farr, Part II).

In terms of risks, almost all tuberculosis patients died from their disease (mortality risk = 90–100%), whereas less than half of the sick died from cholera (mortality risk = 46%). Tuberculosis was more dangerous. Why did it excite less terror? Farr explained that this was because:

> *"cholera destroys in a week more than phthisis consumes in a year"* (Farr, Part II).

Indeed, the average duration of the disease was 2 years for tuberculosis and 7 days for cholera. When time was taken into consideration, tuberculosis appeared less frightening than cholera. Farr was able to express this nuance by using a mortality *rate*, which related the death *risk* and the average duration of the disease. The death rate for tuberculosis was small (less than 1 death per hundred patients per week) compared to the death rate of cholera (about 46 deaths per hundred patients per week). Farr concluded that it was the high mortality rate of cholera which excited terror. Both risks and rates were needed to describe, compare and understand the patterns of occurrence of cholera *vs.* tuberculosis.

The historical or scientific contexts in which innovation occurs may therefore be unique to understand the purpose of new approaches. As time goes by, successful innovations are formalized, become more abstract and their original purpose can sometimes be lost sight of in the process.

An antidote to dogmatism

There is another reason why this book can be useful for teaching epidemiology. Visualizing the evolution of methods can confer a protection against dogmatism, that is, a tendency to rigidly protect a partially understood theoretical heritage. Here is an example. Imagine that you present to a class of epidemiology students one of the analyses of the 1950 case-control study by Doll and Hill, in which 99.7% of the lung cancer cases and 95.8% of the controls free of lung cancer had ever smoked in their lifetime (Doll and Hill, 1950). Almost invariably, students who have already been exposed to the analysis of case-control studies immediately compute an odds ratio of [(99.7 ÷ 0.3) : (95.8 ÷ 4.2) =] 14.6 and interpret it as ever smokers having a 14.6 times greater risk of developing lung cancer than never smokers. No consideration is given to the primary finding of this analysis: the extremely high proportion of smokers in both groups. Moreover, few students can explain the conceptual background that legitimates this almost magic transformation of two exposure percentages (99.7% and 95.8%) into an impressive relative risk of 14.6. Replacing this case-control study in its context may help students to appreciate that the exposure percentages are the primary results of the case-control study. The first publications by Doll and Hill did not use odds ratios. Students are also more likely to catch the rationality of using odds ratios and interpreting them as relative risks when they visualize how the theory relating case-control studies to cohort studies has been developed over several decades.

There is a third reason for which the history of epidemiologic methods and concepts has its place in the epidemiology curriculum. Concepts and methods that evolve cannot, by definition, be carved into stone. Students may therefore realize that their role, as future epidemiologists, will also be to adapt and refine the methodological and conceptual corpus relative to the new, emerging challenges humanity faces.

How to use this book?

In order to facilitate the usage of this book for teaching purposes, an index of keywords is provided, which connects the entire content of the volume. In addition, the references of the two parts of the book have been grouped into a single bibliography section. I will try to make available additional material, including historical datasets, on *www.epidemiology.ch*, choose history, either directly or through web links.

Acknowledgements

I am indebted to Dr. Fang F. Zhang for her help with the bibliographic search and checking, to Professors Michael C. Costanza and Ulrich Troehler, to Roger H. Bernier as well as Sigrid Beer and Maurice Jacob for their careful reading of previous versions of this manuscript, to Séverine Schusselé Filliettaz for her editorial help, and to Joëlle Paratte and Catherine Zarola for the secretarial support.

I dedicate this book to the Epistemology Group of the Wade Hampton Frost Reading Room, at The Johns Hopkins University School of Public Health, who met regularly between 1986 and 1989. Its core members were Gail Geller, Steven Goodman, Camara Phyllis Jones, Ruth Levine, Scott Zeger and me. A wonderful experience. Discussions were lively!

Part I
Epidemiology: An epistemological perspective

Epidemiology: An epistemological perspective

Alfredo Morabia

To the Epistemology Group of the Wade Hampton Frost Reading Room, Baltimore, 1986–1988

1. Introduction

1.1. A contextual name

The term "epidemiology" is a source of confusion about the nature of this discipline. For the public, "epidemiology" evokes a medical discipline that deals with large-scale outbreaks of infectious diseases. This was indeed its meaning in the first treatises which included "epidemiology" in their titles. In the 16th century the Spanish physician Angelerio published a study on plague entitled "*Epidemiología*" and in 1802 another Spanish physician, Villalba, wrote a compilation of epidemics and outbreaks over 13 centuries entitled "*Epidemiología Española*" (meaning Spanish epidemiology) (Pan American Health Organization, 1988, p. 3–4).

The term epidemiology was also quite accurate when the discipline made its first steps. It reflected the particular historical context in 19th century England, when epidemics of infectious diseases, and in particular cholera, were the main scourges whose causes had to be identified. The *London Epidemiologic Society*, created in 1850, assembled scientists, public health practitioners and physicians to unite their efforts in the fight against "epidemics". Today, epidemiology is still associated with the fight against infection, in all types of contexts, including emerging diseases (e.g., severe acute respiratory syndrome or SARS), bioterrorism (e.g., criminal dissemination of anthrax bacteria), and even digital viruses! Isn't it meaningful that a bioinformatician, Alberto-Laszlo Barabasi, describes "computer security experts" as "a new breed of epidemiologists who vigilantly monitor the health of our online universe", protecting it from international viruses capable of causing life-threatening emergencies (Barabasi, 2002, p. 141)?

Even though the name continues to evoke the fight against infectious plagues, the domain of epidemiology has enormously expanded and is not restricted to specific types of diseases. If we had to name the discipline today, we would probably give it a different name. Physics, chemistry, or medical specialties such as cardiology or neurology have names that are unambiguous, because they describe the subject of the discipline. The name "epidemiology", on the other hand, has more to do with the circumstances in which the discipline was born than with the substance of the discipline in its present state.

What is then the subject of epidemiology? We can rephrase the question and ask: Why would one hire an epidemiologist today rather than a statistician, a sociologist, a clinician, etc.? An epidemiologist is expected to have learned a particular set of methods and concepts taught in epidemiology classes which are needed to identify determinants of health and disease: describe states of health in populations, investigate outbreaks of diseases, compare groups, use, with increasing degrees of complexity, the concepts of bias, confounding and interaction and be familiar with the epidemiologic approaches to causal inference. This would however still be an insufficient reason. It is like saying that we need cardiologists because they know how to use a stethoscope. Most physicians use stethoscopes and most public health professions are familiar with basic epidemiology and use it. However, they do not necessarily master it. Thus, what defines an epidemiologist is probably the ability to *adapt* this particular set of methods and concepts to specific research questions. This ability allows them, in more exceptional circumstances, to make methods and concepts *evolve* when encountering new types of problems.

The subject of epidemiology is therefore the investigation of causes of health-related events in populations. A name more closely reflecting this subject would be "population health etiology", etiology meaning "science of causation".

1.2. Historical contribution of epidemiology

Science allows us to understand how our world is and how it works. We identify causal links and these indicate ways to act upon the world and modify it. What is then the historical contribution of epidemiology to knowledge?

Epidemiology is a recent scientific discipline. It has roots in the 17th century but it is really a 19th century science. Its mission has historically been to identify determinants of human diseases (and later health), mostly at the population level. Epidemiologic discoveries can be used for improving human health. Probably one of the most important discoveries, for its scientific and public health impacts, has been the demonstration that cigarette smoke *caused* lung cancer in smokers, and that preventing exposure to cigarette smoke could prevent occurrence of lung cancer.

To identify causes we can act upon, we need methods, that is, strategies or experiments, which are organized in such a way that their results can reveal stable relations and laws. Experiments can be of different sorts. In some (typically laboratory) experiments, the researcher can manipulate exposure to assess changes in outcome. This is not the main type of experiments in epidemiology. Epidemiologists usually compare groups of people differing on carefully selected characteristics, but they cannot manipulate exposure. For example, they cannot allocate a certain number of cigarettes to be smoked per day. The fundamental observation establishing that cigarette smoke caused lung cancer was that smokers tended to develop lung cancer *more* frequently *than* non-smokers. Because they are mostly based on observations (as opposed to interventions), epidemiologic experiments have considerable complexity. If lung cancer is more common in smokers than in non-smokers, this does not mean yet that smoking causes lung cancer. Smokers and non-smokers could differ on one or several characteristics, which are the true causes of lung cancer (i.e., confounding). The disease could have multiple causes, whose pathways overlap with other pathways (i.e., interaction). The experiment itself is prone to errors, which can interfere with the sound interpretation of its results (i.e., biases). Therefore comparing groups would be a very naive endeavor if it were not supported by a theory that allowed epidemiologists to design experiments, organize the facts and interpret the observations in a way that takes into account the complexity of the matter studied. I will refer to the elements of this theoretical framework as *concepts*. We will see that confounding, interaction and bias are examples of concepts. We did not simply observe them. They are intellectual constructions that were (and are) refined over time.

Thus, historically, the specific contribution of epidemiology has been the progressive constitution of a coherent ensemble of methods and concepts, aimed to assess health determinants. We will see that it was based on two principles: population thinking and group comparisons.

1.3. Theme of this essay

This essay is about the genesis of epidemiology as a scientific discipline. Its theme is that current epidemiologic concepts and methods have evolved since the 18th century in a series of relatively well-defined steps to constitute an integrated theory based on two essential principles: 1) population thinking and 2) group comparisons.

Population thinking, as opposed to individual thinking, is a mode of conceptualizing issues for a whole group of people defined in a specific way (e.g., geographically, socially, biologically). The entire group is the population. In 1950, John E. Gordon, Professor of Epidemiology and Preventive Medicine at the Harvard School of Public Health, expressed the essence of population thinking when he stressed that each population has its own individuality:

> *"The study of disease as a mass phenomenon differs from the study of disease in the individual primarily in respect to the unit of investigation. It is early appreciated that the herd, the crowd or the community is not a simple aggregate of the persons comprising that grouped population, but that each universe of people is an entity, a composite that possesses as much individuality as does a person."* (Gordon, 1950, p. 198).

The second principle, *group comparison*, consists in contrasting what is observed in the presence of exposure to what would have occurred had the group of interest not been exposed to the postulated cause. Differences in event occurrence between groups can logically be interpreted as being caused by the exposure. This is the main mode of knowledge acquisition in epidemiology. It relies on population thinking.

This essay addresses questions such as: how did epidemiologists integrate into their population thinking measures of disease occurrence of growing theoretical complexity and abstraction? How did simple ratios and proportions evolve into risks and rates, and later cumulative incidences and incidence densities? How did simple group comparisons eventually lead to a unified theory of study designs distinguishing cohort from case-control studies? Historical examples of the theoretical innovations and refinements illustrate the answers.

Even though there is a historical thread to its argument, this essay is more about the *epistemology* than about the history of epidemiology. Epistemology is a discipline that deals with the evolution of knowledge. This essay focuses more on how epidemiologic ideas evolved than on the description of the historical contexts in which these evolutions occurred or the identification of the exact moments at which they occurred, who had the original idea or published it first, etc. This approach is, I believe, analogous to annotated anthologies of articles and books (Pan American Health Organization, 1988; Greenland 1987a) or to the James Lind Library enterprise (http://www.jameslindlibrary.org).

Taken in isolation, population thinking and group comparisons can be found in other disciplines. Population thinking belongs to demography, statistics, and biology (Mayr, 1985). Group comparisons can be found in sociology or anthropology. But the blending of population thinking and group comparisons in an integrated theory to appraise health-related causal relations characterizes epidemiology. Indeed, the juncture of population thinking and group comparisons was the critical element that led to the birth of epidemiology in the 18th century. Over a period of less than 300 years, the theory of epidemiology has become quite rich. It comprises methods for group-comparisons (i.e., contrasts of exposed *vs.* unexposed to potential risk factors, and affected *vs.* unaffected by specific conditions) and two sets of concepts. One set rigorously expresses health-related phenomena occurring at the population level (e.g., prevalence, incidence, risks or rates). Another set of concepts is related to the design and interpretation of group-comparisons (e.g., confounding, interaction, bias, causal inference).

The material assembled in this essay demonstrates that epidemiology is a dynamic scientific discipline. Its methods and concepts have evolved across time, and will most likely continue to do so. This thesis would be refuted if it was shown that 1) the apparent evolution described below is a fallacy, that is, the whole corpus was present from the inception of epidemiology and has only been repeatedly re-invented; 2) epidemiology has now reached its definitive form and will not evolve beyond its current state of formalization.

2. Population thinking

2.1. Definitions

Predicting the experiences of a whole group of people distinguishes population thinking from other modes of reasoning. Under certain assumptions, population predictions can be made with a measurable degree of certainty. We can predict the number of new cases of disease in a population, but we cannot predict if a given individual will become sick. What will happen to an individual or the way an individual will behave in the future cannot be predicted with certainty.

Population thinking leads, however, to reliable predictions at the population level, which can then be applied to individuals. Suppose that 150 cases of breast cancer occur per 100,000 women and per year in a population of 200,000 women. We can predict with certainty that, if the rate remains constant, 300 new cases of the disease (plus or minus a certain number of cases reflecting the imprecision of the estimate) would be diagnosed each year. We cannot however precisely predict whether a specific woman, among the 200,000 women "at risk" for the disease, will develop breast cancer. At the individual level we can formulate "probabilities": each woman in this population has an annual risk of $[300 \div 200,000] = 0.15\%$. This probability statement is based on what we observed for the group to which the woman belongs.

The relevance of population thinking to medical practice is not straightforward. Clinicians have opposed it in the past and still tend to avoid it. Medicine is the art of individual thinking. A skilled physician is one who is able to make the best prediction in terms of diagnosis and prognosis for the individual patient and adapt the management and treatment to the unique characteristics of an essentially unpredictable person. Because medicine is the art of individual thinking, we need physicians and cannot replace them by computers. But it has been a major and difficult conceptual leap for physicians to realize that something useful could be learned for the individual from populations.

Thus, there is a contradiction between population and individual thinking. For all of us, it takes a certain change in perspective to realize that populations don't behave as if they were simply the collection of unique and unpredictable individuals. Even though we don't understand exactly why that is so, populations have, to use Gordon's expression, their individuality. For example, heavy drinkers represent a larger fraction of some populations than others. When heavy drinking is common, the whole population tends to drink, on average, more alcohol compared to populations in which heavy drinking is less common. Heavy drinkers do not appear to be a well-defined, proportionally constant subgroup of people in every society. Their frequency varies and can even be predicted from the average alcohol intake of the population they belong to. This phenomenon was first reported by the French demographer Sully Ledermann in the 1950s (Ledermann, 1956) with respect to alcohol consumption. It has been popularized in epidemiology by Geoffrey Rose (1926–1993), Emeritus Professor of Epidemiology at the London School of Public Health and Tropical Medicine, in a paper entitled: "The population mean predicts the number of deviant individuals" (Rose and Day, 1990).

From where do populations get their individuality? How does the community influence individual behaviors? There are probably no simple answers to these questions but it is clearly established that populations are more than collections of individuals. Some populations tolerate more obesity, excess alcohol intake, smoking, etc. in society. Some populations are physically more active than others. Some societies are more egalitarian than other. The crucial point is that the statistical laws that govern populations provide information that can be useful for the individuals belonging to these populations.

2.1.1. Ratios, risks, rates and odds

In order to think at the population level, we need to be able to describe the occurrence and evolution of events in populations. This requires appropriate measures. How frequent is the disease? How will it evolve in the future? At what speed will this evolution take place?

We will review how the intuitive adoption of population thinking eventually became a theory comprised of a set of well-defined concepts. This will take us from the 17th century to modern times. But before we get to these examples, we need to define some of the terms that are indispensable for exploring epidemiology's past. The number of concepts used in epidemiology is relatively limited, but the wealth of terms found in the epidemiologic literature can be confusing. An astounding effort of homogenization has been made by the *International Epidemiology Association* (Last, 2001), but we are still far from a consensual usage of a minimum terminology.

The words risk, rate, ratio, and odds are measures of event occurrence that differ by the nature of their numerator and denominator. I will use the definitions of these terms that Regina C. Elandt-Johnson, statistician from the Department of Biostatistics, University of North Carolina, gave in the very influential commentary she wrote in the October 1975 issue of the *American Journal of Epidemiology* (Elandt-Johnson, 1975).

Rates, risks, ratios and odds are measures (M) computed by dividing one quantity by another. The dividend is the numerator and the divisor is the denominator.

$$M = a \div b, \text{ where } M = measure, a = numerator \text{ and } b = denominator$$

In a *ratio*, the numerator and denominator are two separate and distinct quantities, which are not included in one another. For example, dividing the number of deaths (numerator) by the number of births (denominator) is a ratio. The etymology of the word "ratio" is interesting. In Latin, it means "reason". Its original usage in mathematics may be related to the fact that a ratio yielded a rational (an integer divided by another, e.g., 4 ÷ 2, as opposed to an irrational, e.g., square root of 2) number. But the term ratio now relates more to the principle of *comparing* two quantities.

A *risk* is a proportion, that is, a measure in which the denominator includes the numerator. For example, the risk of developing lung cancer is the proportion of a group of people at risk (denominator) who newly develop lung cancer (numerator) over a specified period of time (e.g., the risk of lung cancer can be 10% over 20 years in heavy smokers).

A *rate* is a measure of change in one quantity per unit of another quantity. In epidemiology, a rate is often used as synonym for incidence rate, which is the change in risk per unit of time. For example, a risk of 10% over 20 years can, if constant, be expressed as a rate of 0.5 per 100 and per year [rate = risk ÷ time = 10% ÷ 20 years = 0.5% per year].

To contrast the frequency of occurrence of an event to that of nonoccurrence we use the *odds*. The *odds of disease* are computed by dividing the risk by its complement: a risk of 10% over 20 years corresponds to the odds of 1 to 9 [odds = risk ÷ (100%-risk) = 10% ÷ 90% = 1 over 9]: the disease has 1 chance to occur *vs.* 9 not to occur. Similarly, the *odds of exposure* is obtained by dividing the percentage of exposed by the percentage of unexposed.

2.1.2. Prevalence, incidence, mortality, case fatality

Different concepts express whether a count (usually of people) is the result of past events or if it is a prediction for the future. In this essay I shall use the following terminology. The *prevalence* is the proportion of people in the total population suffering from a given disease (or exposed to a given factor) at a given point in time. The trait (disease, exposure, etc.) may be long existing or recent. Thus, prevalence measures a state of health resulting from events that occurred in the distant or recent past. The *incidence* is the proportion of *new* cases occurring in a population *at risk* of disease over a specified period of time (i.e., excluding prevalent cases or people not susceptible of contracting the disease). It is a synonym of risk. In contrast to prevalence it is a predictive statement about cases-to-be in a population still free of the disease. *Mortality* indicates the proportion of deaths in general, whereas *case fatality* is reserved for the deaths occurring among people who are diseased.

When incidence, mortality and case fatality are expressed per *unit of time*, they will be called incidence rate, mortality rate and case fatality rate.

2.2. Origin of population thinking

At the dawn of the 17th century, emerging modern European states became interested in collecting population data and using them to guide their policy. The wealth and power of modern states depended on the education, health, income, political involvement and other characteristics of the population they governed. In England and France, the devastations of plague epidemics stimulated the process of population data collection, in which health indicators represented an important component. Hence, the etymology of the word "statistics": systematic data collection for the state. As the historian of public health, George Rosen (1910–1977) has put it,

> *"Initially, those who undertook to use the statistical approach concerned themselves chiefly with what might be called the bookkeeping of the state. Efforts were made to ascertain the basic quantitative data of national life in the belief that such knowledge could be used to increase the power and prestige of the state (…) The father of "political arithmetic" was William Petty (1623–1687), physician, economist and scientist, who invented the term and was keenly alive to the importance of a healthy population as a factor in national opulence and power. Repeatedly, Petty urged the collection of numerical data on population, education, diseases, revenue and many other related topics."* (Rosen, 1958, p. 111).

To the best of our current knowledge, the book of John Graunt (1620–1674) entitled *"Natural and Political Observations made upon the Bills of Mortality"* (Graunt, 1662) may be the first solid contribution to "public health statistics". According to a 17th century biographer (Aubrey, 2004), John Graunt was by profession a haberdasher, who eventually went bankrupt. He was also admitted as fellow of the Royal Society and pioneered the analysis of the Bills of Mortality (ancestors of the death certificates, systematically collected in England since 1603) to find uniform and predictable mass phenomena.

Kenneth J. Rothman, Professor of epidemiology at Boston University, has written a laudatory commentary on Graunt's contribution:

> *"With this book Graunt added more to human knowledge than most of us can reasonably aspire to in a full career. Graunt was the first to report, and to document, that more boys than girls are born. He presented one of the first life-tables. He reported the first time-trends for many diseases, taking into account changes in population size. He described new diseases, and noted others that seemed to increase over time only because of changes in classification. He offered the first reasoned estimate of the population of London, demonstrating its rapid growth and showing that most of the growth came from immigration. He proffered epidemiologic evidence refuting the theory that the plague spreads by contagion. (He also refuted the notion that plague epidemics are coincident with the reign of a new king.) He showed that the large population decreases in plague years were offset by large increases in births in subsequent years. He showed that physicians have twice as many female as male patients, but that more males than females die. He produced the first hard evidence about the frequencies of various causes of death.*

And, presaging our present-day paranoia, he tried to allay unwarranted anxiety about risks that were feared far out of proportion to their likelihood of occurrence." (Rothman, 1996, p. 37).

It should be kept in mind that the history of English "statistics" has apparently been more studied than that of other countries, even in Europe. Thus, it is much less known that the Swiss physician Felix Platter (1536–1614) had shown, before Graunt, that the plague appeared to regulate the population size of the City of Basel in the northern part of Switzerland (Mattmueller, 2004).

The growing interest in population data, probabilities and population thinking reached medicine too. Compiling the mass of data generated by the activity of hospitals and infirmaries could be used to improve medical activity (Troehler, 2000, p. 15). We find in 18th century England early attempts to evaluate the *average* effect of specific therapies in groups of patients. In the 19th century, some physicians clearly expressed the need for aggregated data:

"... that it is impossible to appreciate each case with mathematical exactness, and it is precisely on this account that enumeration becomes necessary."
(Louis, 1836, p. 60).

And for population thinking:

"To ascertain the cause of cholera, we must consider it not only in individual cases but also in its more general character as an epidemic." (Snow, 1849, p. 746).

Population thinking in the domain of health first appears in the 18th century and is unambiguously expressed by scientists of the 19th century. Let us review now the evolution of the measures and concepts which have contributed to population thinking in epidemiology.

2.3. Early ratios, proportions and rates

The first measures used to express the occurrence of disease in populations were ratios, proportions and probably primitive mortality rates.

2.3.1. Eighteenth century

Plague, a lethal disease caused by *Tersinia Pestis* and propagated by fleas and rats, has constituted a significant demographic factor in late medieval and early modern times in all parts of Europe (McNeil, 1976, p. 151). The data in Table 1 are from chapter IV ("Of the plague") of John Graunt's *"Natural and Political Observations Made upon the Bills of Mortality"*(Graunt, 1662). The table shows the overall num-

Table 1 – Proportions and ratios in the work of John Graunt. The data are extracted from chapter IV ("Of the plague") of John Graunt's "Natural and Political Observations upon the Bills of Mortality" (Graunt, 1662, pp. 33–36).

Year	Deaths ("Died" or "buried")	"Whereof plague"	Other causes	Plague mortality "proportion"	Births ("christened")	Death to birth ratios
1592	25,886	11,503	14,383	2 to 5	4,277	6 to 1
1603	37,294	30,561	6,733	4 to 5	4,784	8 to 1
1625	54,265*	35,417	18,848	7 to 10	6,983	8 to 1
1636	23,359	10,400	10,400	2 to 5	9,522	5 to 2

* The table in Graunt's book says 51,758, which is probably a typographical error. The "Table of burials and christenings", appended in page 75 of the *Observations,* indicates a total of 54,265 deaths. Graunt uses sometimes 54,265, and sometimes 51,758, in his calculations.

bers of deaths, deaths due to the plague and the number of "christened", that is, births, in London for the years 1592, 1603, 1625 and 1636. The table also reports the "proportions" of all deaths due to plague, and the ratios of "buried to christened", that is, deaths to births. Graunt assembled the numbers and made the calculations in Table 1 to address the following question:

> "In which of [these years] was the greatest Mortality of all Diseases in general, or of the Plague in particular?" (Graunt, 1662, p. 33).

a) Proportions
Graunt uses proportions (column 5 of Table 1) to show that the greatest mortality from plague occurred in 1603, as 80% (4 to 5) died of plague, which is greater than the 70% (7 to 10) which occurred in 1625.

> "For if the Year 1625 had been as great a Plague-Year as 1603 there must have died not only 7 to 10 but 8 to 10 which in those great numbers makes a vast difference (…) We must therefore conclude the Year 1603 to have been the greatest Plague-Year of this age." (Graunt, 1662, p. 34).

b) Ratios
Graunt notes some inconsistency in the Bills. The year of greatest mortality from the plague (1603) is different from the year of greatest overall mortality (1625). For that purpose, Graunt computes the ratio of the number of deaths (i.e., burials) over the number of births (i.e., christenings) (last column of Table 1). This ratio is 8 to 1 both

in 1603 and 1625. There was apparently no "errour in the Accompts" for the overall mortality in 1625. However, compared to the years before (1622) or after (1626) the plague, there was in 1625 an excess of 11,000 deaths from causes other than the plague. This excess could be explained by misclassification of plague deaths into deaths from other causes. Graunt thus added 11,000 to the 35,417 plague deaths of 1625, making a total of 46,417, which is about "four to five" of the whole 54,265, almost the same as 1603

> "... thereby rendering the said year 1625 to be as great a Plague-year as that of 1603 and no greater, which answers to what we proved before, viz. that the Mortality of the two Years was equal." (Graunt, 1662, p. 35).

c) Rates
Graunt observes that the mortality from plague varies from one epidemic to another and makes "sudden jumps" within the evolution of the same epidemic. In order to describe this mortality variation, Graunt uses a primitive form of mortality rates. The time unit is *year* to compare one epidemic with the other

> "The Plague of 1636 lasted twelve Years, in eight whereof there died 2000 per annum one with another, and never under 300." (Graunt, 1662, p. 36).

The sudden jumps of deaths occurring within the same epidemic are given per *week*:

> "...the sudden jumps, which the Plague hath made, leaping in one Week from 118 to 927: and back again from 993 to 258: and from thence again the very next Week to 852." (Graunt, 1662, p. 36).

Of course, deaths are not divided by the number of people at risk, and these rates may not have been accurate if the population of London varied substantially during plague years, when the wealthiest fled out of the city. But these deaths per year or per week play the role of mortality rates. On their basis, Graunt can go beyond the mere description of the overall burden of deaths due to each plague epidemic. Deaths per year or per week decompose the overall mortality from plague into small units of time allowing Graunt to describe the variation in intensity of the epidemic. Indeed, Graunt concluded that such sudden changes in mortality had to be determined by some external causes, related to the environment, and could not be due to causes internal to the human constitution:

> "The which effects must surely be rather attributed to change of the Air, then of the Constitution of Mens bodies, otherwise then as this depends upon that." (Graunt, 1662, p. 36).

Table 2 – Mortality after 7 weeks. London, 1854: "The following is the proportion of deaths to 10,000 houses, during the first seven weeks of the [1854] epidemic, in the population supplied by the Southwark and Vauxhall Company, in that supplied by the Lambeth Company, and in the rest of London." Source: Table IX, in (Snow, 1855, p. 53).

	Number of houses	Death from cholera	Deaths in each 10,000 houses
Southwark and Vauxhall Company	40,046	1,263	315
Lambeth Company	26,107	98	37
Rest of London	256,423*	1,422	59**

* There seems to be some inconsistency between the table and the text relative to the number of households in the rest of London. *"The number of houses in London at the time of the last census was 327,391. If the houses supplied with water by the Southwark and Vauxhall Company, and the deaths from cholera occurring in these houses, be deducted, we shall have in the remainder of London 287,345 houses ..."* (Snow, 1855, p. 50). Thus, [327,391–40,046 –26,107 =] 261,238, which is different from the 287,345 given elsewhere in the text and from the 256,423 in the table.

** [1,422 ÷ 256,423 =] 55 per 10,000, not 59 as reported by Snow.

2.3.2. Nineteenth century

Cholera had long been endemic in Bengal, India. It was a frightening disease, which killed its victims sometimes within hours, by radical dehydration from diarrhea, vomiting and fever. Ruptured capillaries made the skin turn black and blue, hence the popular name of the disease: the blue death or, in French, *la mort bleue*. In the early 19th century, cholera made recurrent world excursions, which brought it several times to London.

John Snow (1813–1858) was an English anesthesiologist, convinced that cholera was a contagious disease. He had been studying the recurring outbreaks of cholera in England and published in 1849 the hypothesis that polluted water was one of the means of cholera transmission (Vinten-Johansen et al., 2003; Shephard, 1995). When cholera returned to London in July 1854, John Snow used the opportunity to test his hypothesis. I will describe the study itself in detail later (section 3.3.2), but focus here on the measures of disease occurrence used by Snow.

a) Ratios

Table 2 reproduces the most famous results of John Snow's investigation on the mode of transmission of cholera from the 1855 edition of his book *"On the Mode of Communication of Cholera"* (Snow, 1855). They were collected during the first seven weeks of the epidemic of cholera that hit London in July 1854. Snow uses a ratio to

Table 3 – Mortality after 14 weeks. London, 1854: "By adding the number of deaths, which occurred in the first seven weeks of the epidemic, we get the numbers in the subjoined table (No. XI), where the population of the houses supplied by the two water companies is that estimated by the Registrar General." Source: Table XI, in (Snow, 1855, p. 55).

	Population in 1851	Death by cholera in 14 weeks end Oct 14 [1854]	Deaths in 10,000 livings
Southwark and Vauxhall Company	266,516	4,093	153
Lambeth Company	173,748	461	26
London	2,362,236	10,367	43

quantify the impact of the epidemics on, respectively, the clients of two water supply companies, the Southwark and Vauxhall Company, and the Lambeth Company, and the rest of London. The numerators are the numbers of deaths observed in each of the three groups. The denominators are the numbers of households supplied by water companies. Snow refers to this ratio by saying, inappropriately, that it is "the proportion of deaths to 10,000 houses" (Snow, 1855, p. 86).

However, to interpret the ratio of deaths to households as a proportion or a risk, Snow would have had to assume that the average size of the households was similar across London. Let us imagine that the Southwark and Vauxhall Company supplied poor and crowded house blocks, in which the average household was 8.4 times larger than in the more well off house blocks supplied by the Lambeth company. In that situation, the actual mortality risk from cholera would be identical for the two companies, as [1263 ÷ (40,046 × 8.4)] is equivalent to [98 ÷ 26,107]. Indeed, According to John Eyler (Eyler, Part Ia), the fact that Snow did not know the number of clients at risk of cholera fed the initial skepticism towards his conclusions.

b) Proportions
In Table XI of "*On the Mode of Communication of Cholera*" (see Table 3 above), Snow does present real proportions. The numerator is the number of deaths while the denominator is the number of people living in the houses supplied by the companies. This denominator had its own limitations as it was based on an already three-year old census. The office of the Registrar General computed these proportions.

Note that apparently 6 to 7 people lived in each household supplied by both companies. The deaths had tripled for the Southwark and Vauxhall, almost quintupled for the Lambeth company in seven weeks. Still, mortality over 14 weeks (Table 3)

Table 4 – Duration, mortality (i.e., risk) and force of mortality (i.e., rate) for cholera and phthisis. Source: (Farr, Part II).

Disease	Mean duration (in days)	Mortality (% of all the sick)	Force of mortality (= Mortality rate per 100 sick a year)
Cholera	7	46	2415
Phthisis	730	90–100	50

was almost half of that over 7 weeks based on households (Table 2) and differences were less important.

2.4. Risks and rates

It has taken about 150 years to sort out the properties of risks and rates, clarify their interpretation and produce a theory of their mathematical relationships. We will review here three episodes of this process.

2.4.1. Burden of life destruction and force of mortality

As Superintendent of the General Register Office, England's center for vital statistics, William Farr (1807–1883) was responsible for collecting and reporting information on causes of death (Susser and Adelstein, 1975). In the pamphlet entitled "*On Prognosis*", reproduced *in extenso* in this book (Farr, Part II), Farr illustrates the need for different types of measure of disease occurrence by contrasting an acute infectious disease, cholera, with a chronic infectious disease, phthisis (i.e., tuberculosis). He invokes the following paradox:

> "*Cholera destroys in a week more than phthisis consumes in a year. Phthisis is more dangerous than cholera; but cholera, probably, excites the greatest terror.*" (Farr, Part II).

Table 4 shows that almost every tuberculosis patient will die from the disease. The case fatality risk of phthisis is 90–100%. Cholera kills only one of two persons who are affected: its case fatality risk is 46.2%.

Half of the people who get cholera but almost none of those with phthisis will survive. Between cholera and phthisis, it would seem reasonable to prefer cholera, but people fear cholera more than tuberculosis. Why is it so? Farr notes that mortality is insufficient to characterize the "form and nature of diseases". We need two different measures of disease occurrence:

"Diseases may be examined (1) in their tendency to destroy life, expressed by the deaths out of a given number of cases; and (2) in their mean relative 'force of mortality', expressed by the deaths out of a given number sick at a given time."
(Farr, Part II).

Let us consider each of these two ways of examining a disease. For the first parameter, "the tendency to destroy life", Farr gives as synonyms the "probability of death", "mortality" and "death percent". If 990 patients died out of 2,142 cases of cholera, "mortality" is 46.2%. Farr does not use the word "risk", but risk is the term that we would commonly use today. More specifically, this is a "case fatality risk". It expresses the probability that patients with cholera will *die* from their disease. Deaths are in the numerator and sick people are in the denominator.

The second parameter, "force of mortality", is the "quantity eliminated daily by death out of a given constant quantity (e.g., 100) sick". Farr also refers to it as the "mean *rate* of dying per unit of sick time". To compute the force of mortality, Farr divides the number of deaths by the product of the number of persons sick and the average duration during which they were sick. If 2,142 cases of cholera have been sick an average of 7 days each, this corresponds to a total of [7 × 2,142 =] 14,994 days of sickness, or sick person-days. Sick-person days divided by 365 days in a year gives 41 years of sickness or 41 sick person-years. Thus, if 990 die out of 41 sick person-years of cholera, the "force of mortality" is [(990 ÷ 41) × 100) =] 2,415 per 100 sick person-years. The modern synonym of "force of mortality" is mortality rate, and in this example specifically, it is a "case fatality rate". It is the proportion of the cases that will die from their disease *per unit of time*: 2,415 per 100 patients per *year* or 6.6 per 100 patients per *day*.

Distinguishing these two measures of death occurrence allows Farr to explain the paradoxical terror generated by cholera. The data are shown in Table 4. Almost all patients died from tuberculosis (mortality risk = 90–100%), but the death rate is small (50 per 100 per year) and the average duration of the disease is long (2 years). Tuberculosis kills slowly. On the other hand, less than half of the sick will die from cholera (mortality risk = 46%), but the death rate is huge (2,415 per 100 per year) and the average duration of the disease is short (7 days). Cholera appears abruptly, kills rapidly and disappears. Viewed as such, cholera is more frightful.

Why did Farr use the word "force" to characterize a rate? We can speculate that this is in relation to the concept of physical force. Farr must have been familiar with the concept of force defined by the physicist Isaac Newton (1643–1727) in his *"Principia"* (Newton, 1687):

"An impressed force is an action exerted upon a body, in order to change its state, either of rest, or of moving uniformly forward in a right line. This force con-

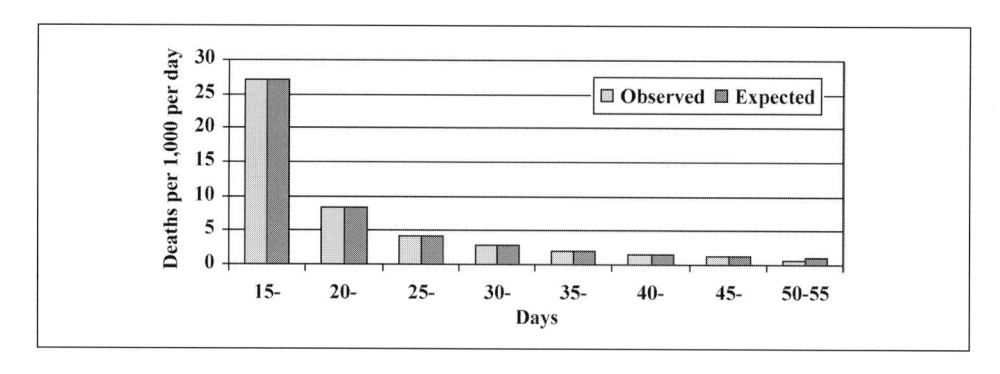

Figure 1
Evolution of the observed and expected death rates from smallpox. Source: William Farr, On Prognosis (Farr, Part II).

sists in the action only; and remains no longer in the body when the action is over." (Cited by Einstein and Imfeld, 1966, p. 11).

A force can be represented by a vector, which has a direction and a velocity. The velocity, that is, the distance covered per unit of time, is by definition a rate. The force of mortality, like a vector, has a velocity and a direction. Mortality rates can go up or down.

Farr notes that predicting the direction in which mortality will evolve is crucial for prognosis. The sign of the force indicates whether the rate increases or decreases over time. Indeed, Farr gives the data needed to compute the force of mortality on the 18th, 19th day, etc. of duration of smallpox (Gerstman, Part II). Using the word "*rate*", Farr notes that:

"*The rate of mortality [from smallpox] increased from the 5–10 days to 10–15 when it attained a maximum (31.18); it decreased in a determined progression from the next period (15–20 days) to the end.*" (Farr, Part II).

Farr was mostly interested in the declining part of the rate curve (see Figure 1), which demonstrated some mathematical regularity:

"*The decrease begins to take place in geometrical progression; but the tendency to decrease is met by another force that neutralizes part of its effect.*"
(Farr, Part II).

Again, the use of the force of mortality had a very important clinical implication. In the case of cholera, early treatment was essential because half of the deaths happened in the first 24 hours:

"What the practitioner does he should do quickly."
(Farr, Part II).

2.4.2. The fallacy resulting from neglect of the period of exposure to risk

We speak of a 5-year-risk or a 10-year risk. Whether the risk is over 5 or 10 years is critical for its interpretation. Neglecting the period of exposure to risk can also lead to invalid interpretation of a study result. The British epidemiologist Austin Bradford Hill (1897–1991) described the potential fallacy resulting from neglect of the period of exposure to risk in his textbook *"Introduction to medical statistics"* (Hill, 1939). As it is difficult to write more clearly than Hill, I will quote him here extensively.

"Suppose on January 1st 1936 there are 5,000 persons under observation, none of whom are inoculated; that 300 are inoculated on April 1st, a further 600 on July 1st, and another 100 on October 1st. At the end of the year there are, therefore, 1,000 inoculated persons and 4,000 still uninoculated. During the year there were registered 110 attacks amongst the inoculated persons and 890 amongst the uninoculated. If the ratio of recorded attacks to the population at the end of the year is taken, then we have rates of 110 ÷ 1,000 = 11.0 per cent amongst the inoculated and 890 ÷ 4,000 = 22.3 per cent amongst the uninoculated, a result apparently very favorable to inoculation. This result, however, must be reached even if inoculation is completely valueless, for no account has been taken of the unequal lengths of time over which the two groups were exposed. None of the 1,000 persons in the inoculated group were exposed to risk for the whole of the year but only for some fraction of it; for a proportion of the year they belong to the uninoculated group and must be counted in that group for an appropriate length of time.

The calculation should be as follows:

All 5,000 persons were uninoculated during the first quarter of the year and therefore contribute (5,000 × 1/4) years of exposure to that group. During the second quarter 4,700 persons belonged to this group – i.e., 5,000 less the 300 who were inoculated on April 1st – and they contribute (4,700 × 1/4) years of exposure to the uninoculated group. During the third quarter 4,100 persons belonged to this group – i.e.. 4,700 less the 600 who were inoculated on July 1st – and they contribute (4,100 × 1/4) years of exposure. Finally in the last quarter of the year there were 4,000 uninoculated persons – i.e., 4,100 less the 100 on October 1st – and they contribute (4,000 × 1/4) years of exposure. The "person-years" of exposure in the uninoculated group were therefore (5,000 × 1/4) + (4,700 × 1/4) + (4,100 × 1/4) + (4,000 × 1/4) = 4,450, and the attack-rate was 890 ÷ 4,450 = 20 per cent. – i.e., the equivalent of 20 attacks per 100 persons per annum. Similarly the person-years of exposure in the inoculated group are (0 × 1/4) + (300 × 1/4) + (900 × 1/4) +

Table 5 – Hypothetical example illustrating the fallacy resulting from neglect of the period of exposure to risk. Source: Table XVII, in (Hill, 1939, p. 130).

Inoculated at each point of time	Inoculated Exposed to risk in each quarter of the year [A]	Attacks at 5 per cent per quarter [B = A × 0.05]	Uninoculated Exposed to risk in each quarter of the year [C]	Attacks at 5 per cent per quarter [D = C × 0.05]
Jan. 1st, 0	0	0	5,000	250
April 1st, 300	300	15	4,700	235
July 1st, 600	900	45	4,100	205
Oct. 1st, 100	1,000	50	4,000	200
Total at end of the year	1,000	110	4,000	890

$(1,000 \times 1/4) = 550$, *for there were no persons in this group during the first three months of the year, 300 persons during the second quarter of the year, 900 during the third quarter, and 1,000 during the last quarter. The attack-rate was, therefore, 110 ÷ 550 = 20 per cent, and the inoculated and uninoculated have identical attack-rates. Neglect of the durations of exposure to risk must lead to fallacious results and must favor the inoculated. The figures are given in tabulated form (Table XVII).*

Fallacious Comparison – Ratio of attacks to final population of group. Inoculated 110 ÷ 1,000 = 11.0 per cent. Uninoculated 890 ÷ 4,000 = 22.3 per cent.

True Comparison – Ratio of attacks to person-years of exposure. Inoculated 110 ÷ (300 × 1/4) + (900 × 1/4) + (1,000 × 1/4) = 20 per cent. Uninoculated 890 ÷ (5,000 × 1/4) + (4,700 × 1/4) + (4,100 × 1/4) + (4,000 × 1/4) = 20 per cent." (Hill, 1939 pp. 128–130).

Using the terminology adopted in this book, the risks (number of cases divided by persons at risk) were 11% in the inoculated and 22.3% in the uninoculated. Apparently, inoculation protected. But the period during which cases were ascertained was shorter for the inoculated than it was for those uninoculated, because the inoculation had been done progressively between April and October of the year of observation. Using person-years at the denominator corrected this imbalance and revealed that the rate was 20 per hundred per year, identical in both groups. The valid conclusion was that inoculation is useless.

The important concept was that a risk was always implicitly associated with a period over which it applied. A risk of 20% has a different meaning if it is expressed over 6 months, one year or ten years. There is no doubt that this was understood before Hill. But Hill's example shows how critical this characteristic of risk can be, especially for group comparisons.

2.4.3. Incidence density and cumulative incidence

Olli S. Miettinen, from the Department of Epidemiology and Biostatistics at Harvard School of Public Health, revisited the relation of risk to rate 138 years after Farr in another seminal paper in the history of epidemiologic methods and concepts entitled *"Estimability and estimation in case-referent studies"* (Miettinen, 1976a). The paper addressed a problem very different from Farr's preoccupation with respect to prognosis: it had to do with the relation of case-control (which Miettinen termed case-referent) and cohort studies (see section 3.11).

Miettinen renamed the incidence rate "incidence density", and interestingly, listed as synonyms two of Farr's expressions, "force of morbidity" and "force of mortality". Miettinen also popularized the term "cumulative incidence" instead of "risk". The properties of risks and rates remained those described by Farr, but Miettinen showed that the risk could be expressed as a function of the incidence density (ID). In its simpler formulation:

$$\textit{Cumulative incidence}_{(up\ to\ time\ j)} = \Sigma_{from\ time\ i\ =\ 1\ to\ j}\ ID_i$$

For example, suppose that the incidence rate of a relatively rare disease (e.g., breast cancer) changes at each year of age and that there is no cohort effect (see section 3.4.3). The risk of a woman to develop breast cancer before age 75 is the sum of the 74 age-specific incidence rates between birth and age 74. In Western societies, this cumulative incidence is about 7%. The formula found in Miettinen's paper (Miettinen, 1976a) allows for the possibility that incidence rates are stable over specific time periods, Δt (e.g., $\Delta t = 5$ for a 5-year risk). In this situation:

$$\textit{Cumulative incidence}_{(up\ to\ time\ j)} = \Sigma_{from\ time\ i\ =\ 1\ to\ j}\ ID_i \times \Delta t_i$$

Miettinen's innovative concepts have reached a much larger audience than the papers in which he developed them. The original papers can be arduous for someone who is not already familiar with epidemiologic concepts and methods and does not have some mathematical background. Therefore, his concepts have usually been disseminated through the work of people who wrote didactic translations of his ideas. We owe to a group of epidemiologists and statisticians at the School of Public Health of the University of North Carolina and Yale University, Hal Morgenstern, David G. Kleinbaum and Lawrence L. Kupper a paper that translates Miettinen's 1976 *"Estimability"* paper into a more universally accessible prose (Morgenstern et al., 1980).

The paper reminded first that:

> "(...) the concept of risk requires a specific period referent, – e.g., the 5-year risk of developing lung cancer." (Morgenstern et al., 1980, p. 97).

When computing the risk, that is, the proportion of all the subjects at the onset who developed the disease during a given period, we assume that all subjects have been followed during the full period. What happens when this condition of complete follow-up is not met? William Farr and Bradford Hill had shown that we could avoid a bias by computing incidence rates based on person-times, instead of risks. Miettinen proposed the following solution: divide the duration of follow-up, t, into short time intervals; compute a risk for each short interval and call it incidence density (ID); sum the incidence densities over all time intervals and you get the cumulative incidence (CI) over the period t. The cumulative incidence is a measure of the risk over period t. Using Miettinen's formula given above, we can compute the cumulative incidence (= risk) as the sum of incidence densities. This measure of risk is not affected by the fact that some observations had incomplete follow-up.

Morgenstern, Kleinbaum and Kupper illustrated the relation of risk (CI) and rate (ID) by the example described in Table 6.

The question is: what is the risk of a 35-year old woman to develop breast cancer before age 55? If we take the 60,000 women in age group 35–39 followed 3 years,

Table 6 – Illustration of the estimation of risk in a dynamic population of 250,000 women free of breast cancer, aged 35 to 55y, followed up for 3 years (on average). Source: Table 1, in (Morgenstern et al., 1980).

Age (yr)	Women at risk [N]	No of incident cases [I]	Person-years [PY = N × 3]	Incidence density[1] (/100,000/yr)	5-year Risk[2] (/100)
35–39	60,000	90	180,000	50	0.250
40–44	70,000	168	210,000	80	0.399
45–49	65,000	215	195,000	110	0.550
50–54	55,000	227	165,000	138	0.686
					20-year Risk[3]
35–54	250,000	700	750,000	–	1.871

[1] Incidence density = I ÷ Person-years.
[2] Estimate of the Δt = 5-year risk for a woman at the beginning of each age category, $R_{\Delta t} \cong 1 - \exp[-ID \times \Delta t]$.
[3] Estimate of the 20-year risk for a 35 year-old woman, $R_{\Delta t} \cong 1 - \exp[-\Sigma_j ID_j \times \Delta t_j] \cong 1 - \Pi_j (1 - R_{\Delta tj})$.

they represent altogether 180,000 person-years (column 4). The incidence density in this age category is therefore [90 ÷ 180,000 =] 50 per 100,000 per year. Now, the risk of developing breast cancer for a women aged 35 before she reaches 40, that is, over a period of 5 years, is obtained, grossly, by multiplying the incidence density by 5 years, that is, 250/100,000 or 0.25% over 5 years (last column). These 5-year risks increase with age. Thus, the 20-year risk for that same woman aged 35 corresponds, grossly, to the sum of the 5-year risks across the four age categories: [0.0025 + 0.00399 + 0.0055 + 0.00686 =] 1.885%, which is close to the 1.871 per 100 obtained using the appropriate formula mentioned in the Table 6. The answer to the question is: the 20-year risk is about 1.9%.

Note that the formula used to compute the cumulative incidences is more complicated than the simple sum of incidence densities, and should be preferred if the disease is not rare. This example underlines the conceptual evolution between Farr and Miettinen, but does not fully reflect the richness of the theory developed underneath.

2.5. Prevalence and incidence

We have seen that *prevalence* measures the accumulation in the population of events (exposures or diseases) that occurred in the distant or recent past, while *incidence* is a predictive statement about cases-to-be in a population still free of the disease. The two concepts are closely related and their relationships have been explored at least under two different perspectives: a) the relation of incidence to prevalence of disease; b) the relation of (excess) incidence to prevalence of exposure.

2.5.1. Disease prevalence divided by incidence

It has been suggested that Farr had made the first description of the relation between prevalence and incidence, as follows:

> "... in estimating the prevalence of diseases, two things must be distinctly considered; the relative frequency of their attacks, and the relative proportion of sick-time they produce. The first may be determined at once, by a comparison of the number of attacks with the numbers living; the second by enumerating several times the living and the actually sick of each disease, and thence deducing the mean proportion suffering constantly. Time is here taken into account: and the sick-time, if the attacks of two diseases be equal, will vary as their duration varies, and whatever the number of attacks may be, multiplying them by the mean duration of each disease will give the sick-time." (Cited by Lilienfeld, 1978, p. 515).

Table 7 – Prevalence, incidence and duration of acute and chronic leukemia. Brooklyn, New York, 1948–1952. Source: Table 6, in (MacMahon et al., 1960, p. 60).

Abbreviations		Acute leukemia	Chronic leukemia
[P]	Prevalence (per million)	6.7	56.1
[I]	Incidence (per million per year)	32.4	29.0
[P/I]	Duration (in years)	0.21	1.93

But this citation seems to only reiterate the distinction between death risk and death rate. Farr says that the number of deaths divided by the number of living cases gives the risk, and divided by sick person-times gives a rate. Farr uses the word prevalence as a synonym for disease occurrence. The key sentence, "time is here taken into account", is related to the computation of person-times.

The first time I found the relation of prevalence to incidence clearly described was in the textbook of epidemiology "*Epidemiology: Principles and Methods*" by Brian MacMahon, Thomas F. Pugh (1914–1973) and Johannes Ibsen (no dates found) (MacMahon et al., 1960, pp. 60–61) from the Department of Epidemiology at Harvard School of Public Health. The relation of prevalence to incidence is quite straightforward:

> "... *a change in point prevalence from one period to the next may be the result of changes in (1) incidence, (2) duration, or (3) both incidence and duration.*" (MacMahon et al., 1960, p. 61).

Prevalence may increase because patients survive longer with their disease. At a given moment, if incidence and duration can be deemed constant, their relation to prevalence seems to come out straight from a textbook of mechanical physics:

Prevalence = Incidence × Average duration of disease

Both incidence and duration need to be expressed in the same time units (e.g., years). Table 7 shows that both acute and chronic leukemia have similar incidence rates (about 30 per million per year), but that chronic leukemia is eight times more prevalent than acute leukemia.

Using the formula above, we can compute the average duration of the disease (D) by dividing the prevalence (P) by the incidence (I):

For acute leukemia: D = P ÷ I = [6.7 ÷ 32.4] = 0.21 years or 2.5 months
For chronic leukemia: D = P ÷ I = [56.1 ÷ 29.0] = 1.93 years or 23 months

These durations were close to the values of 2.4 months for acute leukemia and 20 months for chronic leukemia derived from independent follow-up of these same patients.

The conceptual link between prevalence, incidence rate and duration is perfectly illustrated in this example. It was to be shown later that the full theory was a bit more complicated. The P = I × D relation can only be assessed in populations that are stable in terms of risk and balanced in terms of in- and out-migration (Freeman and Hutchison, 1980; Miettinen, 1985). The exact relation is with the prevalence odds [P ÷ (1-P)] rather than with the simple prevalence (Miettinen, 1985; Rothman, 1986).

2.5.2. Exposure prevalence multiplied by (excess) incidence

Geoffrey Rose introduced a new dimension of population thinking when he computed and interpreted the product of prevalence and (excess) incidence. In the previous examples, population thinking consisted in applying to an individual, information gathered in the population such as the risk of dying from cholera. If, on average, 46% of the cholera patients die from the disease in the population, we would say that any individual in this population had a 46% risk of dying when infected by *Vibrio cholerae*. In his seminal paper entitled "*Strategy of prevention: lessons from cardiovascular disease*" (Rose, 1981), Rose approached the question of the risk impact at the *population* rather than at the *individual* level:

> "What we may call "population attributable risk" – the excess risk associated with a factor in the population as a whole – depends on the product of the individual attributable risk (the excess risk in individuals with that factor) and the prevalence of the factor in the population." (Rose, 1981, p. 1849).

Rose demonstrated that, for diseases such as coronary heart disease or stroke, the majority of the cases occur among subjects at low risk of disease. Why is this so? Because low-risk constitutions for chronic diseases are usually much more common than high-risk constitutions. The histogram in Figure 2 (corresponding to Figure 3 of Rose's paper) shows the prevalence of various categories of serum cholesterol levels in 246 men aged 55–64 at the baseline examination of the Framingham Heart Study.

The way the numbers were obtained is shown in Table 8.

If we set, as Rose did, the point for hypercholesterolemia at 310 mg/dl (or 8 mmol/l), 3% of the population is hypercholesterolemic. If the cutoff is set at 250 mg/dl (6.5 mmol/l) as recommended today, about 25% of the population is hypercholesterolemic. The figure and the table show the mortality rates from coronary heart disease corresponding to each of the categories of serum cholesterol concentration. For example, the mortality rate is 11.19 per 1,000 per year in those with serum cholesterol of 310 mg/dl (8 mmol/l) or more. The excess mortality rate attributable to high cholesterol is obtained by subtracting the absolute mortality rate in

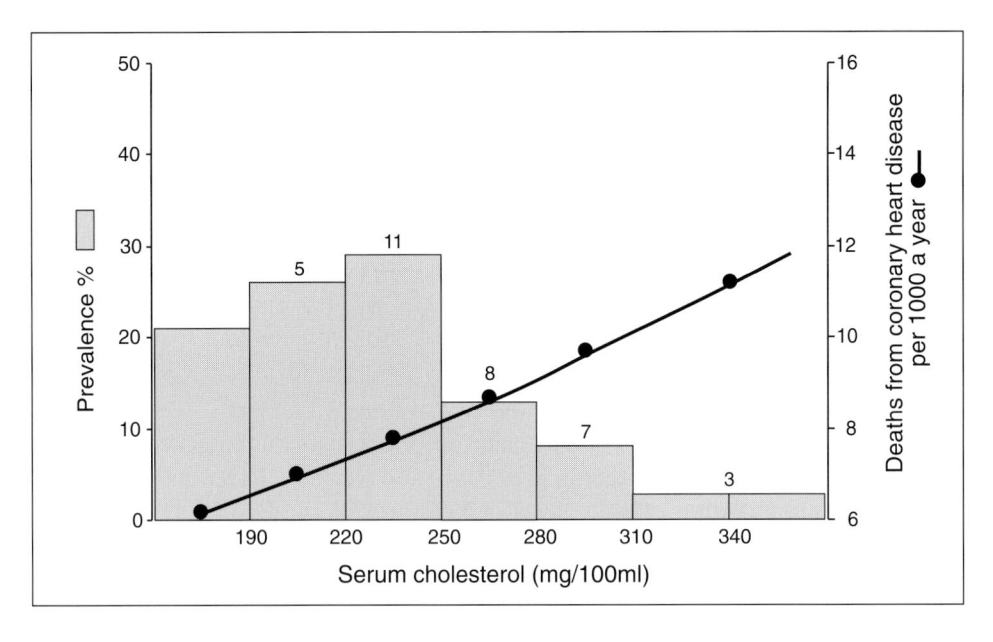

Figure 2
Prevalence of cholesterol levels, and corresponding mortality rates and excess cases. The Framingham Heart Study. Exam 1. Men aged 55–64 years. Source: Figure 3 in (Rose, 1981, p. 1849).

the subgroup with hypercholesterolemia from that with serum cholesterol below 190 mg/dl (4.92 mmol/l), that is, [11.19 – 6.22 =] 4.97/1,000 per year. The attributable risk over 10 years is therefore ten times larger, that is, 49.7/1,000. The 10y-attributable risk applied to 7 men (3% of 246 men) yields [7 × 0.0497 =] 3 deaths per 10,000 men over 10 years. If we do a similar calculation for the subgroup with total cholesterolemia between 220 and 250, we get 11 excess deaths for 10,000 at risk over 10 years. Altogether, 31 of the 34 (91%) excess deaths in 10 years will occur among people with total cholesterol <8 mmol/l, or 16 out of 34 (47%) among people with total cholesterol <6.5 mmol/l. Most cases occur in people without hypercholesterolemia.

Rose's description of Figure 2 reads like this:

> "The risk rises fairly steeply with increasing cholesterol concentration; but out on the right, where the risk to affected individuals is high, the prevalence is fortunately low. If we want to ask, 'How many excess coronary deaths is the cholesterol-related risk responsible for in this population?' we simply multiply the excess risk at each concentration by the number of people with that concentration that are exposed to that risk. In figure 3 [Figure 2 above] these attributable deaths

Table 8 – Prevalence of cholesterol levels, and corresponding mortality rates, excess risk, excess deaths and cumulative proportions of excess deaths. The Framingham Heart Study. Exam 1. Men aged 55-64 years. Source: Tables 13-3-A and B, in (Kannel and Gordon, 1970).

Cholesterol	N [A]	Prevalence (%) [B = A ÷ 246]	Mortality rate (/1,000/ year) [C]	Excess mortality risk (/1,000) over 10y [D = (C – 6.22) × 10]	Excess deaths/ 10,000 over 10 y* [E = (D × A) ÷ 100]	Cumulative proportion of excess deaths [F = Σ (E ÷ 34)]
Less than 190	52	21	6.22	0	0	0
190 to 219	63	26	7.00	7.80	5	14.71
220 to 249	71	29	7.80	15.80	11	47.06
250 to 279	33	13	8.68	24.60	8	70.59
280 to 309	20	8	9.67	34.50	7	91.18
310 or more	7	3	11.19	49.70	3	100
	246	100			34	

* Rose wrote "extra deaths per *thousand* of this population over a 10-year period" but calculations based on the data he used indicate extra deaths per *ten thousand* over 10 years.

are shown as the numbers on top of bars. They add up to 34 extra deaths per 1,000 in this population over a 10-year period, of which only three arise at concentrations at or above 310 mg/100 ml (8 mmol/l) – which would be called high ("outside the normal range") by conventional clinical standards. The rest (90%) arise from the many people in the middle part of the distribution who are exposed to a small risk." (Rose, 1981, p. 1849).

Rose concluded that

"this illustrates a fundamental principle in the strategy of prevention. A large number of people exposed to a low risk are likely to produce more cases than a small number of people exposed to a high risk." (Rose, 1981, p. 1849).

In this same seminal paper, Rose made another key observation, which he called the "prevention paradox":

"A measure that brings large benefit to the community offers little to each participating individual." (Rose, 1981, p. 1850).

This paradox leads to another way of expressing the population attributable risk. Rose noted for example that

> *"when mass diphtheria immunization was introduced in Britain 40 years ago, even then roughly 600 children had to be immunized in order that one life would be saved – 599 "wasted" immunizations for the one that was effective."*
> (Rose, 1981, p. 1850).

How does this relate to the population attributable risk? Rose also could have said that the attributable (death) risk in non-vaccinated children was 17 per 10,000 non-vaccinated children. Hence, the vaccine would have prevented 17 deaths per 10,000 vaccinated children. Instead, he took the inverse of the attributable risk (that is, 1 over the attributable risk) to express the number of children that needed to be vaccinated in order to prevent one death: the number was [1 ÷ 0.0017 =] 588 children. The inverse of the attributable risk (1 ÷ AR) eventually became extremely popular in clinical epidemiology when repackaged under the acronym of NNT (Number needed to treat). Simple rule of thumb: NNT = 1 ÷ AR (Laupacis et al., 1988).

2.6. Risk and strength of association

In 1976 Kenneth Rothman proposed a "conceptual framework for causes" which offered the possibility of expressing the notion of risk in terms of conditions for disease causation.

> *"A cause is an act or event or a state of nature which initiates or permits, alone or in conjunction with other causes, a sequence of events resulting in an effect."*
> (Rothman, 1976, p. 588).

Rothman defined as a *sufficient* cause a *set* of causes, each of which, alone, was not sufficient to produce an effect. Figure 3 (Figure 1 of the paper), classically known today as "Rothman's causal pies", depicts three sufficient causes, each of which comprises 5 component causes.

In the paper, the different letters associated with each component cause served to explain a multitude of epidemiologic concepts, such as etiological fraction or interaction, which I do not describe here. But the contribution of the pies to the evolution of population thinking lies in their ability to conceptualize, and therefore bring to an even higher level of abstraction, the notions of "risk" and "strength of a causal risk factor". Consider that each component cause (which we may also call "risk factors") has a life of its own, and that it is only under some specific circumstances that it is united with other risk factors to form a sufficient cause, and therefore produce disease. Then:

> *"...the mean risk for a group indicates the proportion of individuals for whom sufficient causes are formed."* (Rothman, 1976, p. 589).

This formulation of the notion of risk is tautological. If you accept the definition of the sufficient cause, then of course the risk is the probability that sufficient causes are formed. But the implication of this definition of risk opened the way to a new degree of understanding of the relation between the prevalence of risk factors, and the magnitude of the risk change they potentially incur in the population when a sufficient cause is completed:

> *"A component cause which requires, to complete the sufficient cause, other components with low prevalence is thereby a "weak" (component) cause. (...) On the other hand, a component cause which requires, to complete the sufficient cause, other components which are nearly ubiquitous is a "strong" (component) cause."* (Rothman, 1976 p. 590).

Thus, the strength of a risk factor depends on the prevalence of the complementary risk factors needed to create a sufficient cause. This result has truly insightful implications with respect to population thinking:

> *"The characterization of risk factors as "strong" or "weak" has no universal basis (...) the strength of a causal risk factor (...) is dependent on the distribution in the population of the other risk factors in the same sufficient cause."* (Rothman, 1976, pp. 589–590).

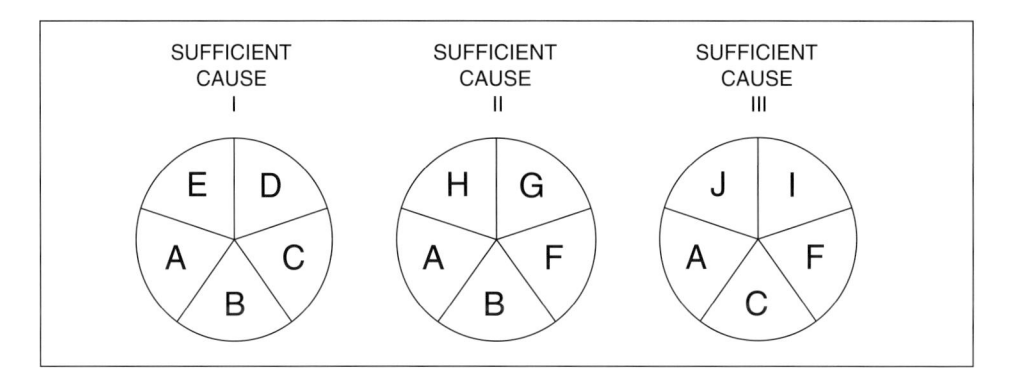

Figure 3
Conceptual scheme for the causes of a hypothetical disease. Source: Figure 1 of (Rothman, 1976).

The same risk factor can be strong in one population if its complement causes are common, and weak in another if its complement causes are rare. The textbook by Rothman and Sander Greenland, epidemiologist at University of California, Los Angeles (Rothman and Greenland, 1998, pp. 9–11) provides a numerical example, which is very useful for illustrating these concepts.

2.7. Evolution of population thinking in epidemiology

Let us at this point synthesize the lessons of the examples reviewed above. Population thinking in epidemiology has its roots in the 17th century. The premises of most measures of occurrence of disease are present in the probably first substantial contribution to population thinking (section 2.3.1). Graunt computed the proportion of deaths from the plague and the ratios of the number of births to the number of deaths. He also computed primitive weekly "rates" of plague mortality in order to compare the mortality during outbreaks of plague that lasted different numbers of years or to describe the evolution over time of a given epidemic. The distinction between rates and risks probably preceded Farr. Both measures are necessary to describe event (e.g., diseases) occurrence in a population.

John Snow used the ratio of the number of cholera deaths to the number of households provided for by each water company (section 2.3.2). This ratio could be an ambiguous measure of risk if the populations compared had different household sizes. This may explain why Farr attempted to relate cholera deaths to the number of people living in the affected neighborhoods as enumerated by the census. Farr's risks were expressed as proportions of inhabitants.

It was probably perceived that risks had to be expressed as percentages of people susceptible to getting the disease but, in public health, there could be problems in getting an appropriate denominator. Analyses in clinical settings did not suffer from this problem. Indeed, medical researchers of the 18th and 19th century commonly used proportions (Troehler, 2000; Morabia, 1996).

Simple proportions have been the most commonly used measures to describe the pattern of occurrence of acute infectious diseases in populations, which occur abruptly and have short average durations. Simple parameters suffice to describe them. The situation is very different for diseases that kill slowly and therefore last a long time. One type of disease kills quickly but lasts only days and does not accumulate in the population (e.g., cholera), while another type kills slowly but lasts for years and cases can accumulate over time (e.g., tuberculosis). Duration of disease is the factor that distinguishes these two types of disease.

Farr therefore divided the risk by the average duration of disease and this yielded a rate measure, that is, an average risk per unit of disease duration (section 2.4.1). The risk of dying from tuberculosis was 100%; the average time to death was 2 years. Thus, the death rate was [100 ÷ 2 years =] 50% per year or < 1% per week, etc.

When using risks instead of rates Farr had expressed the following caveat:

"To determine the mortality of diseases [= risk] they [the patients] should be followed from the beginning to the end; every death or recovery should be recorded; and this, though exceedingly simple, has rarely been done."
(Farr, Part II).

A measure of risk is *implicitly* related to a duration! We can express a risk of the same event over 1 week, 1 year, 10 years, etc. In the 1930s, Hill (see section 2.4.2) demonstrated, using a hypothetical example, the importance of this caveat in the context of a therapeutic trial comparing the ability of a vaccine to prevent disease attacks. By dividing the number of disease attacks by the total number of subjects inoculated during the year, we implicitly compute a risk over one year. However, if some or the entire inoculated group is followed for less than a whole year, the true risk would be underestimated. If this bias has different magnitude among the inoculated and the uninoculated, it may even produce a fallacious association between inoculation and disease risk. The solution was to use person-times in the denominator because it counted everyone's exposure for an appropriate length of time.

Epidemiologists of the 19th century had all the elements to find that the accumulation of cases in the population (prevalence) varied as a function of the incidence rate and the duration of disease. But there may not have been the need to distinguish the risk (the probability of occurrence of new cases) from the prevalence (the proportion of people with the disease in the population) as the diseases studied at that time rapidly ended up in either cure or death.

The spectrum of diseases changed in the 20th century, when major infectious scourges waned and chronic illnesses, such as cardiovascular diseases, cancer or infectious diseases with low case fatality rates surged. Consider the example of tuberculosis. Its incidence rate rapidly declined between 1900 and 1950. Still, a large fraction of the living population had been exposed to the Koch bacillus at some time in their life and had subclinical infections. The risk of getting infected was becoming low, but older people were still dying of infection contracted in the past. To accurately describe this situation, one needed to clarify how prevalence was related to risk. Around 1960, textbooks indicated that prevalence equaled the product of incidence and duration of disease. In the example given by MacMahon et al. (section 2.5.1), chronic and acute leukemia had similar incidence rates, but the prevalence of chronic leukemia was higher because its time to death was on average 2 years *vs.* about 2 months for acute leukemia. In reality, this simple, mechanical physics-looking expression, Prevalence = Incidence × Duration ($P = I \times D$), serves more heuristic than practical purposes. Its exact formulation is more complicated, and it is based on the assumption that the composition and disease experience of the population remains relatively stable.

Dividing a *risk* by the *duration* of disease yielded a rate. Multiplying an incidence *rate* by the *duration* of disease yielded a *prevalence*. What about the product of *prevalence* and incidence *rate*? Geoffrey Rose systematically explored this path and his findings were astonishing (section 2.5.2). They showed, contrary to what we would intuitively expect, that most of the cases of some chronic diseases, such as coronary heart disease, originate from the majority of the population who are at low risk for the trait. The rule was that a small risk applied to a large number of people generates an abundance of cases. The fraction of these cases that can be attributed to a given risk factor was obtained by computing the product of prevalence of exposure and the attributable (or excess) risk. This finding had a major implication for prevention: an efficient prevention strategy should consider targeting the mass of the population and not only the minority that is at high risk for the trait (Rose, 1981).

By the end of the 1960s, the distinction between risks and rates remained essentially conceptual: the number of incident cases was either divided by the number of persons at risk to form a risk, or it was divided by the number of person-times to form an incidence rate. This distinction was sufficient in practice but lacked mathematical rigor. The latter came from Miettinen's expression stipulating, in its simpler formulation, that the cumulative incidence over a time interval was the sum of the incidence densities computed over all the time sub-sections within the whole time interval (section 2.4.3). Considering that cumulative incidence is a synonym for risk and incidence density a synonym for incidence rate, we must acknowledge that quite a theoretical distance had been covered between Farr's *On Prognosis* (Farr, 2003) and Miettinen's *Estimability* (Miettinen, 1976a).

The developments have allowed epidemiologists to study more complex questions, more rigorously too. The future chapters of the evolution of population thinking in epidemiology are currently being written. A likely scenario is that the new concepts will become increasingly abstract and therefore difficult to illustrate using simplified examples as I have done here.

3. Group comparisons

3.1. Definition

Population thinking is indispensable for comparing groups, which is, as I will argue later, the main mode of knowledge acquisition in epidemiology. To compare groups we use measures of occurrence of events in populations. We compare prevalence, risks, rates, and odds.

The role of the comparison is to contrast what is observed in the presence of exposure to what would have occurred had the group of interest not been exposed to the postulated cause. Differences in frequency of disease occurrence between groups can be interpreted logically (albeit not always correctly) as being caused by the exposure. There are two main study designs used in epidemiology to reach this goal.

In the first design, the groups differ in their exposure to the postulated cause (e.g., smoking). The occurrence of disease (e.g., risks or incidence rates) is the compared variable. I use three different terms for this type of study design: 1) exposed *vs.* non-exposed comparisons, because this is what it consists of; 2) cohort studies, because this is their most common current term, although the name was only coined around 1960 (MacMahon et al., 1960) and can hardly be used to describe earlier experiments; cohort studies are further divided, following the terminology used in the paper on the history of cohort studies (Doll, Part II), into a) *prospective* cohort studies, when cohorts are followed as they age; and b) *retrospective* cohort studies, when a substantial part of the follow-up is performed in the past, using historical data; 3) randomized controlled trials, which are a subform of cohort studies in which exposure (usually to a treatment) has been allocated in a random manner.

In the second design, the groups are either affected or non-affected by the studied outcome (e.g., lung cancer). Past exposure to the postulated cause (e.g., cigarette smoking) is the compared variable. I use again three different terms for this type of study design: 1) affected *vs.* non-affected comparisons, because this is what the comparisons consist of; 2) case-control studies, because this is their most common current denomination, although the name was only coined around 1960 (Morris, 1964) and can hardly be used to describe earlier experiments; 3) *nested* case-control studies, which are case-control studies designed within fully enumerated populations under investigation in a cohort study.

Let us consider examples of group comparisons that illustrate the evolution of epidemiologic concepts and methods over time.

3.2. Eighteenth century

The demonstration by James Lind (1716–1794), a Scottish naval physician, that (Lind, 1753) consumption of oranges and lemons could cure scurvy is an important step in the history of epidemiologic methods (Lind, 1753). It is a very early (if not the earliest) description of a group comparison to identify the treatment of a disease.

In the 18th century, scurvy was perceived as a terrible, rapidly fatal epidemic disease, which hit seamen on long voyages, campaigning armies, besieged cities and migrant populations. Scurvy is said to have eliminated 65% of Vasco de Gama's crew in 1498. An attack of scurvy could bring down in a few days seamen and soldiers in apparently good health. Affected persons became weak and had joint pain. Black-and-blue marks appeared on the skin. At the first visible signs of scurvy, red spots around the hair follicles covered the legs, buttocks, arms and back. Gums hemorrhaged and their tissue became weak and spongy. Teeth loosened and eating became difficult and painful. Stupor and death followed rapidly.

Table 9 – Description of treatment and outcomes in James Lind's 1747 experiment on 6 pairs of seamen suffering from scurvy. Source: (Lind, 1753).

Experimental pairs	Treatment for each pair member	Qualitative outcome
1	"a quart of cider a day"	"improved"
2	"twenty five gouts of elixir vitriol three times a-day, upon an empty stomach, using a gargle strongly acidulated with it for their mouths"	"mouth but not internal improvement"
3	"two spoonfuls of vinegar three times a-day upon an empty stomach, having their gruels and their other food well acidulated with it, as also the gargle for their mouth"	"no remarkable alteration (…) upon comparing their condition with others who had taken nothing but a lenitive electuary and cremor tartar …"
4 "two of the worst patients, with the tendons in the ham rigid (a symptom none the rest had)"	"half a pint of sea water every day, and sometimes more or less as it operated, by way of gentle physic"	"no remarkable alteration (…) compared to those who had taken nothing but a lenitive electuary …"
5	"two oranges and one lemon given them every day. These they eat with greediness at different times upon an empty stomach. They continued but six days under this course, having consumed the quantity that could be spared."	"the most sudden and visible good effects were perceived from the use of the oranges and lemons; one of those who had taken them being at the end of six days fit for duty. The spots were not indeed at that time quite off his body, nor his gums sound; but without any other medicine than a gargarism of elixir vitriol, he became quite healthy before we came into Plymouth, which was on the 16th of June. The other was the best recovered of any in his condition; and being now deemed pretty well was appointed nurse to the rest of the sick."

Table 9 – (continued)

Experimental pairs	Treatment for each pair member	Qualitative outcome
6 Reference group. The electuary and the cremor tartar was meant to *"keep their belly open"* and *"for relief of their breast"*.	*"…the bigness of a nutmeg three times a-day of an electuary recommended by an hospital surgeon made of garlic, mustard seed, rad. raphan., balsam of Peru and gum myrrh; using for common drink, barley-water well acidulated with tamarinds; by a decoction of which, with the addition of cremor tartar, they were gently purged three or four times during the course."*	*"no change"*

Scurvy was an important obstacle for naval supremacy. More seamen died of disease than of shipwrecks, battles, or famine. The diet of the sailors included cheese biscuits, salt beef, dried fish, butter, peas and beans. In retrospect, lack of fresh fruits or vegetables deprived the diet of vitamin C.

In 1731, Lind became a naval surgeon. In 1747, while serving on the 50 gun, 960 ton H.M.S. Salisbury, he carried out experiments on scurvy, which he published in 1753:

"On the 20th May, 1747, I took twelve patients in the scurvy on board the Salisbury at sea. Their cases were as similar as I could have them. They all in general had putrid gums, the spots and lassitude, with weakness of their knees. They lay together in one place, being a proper apartment for the sick in the fore-hold; and had one diet in common to all, viz., water gruel sweetened with sugar in the morning; fresh mutton broth often times for dinner; at other times puddings, boiled biscuit with sugar etc.; and for supper barley, raisins, rice and currants, sago and wine, or the like. Two of these were ordered each a quart of cider a day. Two others took twenty-five gouts of elixir vitriol three times a day upon an empty stomach, using a gargle strongly acidulated with it for their mouths. Two others took two spoonfuls of vinegar three times a day upon an empty stomach, having their gruels and their other food well acidulated with it, as also the gargle for the mouth. Two of the worst patients, with the tendons in the ham rigid (a symptom none the rest had) were put under a course of seawater. Of this they drank half a pint every day and sometimes more or less as it operated by way of gentle physic. Two others had each two oranges and one lemon given them every day. These they

eat with greediness at different times upon an empty stomach. They continued but six days under this course, having consumed the quantity that could be spared. The two remaining patients took the bigness of a nutmeg three times a day of an electuary recommended by an hospital surgeon made of garlic, mustard seed, rad. raphan., balsam of Peru and gum myrrh, using for common drink nearly water well acidulated with tamarinds, by a decoction of which, with the addition of cremor tartar, they were gently purged three or four times during the course." (Lind, 1753, p. 145).

"The consequence was that the most sudden and visible good effects were perceived from the use of the oranges and lemons; one of those who had taken them being at the end of six days fit for duty. The spots were not indeed at that time quite off his body, nor his gums sound; but without any other medicine than a gargarism or elixir of vitriol he became quite healthy before we came into Plymouth, which was on the 16th June. The other was the best recovered of any in his condition, and being now deemed pretty well was appointed nurse to the rest of the sick." (Lind, 1753, p. 146).

"As I shall have occasion elsewhere to take notice of the effects of other medicines in this disease, I shall here only observe that the result of all my experiments was that oranges and lemons were the most effectual remedies for this distemper at sea." (Lind, 1753, p. 128).

Table 9 summarizes the results of the Salisbury experiment as described by Lind.

Note that Lind created comparable conditions of disease presentation, setting and diet before attributing the treatments. He also deliberately did not give any putatively active treatment to one of the groups, which served as control.

In Lind's view, oranges and lemons were *"remedies"* for scurvy. He did not mention scurvy *prevention*. His experiment demonstrated the *in*activity of sulfuric acid, vinegar, etc., which were the treatments officially recommended (Carpenter, 1986, p. 54).

Lind believed that scurvy was caused by both diet and some peculiarity of the air at sea, such as its *"moisture"*(Carpenter, 1986, pp. 60–61). This vision makes no sense to us, but in the 18th century, the hypothesis that some inadequacy in the diet could cause scurvy would have sounded absurd. Causes had to be related to some properties of gas or acid-alkaline reaction (Carpenter, 1986, pp. 40 and 75). We know now that a deficit in vitamin C is the cause of the metabolic disorders leading to the signs and symptoms of Lind's sick seamen. Primates share with guinea pigs the misfortune of not manufacturing their own vitamin C and having to obtain it from fresh food. Ascorbic acid (vitamin C) was isolated and synthesized in 1932.

It was Gilbert Blane (1749–1834), another Scottish physician, who, 40 years after Lind's Treatise, convinced the Lords of the Admiralty to supply a quarter of an ounce of lemon juice or lime to their seamen. English sailors to this day are called "limeys", for lime was the term used at the time for both lemons and limes. Between 1895 and 1914, the Navy consumed 7,300 tons of lime. Epidemics of scurvy disappeared.

The work of Lind raises many fascinating questions. Why did Lind decide to conduct this comparative experiment? Who or what inspired him? Why Lind ? Why in 1740? I have not found answers to these questions. Apparently, seamen were often used as experimentation subjects in these years. Let's note that the sample size was so small that Lind must have been expecting an all-or-nothing answer. Indeed, only the two sailors in the orange and lemon pair became rapidly "fit for duty".

3.3. Nineteenth century

Three hundred years ago, medicine in Europe had to deal with the consequences of the colonial expansion of most of its States. "Fever" was the cardinal symptom of many different disorders:

> *"The 18th century struggle against fever has been compared, mutatis mutandis* [from the Latin: changing what needs to be changed], *with our present day efforts against cancer and arteriosclerosis. Both are the great killers of the times."* (Troehler, 1978, p. 78).

This observation can be extended to the first half of the 19th century. There were septic fevers following amputations but also puerperal, choleric, yellow fever, slow fever, diarrheic fevers, smallpox, malaria, hepatitis, and ophthalmic infections. Fevers were everywhere and physicians did not know how to cure them.

We will review here two episodes in which group comparisons yielded the correct answer about the treatment or the etiology of fevers, one in a clinical setting and the other in public health.

3.3.1. The bloodletting controversy

In the aftermath of the French Revolution, François Joseph Victor Broussais (1772–1838), an influential Parisian physician, a Jacobin, having served in the imperial army, was convinced that he had a solution to the therapeutic nightmare of fevers. He taught that fevers were manifestations of organ inflammation and that bloodletting and leeches were efficient to treat them all. Leeches had to be applied on the surface of the body corresponding to the inflamed organ. For example, the chest of a patient suspected of having tuberculosis was covered with multitudes of leeches. At the apogee of Broussais's influence, France used tens of millions of leeches per year. In 1833 alone, France imported 42 million of these annelid worms (Ackerknecht, 1967, p. 62).

Table 10 – Age, number of bleedings, duration of illness and risk of death according to day of first bleeding in Pierre-Charles-Alexandre Louis's "Researches on the effects of bloodletting ...". Source: (Louis, 1836).

Day of first bleeding	No of subjects	Mean age (years)	Duration of disease (days)	Mortality (%)
1–4	41	41	17.8	44
5–9	36	38	20.8	25
Total	77	40	19.2	35

Pierre Charles Alexandre Louis (1787–1872), another French physician, a contemporary of Broussais, who had had some experience as a clinician in Russia before he started practicing in France, was extremely doubtful about the validity of Broussais' theory. Louis published several monographs against Broussais' views, one of which is the "*Researches on the effects of bloodletting in some inflammatory diseases*". A first version appeared as an article in the 1828 Annales de Médecine Générale (Louis, 1828). This paper, revised and expanded, became a book in 1835 (Louis, 1835). The book was translated and published in English by an American student of Louis in 1836 (Louis, 1836).

In this book, Louis reports the following experiment. He had a large collection of case descriptions, which he had accrued during years of intensive clinical activity and autopsy in the Parisian Hospital La Charité. He found in his clinical records a total of 77 patients who were comparable because they had a well-characterized form of pneumonia (Morabia and Rochat, 2001) and were in perfect health at the time of the first symptoms of the disease. Twenty-seven of them had died. For each patient he computed the duration of illness from disease onset to death or recovery.

Louis compared the duration of disease and the frequency of death according to the time during the course of the disease when the patient underwent the first bleeding (Table 10). Louis grouped those first bled during days 1 to 4 of the disease (*early bloodletting*) and those bled for the first time during days 5 to 9 after the onset of the disease (*late bloodletting*). The two groups of patients were of comparable age. Duration of disease was on average 3 days shorter in those with early bloodletting (17.8 days) than in patients with late bloodletting (20.8 days). However, risk of death was 44% in the patients bled during the first 4 days of the disease compared to 25% among those bled later. These results ruled out the strong protective effect of early bleeding claimed by Broussais.

According to Louis

"*a startling and apparently absurd result*" (Louis, 1836, p. 9).

Louis did not conclude that bloodletting was useless but that it was much less useful than had been commonly believed:

"Thus, the study of the general and local symptoms, the mortality and variations in the mean duration of pneumonitis, according to the period at which bloodletting was instituted; all establish narrow limits to the utility of this mode of treatment." (Louis, 1836, p. 13).

In his view, the validity of the technique was limited to severe cases of pneumonia:

"I will add that bloodletting, notwithstanding its influence is limited, should not be neglected in inflammations which are severe and are seated in an important organ; both on account of its influence on the state of the diseased organ; and because in shortening the duration of the disease, it diminishes the chance of secondary lesions." (Louis, 1836, p. 23).

The data reported by Louis can be revisited with modern analytical tools (Morabia, 1996). They are available on *http://www.epidemiology.ch/index3.htm*. We can compare the prevalence of early bleeding in the group of patients who died with those who survived. Or we can compare the death risk in those bled in the first four days after disease onset *vs.* those bled more than four days after disease onset. Using a survival analysis, the group bled during the first four days of disease tended to do worse, but the difference was not statistically significant ($p = 0.07$). Also, if patients bled later in the course of the disease had a better prognosis, because they had already passed the worst phase of the illness, the bias would have favored late bleeding.

Louis was a meticulous clinician convinced of the importance of population thinking in medicine. He had understood that group comparisons were required to assess, in most situations, the true effect of treatments. His real impact on the practice of medicine is, however, hard to assess. Broussais had been the leader of Paris medicine since 1816 but after 1832, his theories rapidly lost support (Ackerknecht, 1967, p. 67). It took another century of progress in medical knowledge to completely settle the bloodletting controversy.

3.3.2. The London 1854 natural experiment

John Snow and William Farr can be considered as a 19th century English duet between a physician, primarily an anesthesiologist, and a "statistician", that is, someone who collected data for the "state" (Morabia, 2001a). It is thanks to their collaboration that the two fundamental elements of epidemiology, population thinking and group comparisons, merged around 1850 to produce the core of a new scientific discipline.

Most epidemiologists are familiar with John Snow's investigations of the 1854 epidemic of cholera in London and of the now famous outbreak around the Broad Street pump. His successful study of 1854, which I will briefly recall later, was preceded by an indefatigable pursuit of all the indices that might have put Snow on the right track (Shephard, 1995; Vinten-Johansen et al., 2003). In 1849, Snow analyzed the reports of the Registrar-General (i.e., William Farr's office) from September 23, 1848 to August 25, 1849. Using the population in 1841 as denominator, mortality varied between 1.10 per thousand inhabitants in the northern district and 7.95 in the southern districts of London (ratio 7.95 ÷ 1.10 = 7.2). (Shephard, 1995, p. 169).

Note that the ratios are quite large and Snow already suspected that this higher mortality originated from the supply of water polluted by sewage. Nevertheless, Snow still did not have a case for his hypothesis that cholera was transmitted by water, linen or foods contaminated by feces of sick people. First, the mortality rates remained small (between about 1 and 10 per 1,000 inhabitants per year), and skeptical opponents could invoke many alternative reasons for which mortality could be higher south than north of the Thames (Eyler, Part IIa).

The conditions for a rigorous group comparison occurred spontaneously. In 1852, one of the major water suppliers of London, the Lambeth Water Company, in accordance with an Act of Parliament, changed its source of Thames water. Its pumps were moved from near Hungerford Bridge, where the water was certainly soiled by sewage, to a place well outside London, beyond the influence of the tide and therefore out of reach of the London sewage. In contrast, another water supplier, the Southwark and Vauxhall Company, continued to draw its water from Battersea Fields, a seriously polluted area.

"London was without cholera from the latter part of 1849 to August 1853. During this interval an important change had taken place in the water supply of several of the south districts of London. The Lambeth Company removed their water works, in 1852, from opposite Hungerford Market to Thames Ditton; thus obtaining a supply of water quite free from the sewage of London. The districts supplied by the Lambeth Company are, however, also supplied, to a certain extent, by the Southwark and Vauxhall Company, the pipes of both companies going down every street, in the places where the supply is mixed, as was previously stated. In consequence of this intermixing of the water supply, the effect of the alteration made by the Lambeth Company on the progress of cholera was not so evident, to a cursory observer, as it would otherwise have been. It attracted the attention however, of the Registrar-General, who published a table in the 'Weekly Return of Births and Deaths' for 26th November 1853 (...)."
(Snow, 1855, pp. 41–42).

William Farr had noticed that the weekly mortality from cholera in the districts partly supplied by the Lambeth Company (61 per 100,000 inhabitants) was lower than that for those districts entirely supplied by the Southwark and Vauxhall Company (94 per 100,000 inhabitants). Note that the rate (between 0.5 to 1 per 10,000 inhabitants per week) and the ratio ([94 ÷ 61 =] 1.5) imply that these were relatively rare events with a weak association. But it was when the cholera returned to London in July 1854, that John Snow resolved to make every effort to ascertain the exact effect of the water supply on the progress of the epidemic (Snow, 1855, p. 47).

It is key to understand that Snow had to invest an enormous amount of energy to create the conditions for a clear comparison of the mortality from cholera among the clients of either of the two large water suppliers. Farr provided Snow with the addresses of all cases of cholera (Eyler, Part IIa). During the first part of the epidemic, Snow himself went to each house and collected information on the exact provider. Clients often did not know the name of the provider. Snow explained that he had

"to distinguish the water from the two companies with perfect certainty by a chemical test [silver nitrate]" (Snow, 1855, p. 48).

The test may not have been as accurate as Snow pretended (Eyler, Part IIa), but it reflects Snow's concern to clearly separate the exposure to the two sources of water supply. The most cited paragraph of the second edition of *"On the Mode of Communication of Cholera"* stresses the novel idea of *group comparisons* that Snow had striven to achieve:

"The experiment, too, was on the grandest scale. No fewer than three hundred thousand people of both sexes, of every age and occupation, and of every rank and station, from gentlefolks down to the very poor, were divided into two groups without their choice, and, in most cases, without their knowledge; one group being supplied with water containing the sewage of London, and, amongst it, whatever might have come from the cholera patients, the other group having water quite free from such impurity." (Snow, 1855, pp. 46–47).

During the first seven weeks of the epidemics there were 1,361 deaths from cholera in the districts supplied by the two companies (See Table 2): 1,263 (315 per 10,000) occurred in Southwark and Vauxhall districts *vs.* 98 (37 per 10,000) in those of the Lambeth Company. The ratio of [315 ÷ 37 =] 8.5 was of a magnitude comparable with the ratio between southern and northern districts observed in 1849, but in this case the two groups were compared on a specific factor, namely water supply. Skeptics could still argue that the association was caused by a third variable, such as poverty or elevation above sea level. But the argument could be "evacuated" by Snow who also compared the mortality from cholera of the houses supplied by the *same* company in 1849 and 1854, that is, before and after the Lambeth Company had moved its pumps to cleaner areas. Mortality had remained constant for the Southwark and Vauxhall clients but was four times lower for those of the Lambeth:

> *"The table exhibits an increase of mortality in 1854 as compared with 1849, in the sub-districts supplied by the Southwark and Vauxhall Company only, whilst there is a considerable diminution of mortality in the sub-districts partly supplied by the Lambeth Company. In certain sub-districts, where I know that the supply of the Lambeth Water Company is more general than elsewhere, as Christchurch, London Road, Waterloo Road 1st, and Lambeth Church 1st, the decrease of mortality in 1854 as compared with 1849 is greatest, as might be expected."*
> (Snow, 1855, p. 56).

Thus, the experiment offered a double perspective on group comparisons: concurrent differences in mortality, and "before and after" changes in exposure comparisons.

To appreciate this considerable achievement of John Snow, it is important to bear in mind the state of public health at these times, and in particular the work of Farr. Farr had created a unique and innovative system of standardized procedures for the collection, classification, analysis and reporting of causes of deaths. The compiling power of Farr's administration was, in Eyler's words, "herculean" given that there were no machines to treat all the information automatically (Eyler, Part IIa).

The description of the experiments and the extent of the co-operation between Farr and Snow (Eyler, Part IIa) all indicate that Snow would not have been able to perform his epidemiologic investigations without Farr's help. Snow's genius was to recognize the conditions of a natural experiment created when the Lambeth Company moved its water inlet to a less polluted area of the Thames. But it was Farr who first noted in 1853 the potential importance of the arrangement of water supply in South London. The following year, during the epidemic of 1854, Snow carried out his investigations and communicated to Farr his first results about the relation between cholera deaths and source of water supply. Snow writes that

> *"Dr. Farr was much struck with the result and, at his suggestion, the Registrars of all the south districts of London were requested to make a return of the water supply of the house in which the attack took place, in all cases of death from cholera."* (Snow, 1855, p. 47).

The discovery of the mode of transmission of cholera appears therefore as a successful synergy between Snow and Farr, that is, medicine and public health surveillance.

3.4. Evolution of confounding

The term confounding (from the Latin *confundere*, to mix together) characterizes, in epidemiology, situations where the group comparisons cannot distinguish between the effects of multiple causes. The measured association therefore is a mix of the effects of several causes. The mixed causes beyond the one studied are the confounders or confounding variables. The presence of confounding between binary variables, that is, variables that can be categorized as 0 or 1 such as gender, treatment or disease status, can be typically assessed when the measure of the association between one cause and disease yields different results in the full population, or separately across categories of the confounding variable(s).

We will review here four episodes illustrating the progressive refinement of the concept of confounding in the 20th century.

3.4.1. The paradoxical fate of a fallacy

In 1903 the Cambridge statistician G. Udny Yule (1871–1951) first demonstrated the mechanism underlying confounding. His demonstration then almost clandestinely traveled in two major epidemiology textbooks of the twentieth century (Greenwood, 1935; Hill, 1939), and finally received widespread recognition after having been rediscovered or re-baptized as a paradox (Simpson, 1951).

Yule formally described some "fallacies that may be caused by the mixing of records" using the hypothetical example:

> *"Some given attribute might, for instance, be inherited neither in the male line nor the female line; yet a mixed record might exhibit a considerable apparent inheritance."* (Yule, 1903, p. 133).

Table 11A cross-tabulates the presence of the "attribute" (e.g., pipe smoking) in fathers and sons. Indeed, 50% of the sons have the attribute, whether or not their father has it. There is therefore no hereditary transmission in men, but note that the attribute is very common.

Table 11B indicates that 10% of the daughters have the attribute, whether or not their mother has it. There is therefore no hereditary transmission in women either, but the attribute is less common in women than in men.

Table 11A – "On the fallacies that may be caused by the mixing of distinct records." Data about fathers and sons. Source: (Yule, 1903).

Sons	Fathers	
	Attribute present	Attribute absent
Attribute present	25	25
Attribute absent	25	25
Children with attribute	[25 ÷ 50 =] 50%	[25 ÷ 50 =] 50%

Table 11B – "On the fallacies that may be caused by the mixing of distinct records." Data about mothers and daughters. Source: (Yule, 1903).

Daughters	Mothers	
	Attribute present	Attribute absent
Attribute present	1	9
Attribute absent	9	81
Children with attribute	[1 ÷ 10 =] 10%	[9 ÷ 90 =] 10%

However, when considering sons and daughters together (Table 11C), it appears that the attribute is more common in children when one parent has the attribute: children are more likely to have the attribute (43%) when parents have it than when they don't (24%).

Table 11C – "On the fallacies that may be caused by the mixing of distinct records." Amalgamated data, both parents and children*. Source: (Yule, 1903).

Children	Parents	
	Attribute present	Attribute absent
Attribute present	26	34
Attribute absent	34	106
Children with attribute	[26 ÷ 60 =] 43%	[34 ÷ 140 =] 24%

* Yule presented in each cell the percentages of the 2 × 2 table total.

Yule gave the reason for the fallacy. The parent attribute was more common in fathers than in mothers and the children's attribute was more common in sons than in daughters. Gender was associated with having the attribute in children and with having the attribute in parents. His description announced the current definition of a binary confounder: a variable associated with both exposure and outcome. This created in the amalgamated 2 × 2 table a false association between attributes in parents and attribute in children. The situation can be represented using the arrow graphs that were introduced much later in the epidemiologic literature (Susser, 1973).

Interestingly for the fate of his fallacy, Yule suggested that a similar mixing of effect could occur in a trial yielding a fictitious association between "antitoxin" and "cure" if females exhibited a greater case fatality and the antitoxin was attributed more often to the men.

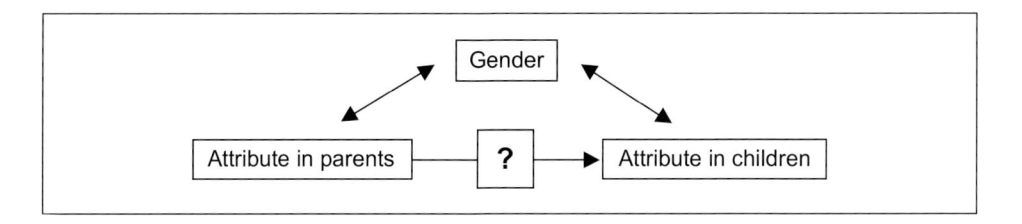

```
┌─────────────────────────────────────────────────┐
│                   ┌────────┐                    │
│                   │ Gender │                    │
│                   └────────┘                    │
│                   ↗        ↘                    │
│  ┌───────────────────┐  ┌───┐  ┌────────────────────┐
│  │Attribute in parents│──│ ? │─▶│Attribute in children│
│  └───────────────────┘  └───┘  └────────────────────┘
└─────────────────────────────────────────────────┘
```

Yule had worked closely with Major Greenwood (1880–1947), eventually the first Professor of Epidemiology in the Department of Epidemiology and Vital Statistics at the London School of Hygiene and Tropical Medicine. Does this explain that 32 years after Yule's publication, an almost identical demonstration of the fallacy was made by Major Greenwood in his 1935 textbook: *"Epidemics and Crowd Diseases"* (Greenwood, 1935)? The example used by Greenwood is shown in Table 12. It refers to a potential "fallacy" that may occur when analyzing results from immunization experiments. It is found in the chapter entitled *"The artificial immunization of man"*. This demonstration has remained, to my knowledge, unnoticed until recently (Zhang et al., Part II).

Table 12 shows that groups differ with respect to both prevalence of inoculation and risk of death. Group 1 has a higher mortality but group 2 has been more inoculated. Inoculation has no effect in groups 1 and 2 taken separately: 50% and 5% of the people, respectively, die. When mixing groups 1 and 2, inoculation becomes spuriously protective (9% of the inoculated *vs.* 46% of the uninoculated die). There is no reference to Yule's work. The whole citation is given as a footnote of Table 12. The relationships between "groups", "inoculation" and death can again be represented using an arrow graph. Note that this time, there is a unidirectional arrow between "group" and "death", as this relationship is likely to be causal:

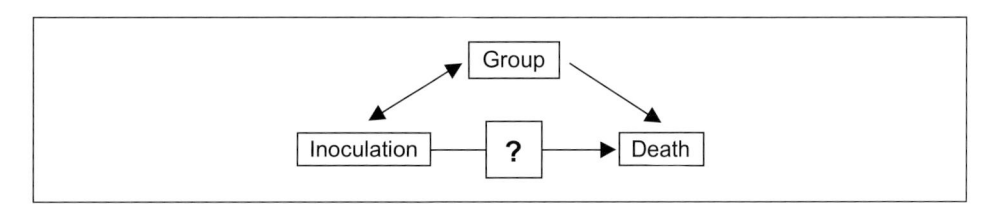

```
┌─────────────────────────────────────────────────┐
│                   ┌───────┐                     │
│                   │ Group │                     │
│                   └───────┘                     │
│                   ↗        ↘                    │
│   ┌────────────┐  ┌───┐   ┌───────┐             │
│   │ Inoculation│──│ ? │──▶│ Death │             │
│   └────────────┘  └───┘   └───────┘             │
└─────────────────────────────────────────────────┘
```

Yule and Greenwood knew Bradford Hill well. Does this explain that 34 years after Yule's publication and 4 years after Greenwood's text, Hill presented an almost identical demonstration of Yule's fallacy in his 1939 textbook *"Principles of medical statistics"*? In Hill's example (Table 13), a treatment has no effect either in men or women, but appears to reduce mortality when the male and female 2 x 2 tables are collapsed. There is no reference to Yule or Greenwood's examples in Hill's text.

Hill's example corresponded exactly to Yule's suggestion: men were more treated and women died more. His explanation was:

Table 12 – Hypothetical example given by Major Greenwood of the potential fallacy resulting from mixing records*. Source: "Epidemics and crowd-diseases" (Greenwood, 1935).

	Group 1		Group 2		All	
	Inoculated	Non inoculated	Inoculated	Non inoculated	Inoculated	Non inoculated
Dead (n)	50	500	50	5	100	505
Alive (n)	50	500	950	95	1,000	595
All (n)	100	1,000	1,000	100	1,100	1,100
Percent dead	50	50	5	5	9	46

* "One has data of the experience of inoculated and uninoculated persons collected over a wide range in space or time, and brings them together in a single statistical summary, which tells us that upon 'n' inoculated persons the attack-rate was 'a' per cent and upon 'm' uninoculated 'b' per cent. If n and m are large numbers, the kind of statistical test I have described may lead to arithmetically overwhelming odds in favour of the inoculated, yet this a priori inference might be quite wrong. It might be that in some of the experiments neither inoculated nor uninoculated ran any serious risk at all; if in these groups there were a great majority of inoculated, the final summary would show a great advantage to them. Suppose in one experiment there were 1,000 uninoculated with a death rate of 50 per cent and 100 inoculated also with a death rate of 50 per cent, while in another experiment there were 1,000 inoculated with a death rate of 5 per cent and 100 uninoculated also with a death rate of 5 per cent. Summarizing, we should find 1100 inoculated persons with 100 deaths, and 1100 uninoculated with 505 deaths, an enormous "advantage" to the inoculated group. No confidence should be placed in odds computed from such summaries." (Greenwood, 1935, pp. 84–85).

> "Superficially this comparison suggests that the new treatment is of some value; in fact that conclusion is wholly unjustified, for we are not comparing like with like (…). There are proportionally more females amongst the controls than in the treated group, and since females normally have a higher case fatality rate than males their presence in the control group in relatively greater numbers must lead to a comparatively high fatality rate in the total sample. Equally, their relative deficiency in the treated group leads to a comparatively low fatality rate in that total sample. No comparison is valid which does not allow for the sex differentiation of the fatality rates." (Hill, 1939, p. 126).

A mysterious aspect of the fate of Yule's fallacy is that it is known today by most of us as "Simpson's paradox". In 1951, E. H. Simpson, for whom I have found no first name or biographical information, used an artificial example to demonstrate that,

Table 13 – Fallacy resulting from mixing of non-comparable records *. Source: (Hill, 1939, p. 126, Table XIV).

	Male		Female		All	
	Treatment	No treatment	Treatment	No treatment	Treatment	No treatment
Dead (n)	16	6	16	24	32	30
Alive (n)	64	24	24	36	88	60
All (n)	80	30	40	60	120	90
Percent dead	20	20	40	40	27	33

"Mixing of non-comparable records: (a) let us suppose that in a particular disease the fatality rate is twice as high among females as it is among males, and that amongst male patients it is 20 per cent. And amongst female patients 40 per cent. A new form of treatment is adopted and applied to 80 males and 40 females; 30 males and 60 females are observed as controls. The number of deaths observed among the 120 individuals given the new treatment is 32, giving a fatality-rate of 26.7 per cent., while the number of deaths observed amongst the 90 individuals taken as controls is 30, giving a fatality-rate of 33.3 per cent. Superficially this comparison suggests that the new treatment is of some value; in fact that conclusion is wholly unjustified, for we are not comparing like with like. The fatality-rates of the total number of individuals must be influenced by the proportions of the two sexes present in each sample; males and females, in fact, are not equally represented in the sample treated and in the sample taken as control. Tabulating the figures shows the fallacy clearly (Table XIV)." (Hill, 1939, pp.125–126).

under certain conditions, the relation of treatment to mortality could appear drastically different if it were analyzed before or after stratification by gender (Simpson, 1951). His example is shown in Table 14.

In Simpson's example, mortality is slightly lower in the treated groups, in both males and females, but this protective effect vanishes in the pooled comparison. In Yule's, Greenwood's and Hill's examples, "amalgamating" the gender-specific 2 × 2 tables fallaciously *produced* an effect. Simpson does not refer to the work of Yule, Greenwood and Hill. Epidemiologists citing Simpson's work do not usually refer to these earlier papers either (Rothman, 1986; Greenland, 1987a). Who was Simpson? Why is it that his paradox received so much visibility while that of Yule, Greenwood and Hill remained almost unnoticed?

The last episode of the saga of Yule's fallacy can be read in the text entitled "*Modern Epidemiology*". To illustrate Simpson's paradox Rothman told the example of

Table 14 – Original numerical example illustrating Simpson's paradox. Source: (Simpson, 1951).

	Male		Female		All	
	Treated	Not treated	Treated	Not treated	Treated	Not treated
Dead (n)	5	3	15	3	20	6
Alive (n)	8	4	12	2	20	6
All (n)	13	7	27	5	40	12
Percent dead	38	43	56	60	50	50

the delusion of a man who goes one day to buy a hat, tests some hats on two different tables and has the consistent impression that black hats fit him in general better than gray ones. The next day, however, hats from the two tables have been mixed together and now gray hats tend to fit him better. The data given by Rothman are shown in Table 15. It is funny that Rothman, who has a high appreciation of John Graunt, the British 18th century haberdasher (Rothman, 1996), invented an example about ... hats, rather than a health-related example as his predecessors.

There were two novelties in Rothman's example. First, pooling the hats from the two tables reversed the association. The best fit has moved from black to gray hat. More black hats fit on each of the tables, but more gray hats do when the content of the two tables is pooled. And second, it was followed by a mature theory of confounding:

> "On the simplest level, confounding may be considered as a mixing of effects. Specifically, the estimate of the effect of the exposure of interest is distorted because it is mixed with the effect of an extraneous factor." (Rothman, 1986, p. 89).

3.4.2. Early analyses of confounding

One of the first analytical adjustments for confounding was performed by Joseph Goldberger (1874–1929) and Edgar Sydenstricker (1881–1936). Goldberger and Sydenstricker provide another example of an intellectual duet comprising a physician and a statistician.

Goldberger, son of Hungarian immigrants, earned an MD at Bellevue Hospital, New York, had a private medical practice in Wilkes-Barre, Pennsylvania and then joined the United States Marine Hospital Service (later the U.S. Public Health Service) in 1899. Sydenstricker was born to missionary parents in Shanghai, received a Master's degree in sociology and economics in Virginia and, in 1907–1908, was a post-

Table 15 – Hypothetical example illustrating "Simpson's paradox". Source: (Rothman, 1986 p. 89).

	Table 1		Table 2		All	
	Black	Gray	Black	Gray	Black	Gray
Fit (n)	9	17	3	1	12	18
Not fit (n)	1	3	17	9	18	12
All (n)	10	20	20	10	30	30
Percent fit	90	85	15	10	40	60

graduate fellow in political economy at the University of Chicago. In 1920 he was appointed as Chief of the Office of Statistical Investigations in the U.S. Public Health Service (Wiehl, 1974).

Goldberger and Sydenstricker studied the causes of pellagra. Pellagra was first identified among Spanish peasants by Don Gaspar Casal in 1735 (Pan American Health Organization, 1988). A loathsome skin disease, it was called "mal de la rosa" and often mistaken for leprosy. In the United States, pellagra has sometimes been called the disease of the four D's – dermatitis, diarrhea, dementia, and death. By 1912, the state of South Carolina alone reported 30,000 cases and a case fatality rate of 40 percent, but the disease was hardly confined to Southern states. The US Congress asked the Surgeon General to investigate the disease. In 1914, Joseph Goldberger led that investigation.

Goldberger's theory on pellagra contradicted the medical opinion at that time. Pellagra was thought to be an infectious disease due to a still unidentified germ. The Thompson-McFadden Pellagra Commission, established under governmental auspices, had concluded in 1914 that pellagra had no relation to diet, based on an original house-to-house survey of pellagra cases in the cotton mill districts in South Carolina. The Commission's findings were interpreted as strong support for an infectious cause of pellagra (Elmore and Feinstein, 1994). But Goldberger had observed that, in mental hospitals and orphanages, the disease hit inmates but never staff. An infectious disease would not distinguish between inmates and employees.

Among all the experiments of various types that Goldberger and his coworkers carried out to study the causes of pellagra, one is especially relevant for this history of epidemiologic methods. In the spring of 1916, they began a methodologically remarkable investigation in some representative communities of South Carolina. Results have been reported in several papers published in 1920. I will focus here on one of them, "*A study of the relation of family income and other economic factors to pellagra incidence in seven cotton-mill villages of South Carolina in 1916*" (Goldberger et al., 1920).

The relation of poverty to pellagra incidence in the textile-mill communities was well established at that time. The typical sharecropper's lot was a wretched cottage, a few corn plants, and a luxurious but not edible growth of cotton (Roe, 1973). The objective of Goldberger's study was to assess whether diet could play a role, irrespective of poverty. They selected seven representative cotton-mill villages, enumerated their populations and sampled 750 households, comprising 4,160 people, exclusively Whites of anglo-saxon origin. It was

"an exceptionally homogenous group with respect to racial stock, occupation, and general standard of living, including dietary custom" (Goldberger et al., 1920, p. 2678).

The homogeneity of the population did not result in being an obstacle in assessing the effect of diet on pellagra. Even villages that were similar in income were different in diet.

Pellagra incidence was assessed by a "systematic biweekly house-to-house search for cases". Cases had "clearly defined, bilaterally symmetrical dermatitis" (Goldberger et al., 1920, p. 2679). The assessment of diet and income was performed between April 16 and June 15, 1916, as this was the period immediately preceding the expected seasonal sharp rise in pellagra incidence in these villages. Food supply to the household was measured using an "accurate record for a 15-day period". The payroll records of the mills provided about 90% of the family income and statements of the housewife or other family members the other 10%. The half-month incomes so recorded were weighted by the number of "equivalent male units" of food requirement within a household. Weights were 1 for an adult male, 0.8 for an adult female, 0.5 for a child 5 to 9 years old, etc. Hence, in the paper, income is expressed as "half-month family income per adult male unit".

Table 16 shows that pellagra incidence declined rapidly as income increased. It is 16 times larger in households with less than 6 dollars (per half month and per adult male unit, adjusted rate: 41 per 1,000) compared to incomes of 14 dollars or more (adjusted rate: 2.5 per 1,000).

The footnote explaining the presence of "adjusted rates" (in the last column) is of great interest. It deals with an adjustment for age. The authors explained that they standardized the pellagra risks for age because age was associated with both income and pellagra incidence:

"Since a marked variation in the pellagra rate according to age and sex was found for the population studied (Goldberger, Wheeler, Sydenstricker, 1920b), and since, ordinarily, differences in the distribution of persons according to age occur in different economic groups, computation of rates adjusted to a standard population was made. The influence of differences in the sex distribution in any age group was insignificant, and practically the same incidence rates were obtained

Table 16 – Number of definite cases of pellagra and risk per 1,000 among persons of different income classes in seven cotton-mill villages of South Carolina in 1926. Pooled men and women. Source: Adapted from Tables V and Va of (Goldberger et al., 1920, p. 2687).

Half-month family income per adult sale unit	Number of persons	Number of cases	Risk per 1,000	Adjusted risk per 1,000
Less than $6.00	1,312	56	42.7	41.0
$6.00–$7.99	1,037	27	26.0	24.8
$8.00–$9.99	784	10	12.8	14.2
$10.0–$13.99	736	3	4.1	5.2
$14 and over	291	1	3.4	2.5
All incomes	4,160	97	23.3	

after making adjustments to a standard age distribution, as is shown in the following table [last column of Table 16]." (Goldberger et al., 1920, p. 2687).

The total population (all incomes) served as standard population. They noted that the agreement between the crude and the adjusted risks ruled out the possibility that "differences in the sex and age distribution in the different income classes might give rise to" the inverse association of income and pellagra (Goldberger et al., 1920, p. 2689). In modern words, they ruled out a confounding effect of sex or age on the income-pellagra association.

Interestingly, they appropriately pooled the data of men and women: the gender-specific rates across income categories were substantially different but, if we compute the relative risks of income and pellagra incidence (which are not shown in the paper), we see that the relative associations are similar in men and women. Gender did not confound or modify the association. Hence, assessing it in the pooled sample was the correct approach.

After having demonstrated the "inverse correlation between pellagra incidence and family income", they showed that income was also strongly related to diet. Actually, both the lower income households and the pellagrous households had a diet rich in corn meal and grits and poor in milk and fresh products (Goldberger et al., 1920, Table VII p. 2692). Income was therefore, in modern terms, a possible confounder of the diet and pellagra association as it was related to both diet and pellagra incidence.

Goldberger and co-workers then proceeded to compare the diet of two villages (out of the seven studied) which showed the two most extreme incidence rates of pellagra: 0 per 1,000 in *Ny* and 64.6 per 1,000 in *In*. Both were poor villages with about half of their households having an income of 8 dollars or below. Note that this is now an affected/non-affected comparison, different from the exposed/non-exposed comparison shown in Table 16. They compared the fresh meat purchases in the two villages, one free from pellagra (i.e., the non-affected group) and the other severely affected. Because the two villages were similarly poor, there could be no effect of poverty in the comparison. In the non-affected village of *Ny*, 58.1% of the households had reported having purchased fresh meat twice or more in the 15 day record, whereas this proportion was only 8.5% in the affected village of *In*. This analysis demonstrated therefore that within homogeneous categories of income, dietary differences determined incidence of pellagra. The effect of diet was not confounded by income.

This study performed in 1916 and published in 1920 reveals therefore a profound understanding of the issue of confounding and familiarity with some analytical tools to adjust for confounding effects. The effect of income was first identified and clearly separated from a possible age effect by *adjustment*. Then the effect of diet was separated from that of income by *restricting* the analysis to two low-income villages with differing pellagra rates. In addition, the authors had used both exposed/unexposed and affected/unaffected comparisons. The summary and conclusions testify to the progress of epidemiologic concepts and methods in observational studies by 1920:

> "4. In general, pellagra incidence was found to vary inversely according to family income ... 5. The inverse correlation between pellagra incidence and family income depended on the unfavorable effect of low income on the character of the diet; but family income was not the sole factor determining the character of the household diet. 6. Differences in incidence among households of the same income class are attributable (...) to the differences among household with respect to availability of food supplies from such sources as home-owned cows, poultry, gardens, etc. 7. Differences in incidence among villages whose constituent households are economically similar, are attributable to differences among them in availability of food supplies (...). 8. The most potent factors influencing pellagra incidence in the village studied were: (a) low family income, and (b) unfavorable conditions regarding the availability of food supplies, suggesting that under the conditions obtained in some of these villages in the spring of 1916 many families were without sufficient income to enable them to procure the adequate diet, and that improvement of food availability (particularly of milk and fresh meat) is urgently needed in such localities." (Goldberger et al., 1920, p. 2711).

Goldberger was right on target. We now know that pellagra is caused by the lack in the diet of a vitamin, niacin or nicotinic acid, belonging to the B complex. Niacin can be found in yeast, organ meats, peanuts, and wheat germ. The disease is most common in areas where the diet consists mainly of corn, which, unlike other grains, lacks niacin as well as the amino acid tryptophan, which the body uses to synthesize the vitamin. Pellagra can be prevented and treated by niacin (Roe, 1973).

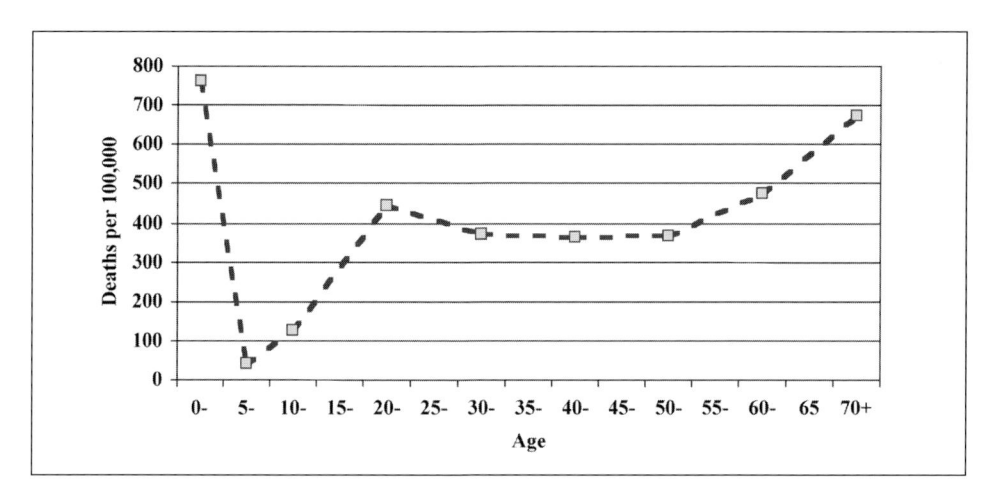

Figure 4
Massachusetts death rates from tuberculosis – all forms – by age, in 1880. Source: (Frost, 1939).

3.4.3. Cohort analysis

Around 1900, investigating the causes of tuberculosis raised new types of group comparison problems. There could be a long latency between exposure to *M. tuberculosis* and the clinical manifestations of the disease. Each population comprised a mixture of people who had been infected at various times in the past and who remained so for decades before they eventually became sick and died of the disease. Infection rates were declining. Therefore, at a given moment in time, older people were more likely to carry the bacillus than younger ones. Vital statistics showed that the mortality from tuberculosis increased with age, but it was unclear whether this was because of an age effect or because of the higher exposure during their youth of the older people.

Wade Hampton Frost (1880-1938), the first Professor and Chairman in the Department of Epidemiology and Public Health Administration at The School of Hygiene and Public Health of the Johns Hopkins University in Baltimore, addressed this question in a paper published after his death (Frost, 1939). He described the fallacy that may occur when naively interpreting cross-sectional changes in death rates with age (Comstock, Part II; Doll, Part II).

Figure 4 presents the change of mortality rates from tuberculosis across age groups in 1880 in Massachusetts. They peak at ages 0–4, are lowest at ages 5 to 9, and then rise across age groups. This apparent age effect was difficult to explain:

"...*nothing that we know of the habits of mankind and the distribution of the bacillus would lead us to suppose that between the first and the second 5 years of*

Table 17 – Key for the interpretation of cohort versus cross-sectional mortality rates.

Age	Calendar year 1880	Calendar year 1890	Calendar year 1900
0–9	$M_{1,1}$ = 1880 mortality rates for those born in 1871 to 1880		
10–19	$M_{2,1}$ = 1880 mortality rates for those born in 1861 to 1870	$M_{2,2}$ = 1890 mortality rates for those born in 1871 to 1880	
20-29	$M_{3,1}$ = 1880 mortality rates for those born in 1851 to 1860		$M_{3,3}$ = 1900 mortality rates for those born in 1871 to 1880

$M_{i,j}$ = mortality rate for people in the ith age group and the jth calendar year.

> *life there is, in general, a diminution in exposure to infection which corresponds to the decline in mortality rate. And there is little, if any, better reason to suppose that the extraordinary rise in mortality from age 10 to age 20, 25 or 30 is paralleled by a corresponding increase in rate of exposure to specific infection."* (Frost, 1939).

Frost therefore proposed to study the age effect using the death rates within the same "cohort" at different ages. The term "cohort" comes from the Latin *cohors*. The antique Roman legions were composed of ten cohorts. The 480 warriors plus 6 centurions of a cohort constituted the basic fighting unit that could be traced during the battle. The term cohort has been imported to epidemiology to define a set of people who are followed or traced over a period of time. Frost showed that the cohort is the appropriate unit in which one can assess an age effect. Table 17 illustrates the rationale of Frost's reasoning. The example is based on the data used by Frost and reproduced by Comstock (Comstock, Part II).

In Table 17, the first column indicates *cross-sectional* age-specific mortality rates in 1880. Differences in mortality rates in the column can be read as the change of mortality rates with age, where each age group corresponds to a different birth cohort, that is, people born at different time points in the past. The numbers on the diagonal indicate the change in mortality rates with age for the 1871–1880 birth cohort, that is, people who were all born between 1871 and 1880. The cross-sectional (e.g., cell $M_{2,1}$) and the cohort ($M_{2,2}$) age-specific mortality rates would be similar if exposure and/or susceptibility (e.g., due to vaccination) to infection did not change between 1871 and 1900. In the absence of a cohort effect, $M_{2,1} = M_{2,2}$, and $M_{3,1} = M_{3,3}$. For a *cohort effect* to take place, mortality at a given age must change over time,

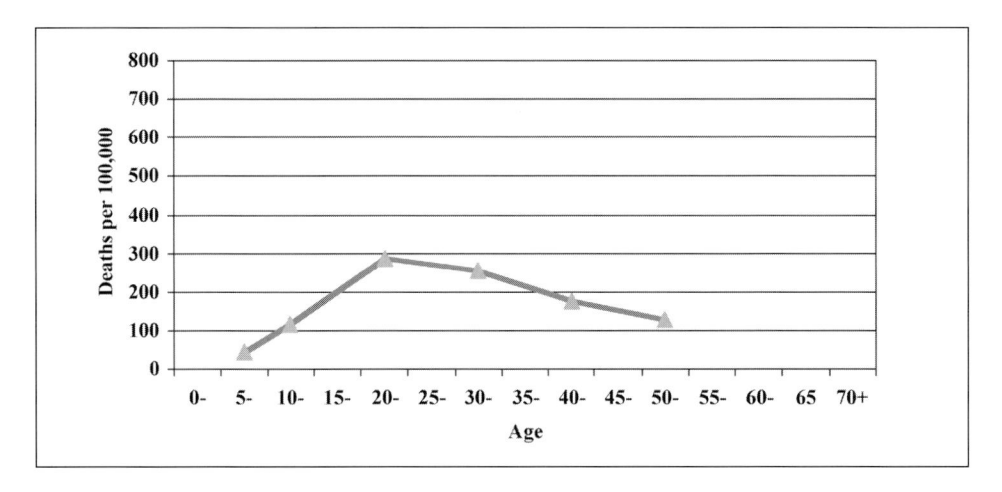

[Figure: graph showing Deaths per 100,000 vs Age, with values rising to ~290 at age 20- then declining]

Figure 5
Massachusetts death rates from tuberculosis – all forms – by age, for the cohort of men who were born in the years 1871 to 1880. Source: (Frost, 1939).

so that the *cross-sectional* age-specific frequency is different from the cohort-and-age-specific frequency: $M_{2,1} \neq M_{2,2}$, and $M_{3,1} \neq M_{3,3}$.

Mortality rates from tuberculosis were changing rapidly across cohorts in the populations studied by Frost. The cohort analysis demonstrated that rates tended to decline with age after age 20, as shown in Figure 5 for the cohort of men born between 1871 and 1880.

Similar observations across several cohorts allowed Frost to conclude that the inexplicable variations of mortality rates with age occurring in the cross-sectional analysis were due to differences in exposure to tuberculosis across birth cohorts. The cohort analysis did not support the hypothesis that a lower exposure to *M. tuberculosis* during infancy resulted in more severe infections in adults. This would have been a major argument against vaccination. Frost concluded that:

> "Present day 'peak' of mortality in late life does not represent postponement of maximum risk to a later period, but rather would seem to indicate that the present high rates in old ages are the residuals of higher [exposure] rates in earlier life." (Frost, 1939).

Actually, Frost had described, without using the term, another manifestation of confounding, between age, birth cohort and mortality from tuberculosis, which could be identified by stratifying on birth cohort.

3.4.4. Alternate allocation of treatment

The contribution of Bradford Hill to the evolution of group comparisons is a major one, in particular for the implementation of a technique to prevent the confounding effects of "disturbing and extraneous factors" in therapeutic trials. It is worth quoting extensively of the section dedicated to "planning and interpretation of experiments".

> "Thus, when the statistician's help is required, it is his task to suggest means of allowing for the disturbing causes, either in planning the experiment or in analysing the results, and not as a rule, to determine what are the relevant disturbing causes." (Hill, 1939, p. 4).

Hill explains in simple terms the foundations of confounding:

> "If we find that Group A differs from Group B in some characteristic, say, its mortality-rate, can we be certain that difference is due to the fact that Group A was inoculated (for example) and Group B was uninoculated? Are we certain that Group A does not differ from Group B in some other character relevant to the issues as well as in the presence or absence of inoculation? For instance, in a particular case, inoculated persons might, on the average, belong to a higher social class than the uninoculated and therefore live in surroundings in which the risk of infection was less." (Hill, 1939, pp. 4–5).

Hill then explains the role of alternate allocations of treatment:

> "The reason why in experiments in the treatment of disease the allocation of alternate cases to the treated and untreated groups is often satisfactory, is because no conscious or unconscious bias can enter in, as it may in any selection of cases, and because in the long run we can fairly rely upon this random allotment of the patients to equalize in the two groups the distribution of other characteristics that may be important. Between the individuals within each group there will often be wide differences in characteristics, for instance, in body-weight and state of health, but with large numbers we can be reasonably sure that the numbers of each type will be equally, or nearly equally, represented in both groups."
> (Hill, 1939, pp. 5–6).

Hill mentions a form of treatment allocation that would be blocked on specific characteristics (e.g., sex) to increase the likelihood of getting comparable groups:

> "If it be known that certain characteristics will have an influence upon the results of treatment and on account of relatively small numbers the distribution of these characteristics may not be equalized in the final groups, it is advisable to extend

Epidemiology: An epistemological perspective

Table 18 – Effect of serum treatment on case fatality in patients with type I or type II lobar pneumonia. Aberdeen, London, Edinburgh and Glasgow, United Kingdom, 1930–1933. Source: (Table III Therapeutic Trial Committee of the Medical Research Council, 1934).

Pneu-monia	Age (years)	Conventional treatment			Serum treatment			
		N	Deaths	% case fatality [A]	N	Deaths	% case fatality [B]	Expected deaths [A × B]*
Type I	20–40	224	25	11.2	140	8	5.7	16
	40–60	77	20	26.0	44	10	22.7	11
						18		27
Type II	20–40	194	44	22.7	111	14	12.6	25
	40–60	111	38	34.2	53	19	35.8	18
						33		43

* The "expected deaths" are those which would have been recorded if the serum-treated groups had died at the same percentage rates as the corresponding controls.

> this method of allocation. For instance, alternate persons will not be treated but a division will be made by sex, so that the first male is treated and the second male untreated, the first female is treated and the second female is untreated. Similarly age may be equalized by treating alternate males and alternate females at each age, or in each broad age-group if individuals whose ages are within a few years of one another may in the particular case be regarded as equivalent."
> (Hill, 1939, pp. 5–6).

Hill cites as example the report of the Therapeutic Trials Committee of the Medical Research Council on the serum treatment of an infection located in lobes of the lung and called lobar pneumonia. Hill had been an investigator in the trial (Therapeutic Trial Committee of the Medical Research Council, 1934). The trial was conducted almost simultaneously in London, Edinburgh, Aberdeen and Glasgow. Patients admitted in Aberdeen, London, Edinburgh for a pneumonia received, alternatively according to the order of admission, either a serum treatment or the conventional treatment, which served as control. In Glasgow, the control group was selected from another hospital without alternate allocation of treatment. The treatment with serum was begun within some hours after admission, but some patients must have been excluded after treatment was allocated as "all patients dying within 24 hours of admission to hospital were taken out of the series". Results of the trial are shown in Table 18.

The mortality risk in the conventional treatment (i.e., controls) was applied to the numbers of people treated with serum to compute the expected number of deaths under the assumption of no serum treatment effect. The analysis was stratified by age. The expected number of deaths was then compared to the number of deaths observed in those treated with serum. Serum appeared to reduce the number of deaths more for type I (18 observed death *vs.* 27 expected) than for type II pneumonia (33 observed *vs.* 43 expected). The effect was stronger in younger subjects. Results were actually very similar when using only the data from the centers, which had used the alternate allocation (London, Edinburgh and Aberdeen).

The example reviewed here paved the way for the development of the modern form of the randomized controlled trial. The James Lind Library provides more elements on this episode and on his place in the history of randomized allocation of treatments (Chalmers, 2004).

3.4.5. Logic of confounding

The logic of confounding received a further boost after the publication, in 1950, of case-control studies showing that smoking was a likely cause of lung cancer. Among those who were skeptical about the link of tobacco to lung cancer stood Ronald A. Fisher (1890–1962), from Cambridge, perhaps the most original statistician of the 20th century (Fisher, 1959; Stolley, 1991). Even though Fisher articulated many criticisms against a causal implication of smoking (Stolley, 1991), his essential argument was that both smoking and lung cancer resulted from genetic predispositions. To support his thesis he presented data shown in Table 19.

Data suggested that some genetic predisposition could explain the habit of smoking. Homozygotic twins (whose genetic constitution is almost identical) were more alike in their smoking behavior than heterozygotic twins (who have only half of their genes in common). Of 51 homozygotic twin pairs, 39 (76%) had similar smoking habits, as opposed to less than half (15 ÷ 31) among heterozygotic twins.

Table 19 – Smoking habits of heterozygotic and homozygotic twins. Source: (Fisher, 1959, p. 40).

Smoking habits	Heterozygotic twins		Homozygotic twins	
	Pairs	Percent	Pairs	Percent
Different	16	52*	12	24
Alike or somewhat alike	15	48	39	76
Total	31	100	51	100

* Fisher's original is 51 but should be 52.

Fisher's idea was that the association between smoking and lung cancer was spurious. Smoking was related to some genetic predisposition, which caused lung cancer. Fisher did not use the word confounding, but his point was that the relation of smoking to cancer was "confounded" by genetic predisposition. The historical interest of this example is that Fisher had articulated the suspicion of confounding in a form that would become typical in epidemiology.

The reason for Fisher's open antagonism is not established. It may well have been another manifestation of the historical dispute between Fisher and his fellow statistician but declared enemy, Karl Pearson (1857– 1936), Galton Professor of Eugenics at Cambridge University. Fisher must have felt that he had to criticize the work of all disciples of Karl Pearson. Fisher died in 1962, before the publication of the US Surgeon General report on Smoking and Health.

3.5. Case-control studies

The principle of the case-control study is the comparison of past exposures between groups of affected and non-affected subjects. The case-control study may be looked upon as a natural extension of the practice of physicians to take case histories as an aid to diagnosis. (Mantel and Haenszel, 1959; Paneth et al., Part II). To get clues about the etiology of the disease, clinicians may have begun the tradition to compare patients suffering from a specific disease with other patients who were free of that disease.

We usually refer to this technique today as a case-control study, but it was first called a "retrospective study". The term "retrospective" meant that the researcher went back from the disease to its potential causes in the past, just as a physician obtains the personal history from a patient.

In 1950, two studies of that type conducted in the United States to assess the relation of smoking to lung cancer were published in the Journal of the American Medical Association (Wynder and Graham, 1950; Levin et al., 1950). Both indicated that exposure to tobacco smoke was more common in lung cancer cases than in controls.

The first study had been led by Morton L. Levin (1904–1995), a student of Frost in the mid-1930s, then hired as cancer epidemiologist at Roswell Park Memorial Institute, Buffalo, New York. Around 1948, Levin and his colleagues identified 1,507 men admitted to Roswell Park Memorial Institute, between 1938 and 1948. The proportion of subjects who had smoked for more than 25 years was 54.1% in lung cancer cases, 34.9% in other cancer controls, 36.9% in lung non tumors, and 29.8% in non-cancer controls (Levin et al., 1950). Levin et al concluded that:

> "The data suggest, although they do not establish, a causal relation between cigarette and pipe smoking and cancer of the lung and lip, respectively. The statisti-

cal association may, of course, be due to some other unidentified factor between these types of smoking and lung and lip cancer." (Levin et al., 1950 p. 474).

Ernst L. Wynder (1922–1999) was still a pre-med student in Saint Louis when he began studying cancer. In 1948 and 1949, supported by Professor Evarts A. Graham (1883–1957), Chairman of the Department of Surgery at Washington University School of Medicine, Wynder (not alone) interviewed 605 men and 25 women with lung cancer (other than adenocarcinoma) from several hospitals and private practices around the United States (Wynder, 1997). Controls were 780 men and 552 women without cancer of the lung admitted to general hospitals. The conclusion of Wynder and Graham's paper was that

"excessive and prolonged use of tobacco, especially cigarets [sic], seems to be an important factor in the induction of bronchiogenic carcinoma" (Wynder and Graham, 1950, p. 336).

The studies by Levin et al. and Wynder et al. had a number of strengths (Paneth et al., Part II), but methodologically they were not different from the studies conducted in the pre-war era. It is once again a study involving Bradford Hill that indicates a methodological watershed. In September 1950, Hill and Richard Doll, at that time a research assistant whom Hill had invited to investigate the causes of lung cancer, published the preliminary report of a study commissioned by the Medical Research Council (Doll and Hill, 1950). This study is now viewed as a model case-control investigation because, for the first time, it had been conceived and designed as such to solve a specific question and generate valid results (Paneth et al., Part II). Doll and Hill were therefore able to answer the question of the relation of smoking to lung cancer more thoroughly and more convincingly.

Twenty hospitals of London informed Doll and Hill of their diagnosed cancer cases (lung, colon, stomach, rectum). Cancers of the colon, stomach and rectum served as "contrasting groups". Research almoners (i.e., social workers) interviewed the cases as well as a patient of the same sex, within the same five-year age group, and in the same hospital at or about the same time, who did not have lung cancer. Attention was paid to the duration of smoking, to histories of starting and stopping smoking, and to the amount smoked. Contrasts were made between cases of lung cancer and matched controls in overall smoking, amount smoked most recently, maximum ever smoked, age of onset of smoking, type of tobacco and duration of smoking. Stratified analyses were used to deal with potential confounders, including urban/rural residence.

Table 20 presents the simplest analysis of the case-control study results. The conclusion that cigarette smoking could cause lung cancer was based on refined analysis of the data, presented in many tables and figures. I like, however, the presentation of the data as in Table 20 because we may not perceive today that 95.8% of the controls had smoked. Even though almost all cases were smokers of some sort, there was

Table 20 – Percentage of ever smokers in cases of lung cancer and hospital controls. Source: (Doll and Hill, 1950).

Smokers	% Cases (n = 649)	% Controls (n = 649)
Yes	99.7	95.8
No	0.3	4.2

space for skepticism. Indeed, it is with skepticism that these results were received in the medical and political community.

The authors firmly concluded that cigarette smoking was

"a factor, and an important factor, in the production of carcinoma of the lung." (Doll and Hill, 1950).

The British Medical Journal wrote a favorable review (Editorial, 1950). But a retrospective account of the events surrounding the publications of these three case-control study articles shows that things had not been easy (Armenian and Szklo, 1996; Wynder, 1997; Terris, 1997; Doll, 1998). Doll has explained how the publication of their study was delayed:

"By the end of 1949 the position was so clear that we had written a paper based on our findings in 709 pairs of lung cancer cases and control patients drawing the conclusion that (I quote) 'smoking is a factor, and an important factor, in the production of carcinoma of the lung'. When, however, we showed the paper to Sir Harold Himsworth, who had by then succeeded Sir Edward Mellanby as Secretary of the Medical Research Council, he wisely advised us to postpone publication until we had checked that similar results would be reproduced outside London. We consequently withheld publication and started to interview similar groups of patients in some of the principal hospitals in and around Bristol, Cambridge, Leeds and Newcastle. Before we had obtained much more data, however, Wynder and Graham (1950), reported very similar findings in their study of patients in the US, and we consequently published ours a few months later (in September 1950) without waiting for the results of the extended study. The latter was published in 1952, relating to 1,465 pairs of patients and controls and showed essentially identical results in all centers – except that heavy smoking by women had not spread outside London." (Doll, 1998, p. 134).

Both the Royal College of Physician's 1962 report entitled *Smoking and Health*, and the US Surgeon General's Report of the same title, published in 1964, relied heavily on case-control studies in their assessment of the evidence. The Royal College of Physicians Committee cited 23 case-control studies, all of which showed a relationship of smoking to lung cancer, and the Surgeon General's Report cited 29 such studies, all but one of which (a study in women) confirmed the association. The powerful consistency of these case-control studies, and the replication of their findings in cohort studies promoted the general acceptance of the case-control study as a scientific research tool.

3.6. Cohort studies

The conclusion that cigarette smoking was an important cause of lung cancer was accepted by

> *"very few other scientists at the time, who were unaccustomed to the idea that firm conclusions about causation could be drawn from case-control studies, and it was clear that if the conclusion was to be widely accepted the conclusions would have to be checked by some other method of enquiry"* (Doll, Part II).

The case-control design was deemed susceptible to all sorts of biases, based either on inaccurate recall or on selection. It was believed that it led more often to erroneous conclusions than to correct ones (White, 1990) and that it was inherently biased (Doll, 1984). In response to the criticisms expressed towards case-control studies, Doll and Hill designed a new type of study based on very different premises. In their 1954 paper on *"The mortality of doctors in relation to their smoking habits"* (Doll and Hill, 1954), they noted that a number of studies had been made of the smoking habits of patients with and without lung cancer and that further studies of the same kind were unlikely to shed new light upon the nature of the association. An entirely new approach was needed, which would be free of the potential flaws of case-control studies. They proposed to call the new approach "prospective", which the Oxford English Dictionary defined as "characterized by looking forward into the future". They sent a short questionnaire eliciting smoking habits to 59,600 British Doctors. The history of the British Doctor Study is told by Richard Doll in this book (Doll, Part II).

In January 1, 1952, E. Cuyler Hammond (1912–1986) and Daniel Horn (1916–1992), respectively Director and Assistant Director of statistical research at the American Cancer Society, launched the U.S. counterpart of the British Doctor Study, but with an almost four times larger sample size. They designed and pretested a questionnaire on smoking habits, trained 22,000 American Cancer Society volunteers and asked each of them

> *"to have the questionnaire filled out by about 10 white men between the ages of 50 and 69 whom they knew well and would be able to trace"* (Hammond and Horn, 1958).

They received 204,547 completed questionnaires from California, Illinois, Iowa, Michigan, Minnesota, New Jersey, New York, Pennsylvania and Wisconsin. The health status of the participants was checked each year and death certificates obtained for men recorded as dead. In 1958, Hammond and Horn published in the Journal of the American Medical Association an analysis of the death rates in relation to the smoking habits of 187,783 men, traced from 1952 through 1955, for an average 44 months and representing 667,753 man-years (Hammond and Horn, 1958). The analysis consisted in comparing the observed number of deaths to

"...the number of deaths which would have occurred among men in each smoking category if their age-specific death rates had been exactly the same as those for men who never smoked. This will be referred to as the 'expected' number of deaths." (Hammond and Horn, 1958, p. 1160).

Hammond and Horn used the observed and expected number of deaths to compute both the mortality ratio (observed divided by expected) and the excess deaths (observed minus expected). Their study was so large that they were able, after a relatively short follow-up, to ascertain the potential associations of tobacco smoke with many causes of death beyond lung cancer. Table 21 presents some of the results of the American Cancer Society cohort study.

A notable aspect of the paper was that it presented both the mortality ratio and the excess deaths. These two measures of effect combined revealed important features of the health effects of smoking. Mortality *ratios* indicated that the strongest association was with lung cancer: smokers had 10.73 times the risk of dying from lung cancer compared to never smokers. The association was weaker with coronary artery disease (mortality ratio = 1.70). The excess deaths indicated, however, that coronary artery disease was, by far, a more common cause of excess deaths, since it accounted for 52.1% of all excess deaths in smokers compared to non-smokers. Both relative (mortality ratio) and absolute causality (excess deaths) were needed to fully understand the effects of smoking on health:

"the relative importance of the association is dependent on the number of deaths attributed to each disease, as well as on their degrees of association with cigarette smoking" (Hammond and Horn, 1958, p. 1308).

A group of American statisticians and epidemiologists, including Hammond (Cornfield et al., 1959), would re-express one year after the publication of Hammond and Horn's study the need for both absolute and relative measures of association in epidemiology:

"Relatively, cigarettes have a much larger effect on lung cancer than on cardiovascular disease, while the reverse is true if an absolute measure is used. Both the

Table 21 – Mortality ratio and excess deaths of various causes among men with a history of regular cigarette smoking. American Cancer Society, 1952 cohort study. Source: (Hammond and Horn, 1958).

Cause of death	Observed deaths	Mortality ratio (observed ÷ expected)	Excess deaths (observed- expected)	Percentage of all excess deaths (%)
Coronary artery disease	3,361	1.70	1,388	52.1
Lung cancer	397	10.73	360	13.5
Other cancer	1,063	1.50	359	13.5
Other heart and circulation disorders	676	1.30	154	5.8
Pulmonary (except cancer)	231	2.85	150	5.6
Cerebral vascular	556	1.30	128	4.8
Gastric and duodenal ulcers	100	4.00	75	2.8
Cirrhosis and liver	83	1.93	40	1.5
All other	849	1.01	11	0.4
Total	7,316		2,665	

> *absolute [attributable or excess risk, risk difference] and the relative measure [relative risk, odds ratio] serve a purpose. The relative measure is helpful in (…) appraising the importance of an agent with respect to other possible agents inducing the same effect (…). The absolute measure would be important in appraising the public health importance of an effect known to be causal."* (Cornfield et al., 1959, p. 194).

The importance of smoking as a cause of coronary artery disease may have been misinterpreted if the association with smoking had only been reported as a mortality ratio, or more generally, as a relative risk. The study stressed the importance of looking at the data under two different perspectives, easily derived from cohort studies. One type is related to the interpretation of relative risks. It is a very intuitive concept; e.g., the risk in the exposed is twofold, threefold, etc. greater (or smaller) relative to the risk in the unexposed. Relative risks are useful to identify risk factors, even when the disease is extremely rare. They do not require population data on prevalence or incidence and, therefore, can be estimated from a case-control study. However, a relative risk of 10 can be obtained from a ratio of 10/1, 100/10, or 10,000/1,000. It does not reflect the public health or clinical importance of the association. In contrast, the various forms of attributable risks (synonymously defined as risk difference, excess risk, absolute risk, or excess deaths in Hammond and Horn's paper) corresponding to the previous relative risks of 10 are, respectively, 9, 90 and 9,000 cases, say, per million over a given time period. They have a straightforward public health or clinical interpretation: the exposure causes an absolute number of cases in excess over a given time period. I have proposed elsewhere to call these two types of perspectives relative and absolute causality (Morabia, 2001b).

3.7. Selection bias

Another opponent of the smoking-lung cancer association was Joseph Berkson, (1899–1982) who graduated (MD and ScD) from The Johns Hopkins University and later became Head of the Biometry and Medical Statistics Division at the Mayo Clinic in Minnesota. It is in that position that he developed a theoretical mechanism of bias, known today as "Berkson's bias" or "Berkson's fallacy", that could plague hospital-based case-control studies (such as those of smoking and lung cancer) and therefore invalidate their findings (Berkson, 1946).

Berkson's argument was that case-control studies comparing hospital patients with different diagnoses – note that the three influential smoking and lung cancer studies known to Berkson were hospital-based – could yield false associations only as a result of a selective process of hospitalization. Conceptually, if a larger fraction of all exposed cases was likely to be hospitalized than that of exposed controls, then a comparison of hospitalized cases and controls would find an association between smoking and lung cancer even if no such association existed in their population. Berkson's paper demonstrated that this was possible mathematically and in doing so probably represented the "first algebraic analysis of an epidemiologic selection bias" (Greenland, 1987b, p. 86).

Berkson's paper starts with explaining the essential difference between a case-control study, which he refers to as the "practical statistics", and the laboratory experiment. The laboratory experiment compares groups of exposed and unexposed animals. The outcome is a true random variable, while in the case-control study, we search for an association between exposure and disease after disease has already occurred:

"all the effects are already produced before the investigation starts"
(Berkson, 1946).

The paper uses the example of a hospital-based case-control study of the association of diabetes (cases) and cholecystitis (exposure). Controls are ophthalmology patients who came to the clinic to get glasses because of refractive errors. Berkson demonstrates that, under specific assumptions, the case-control study may spuriously observe an excess of cholecystitis of 2.32% (± 0.5%) in patients with diabetes than

Table 22 – Population frequency, referral rates, and hospital frequency for exposed and unexposed cases and controls. Source: Table 5.2. in (Schlesselman, 1982, p.129).

Exposure	Disease	Population frequency	Proportion referred	Hospital frequency
Yes	Case	A	s_1	$s_1 A$
	Control	B	s_2	$s_2 B$
No	Case	C	s_3	$s_3 C$
	Control	D	s_4	$s_4 D$

Population odds ratio: $\Psi = AD \div BC$
Hospital odds ratio: $\Psi' = [(s_1 s_4) \div (s_2 s_3)] \, \Psi = \text{bias} \times \Psi$

among controls while there is no such association in the whole population from which cases and controls originate (Berkson, 1946).

The mechanism underlying Berkson's bias was elegantly explicated by the epidemiologist James J. Schlesselman in his 1982 "Case-control Studies" (Schlesselman, 1982). To facilitate a modern interpretation of these data, Schlesselman shows the impact of the bias on the odds ratio, that is, the ratio of the odds of exposure in the cases over the odds of exposure in the controls:

"Differential referral patterns are another source of potential bias in hospital or clinic-based case-control studies. Table 5.2 [Table 22 above] shows that differential rates of hospitalization for exposed and unexposed cases and controls can distort the odds ratio- determined in the hospital from that in the population. Whereas the population odds ratio is $\Psi = AD \div BC$, the odds ratio in hospital is $\Psi' = b \, \Psi$ where the bias term $b = (s_1 s_4) \div (s_2 s_3)$ depends on the (usually unknown) differential referral rates s_1, s_2, s_3, and s_4 defined in Table 5.2 [Table 22 above]." (Schlesselman, 1982, p. 128).

Table 23 presents Berkson's data from a hypothetical hospital-based case-control study of the association of diabetes with cholecystitis, in which cases suffer from diabetes and controls from ocular refractive errors requiring glasses, using Schlesselman's notation defined in Table 22.

Applying Schlesselman's factorization of the cross-product ratio of the sampling fractions to Berkson's data, we get:

Population $\Psi = AD \div BC = (3{,}000 \times 960{,}300) \div (29{,}700 \times 97{,}000) = 1$
Hospital $\Psi' = [(s_1 s_4) \div (s_2 s_3)] \times \Psi = [(0.2087 \times 0.20) \div (0.32 \times 0.069)] \times 1 = 1.89 \times 1 = 1.89$

Table 23 – Example of a hypothetical hospital-based case-control study of the association of diabetes with cholecystitis, in which cases suffer from diabetes and controls from ocular refractive errors requiring glasses. The proportions referred are: 0.05 for diabetes, 0.2 for refractive errors and 0.15 for cholecystitis. All forces of hospitalization are independent of each other. Source: (Berkson, 1946).

Exposure	Disease	Population frequency	Proportion referred*	Hospital frequency
Yes	Case	A = 3,000	$s_1 = 0.2087$	626
	Control	B = 29,700	$s_2 = 0.32$	9,504
No	Case	C = 97,000	$s_3 = 0.069$	6,693
	Control	D = 960,300	$s_4 = 0.20$	192,060
Odds ratio**		Ψ = AD ÷ BC = (3,000 × 960,300) ÷ (29,700 × 97,000) = 1		$\Psi' = [(s_1 s_4) \div (s_2 s_3)] \times \Psi$ = [(0.2087 × 0.20) ÷ (0.32 × 0.069)] × 1 = 1.89 × 1 = 1.89

* The reader should refer to Berkson's paper to understand how these probabilities were computed.
** Computed using the equations of Table 22.

Thus, diabetes is not associated with cholecystitis in the population (odds ratio = 1), but it is in the hospital-based study because of the differential sampling fractions (or forces of hospitalization) of the different categories of cases and controls (odds ratio = 1.89).

Berkson's argument was not based on real data and has never been clearly demonstrated empirically. Some investigators got close though (Vineis, Part IIa; Roberts et al., 1978). There was, however, an element in Berkson's example that was peculiar: the "exposure" was a disease (i.e., cholecystitis), which, alone, could contribute to hospitalization. In case-control studies, exposures are usually risk factors, which are not sufficient motives of hospitalization. e.g., being a smoker does not lead to hospitalization independently of the diseases that smoking causes. Therefore, it was argued that in Berkson's example the bias occurred only because cholecystitis *contributed independently* to hospitalization (Kraus, 1954). Otherwise, there would have been no selection bias (i.e., using Schlesselman's notation, s1 = s3 and s2 = s4). The counterargument therefore was to Berkson's criticism that epidemiologic studies of smoking and cancer could not have been threatened by Berkson's bias.

Berkson's criticism did not end up hurting epidemiology. On the contrary, it stimulated the development of a formal theory of selection (or response) biases, of which Berkson's bias has since become a classic example. It was shown that there were many conditions under which the imbalanced selection of cases and controls would not lead to selection bias:

> "Physicians or self referral are two of many selective factors operating to produce the final case-control series in any hospital-based study. In general, if one regards the terms s1 to s4 as the sampling proportions for the four cells of the 2 × 2 table with population frequencies A, B, C, and D in Table 5.2 [Table 22 above], then a general condition for the absence of bias in the estimation of the odds ratio is that b = 1, implying that $s_1s_4 = s_2s_3$. For example, if among cases one is k times more likely to choose an exposed individual, and if among controls one is also k times more likely to choose an exposed individual, then $s_1 = ks_3$ and $s_2 = ks_4$, resulting in b = 1. Thus, in principle, a biased selection of cases can be compensated by a biased selection of controls. However, one usually strives to choose both cases and controls in a manner that assures that exposed and unexposed individuals have equal probabilities of selection, that is, $s_1 = s_3$ and $s_2 = s_4$."
> (Schlesselman, 1982, p. 128).

The theory of selection bias in case-control studies was later expanded to losses of follow-up in cohort studies and further generalized. About 40 years after Berkson's paper, epidemiologists had arrived at a well-formalized theory of selection and response bias.

3.8. Interaction

The concept of interaction is used in epidemiology to define a situation in which an association differs in subgroups of the population. It implicates at least three elements: an exposure, an outcome and another factor, which is sometimes referred to as the "effect modifier". The interaction between fava bean consumption, hemolytic anemia and the glucose-6-phosphate dehydrogenase genetic deficiency is an extreme example, in which the association between fava beans and hemolytic anemia can be observed when the genetic variant is present but not when it is absent. More commonly, an effect modifier modulates the effect of the studied exposure. There is *synergy* when the effect modifier amplifies the effect of exposure. There is *antagonism* when the effect modifier reduces the effect of exposure.

According to Major Greenwood, the Roman physician Galen (AD129-AD210) considered that ill-health depended on the interaction between *temperament*, *procatarctic* factors and *constitutions*, which correspond grossly to our current genetic, behavioral and environmental risk factors:

> "Let us imagine, for instance, that the atmosphere is carrying diverse seeds of pestilence, and that, of the bodies exposed to it, some are choked with excremen-

titious matters apt in themselves to putrefy, that others are void of excrement and pure. Let us further suppose an obstruction of orifices and resultant plethora in the former, likewise a life of luxury, much junketing, drinking, sexual excess and the crudities which must attend on such traits; in the latter let us suppose cleanliness, freedom from excrementitious matters, orifices unobstructed and uncompressed, desirable conditions, as we may say, free transpiration, moderate exercise, temperance in diet. All this being supposed, judge thou, which class of body is likelier to be injured by the inspiration of putrid air."
(Greenwood, 1935, p. 27).

Thus, for Galen, an environmental risk factor is more likely to affect a debauched than an ascetic person. If the logical content of the epidemiologic concept of interaction can be found in antiquity, the theory of interaction is absent from the epidemiologic literature until the 1960s. The relation between exposure to asbestos, smoking and lung cancer has become the classical example of interaction between several causes.

Asbestos was used on a very large scale during the 20th century, most particularly for construction and public infrastructures (see Stellman, Part II). Its carcinogenic effect was first noted as an occupational disease. During the 1950s, workers exposed to asbestos were more likely to develop lung cancer than the general population (Doll, 1955), but they, as most of the male population, usually also smoked. Whether asbestos had an *independent* contribution to the risk of lung cancer remained to be demonstrated. The group led by Irving Selikoff (1915–1992), Director of the Division of Environmental and Occupational Medicine at Mount Sinaï Hospital, New York, assembled a cohort of the members of a union, *The International Association of Heat and Frost Insulators and Asbestos Workers*, that is, workers exposed to asbestos and working in the United States or Canada.

The cohort comprised 17,800 workers who had filled out a questionnaire in 1966. The causes of death were systematically registered after that. In 1976, 397 cases of lung cancer occurred among the 12,051 workers who had been exposed at least 20 years to asbestos. They contributed 77,391 person-years of follow-up.

As, by definition, members of the *International Association* were all exposed to some degree to asbestos, Selikoff searched for an external cohort of workers who would be comparable in terms of work conditions but essentially unexposed to asbestos. With Cuyler Hammond, they identified a subgroup of the American Cancer Society cohort study described above (Hammond and Horn, 1958), comprising 73,763 men who had blue-collar jobs in environments rich in dust, fumes and vapors but not asbestos. These blue-collar workers had been followed up between 1967 and 1972.

The results of this study comparing a cohort of asbestos workers to a cohort of blue-collar workers are shown in Table 24 (Hammond et al., 1979).

Table 24 – Age-standardized lung cancer death rates (per 100,000 per year) for cigarette smoking and/or occupational exposure to asbestos dust compared with no smoking and no occupational exposure to asbestos dust. Source: (Hammond et al., 1979, p. 487).

Group	Exposure to asbestos	History cigarette smoking	Death rate	Mortality difference*	Mortality ratio**
Control	No	No	11.3	0.0***	1.00***
Asbestos workers	Yes	No	58.4	+47.1	5.17
Control	No	Yes	122.6	+111.3	10.85
Asbestos workers	Yes	Yes	601.6	+590.3	53.24

* Attributable risk.
** Relative risk.
*** Reference group.

The authors interpreted the data in Table 24 as follows:

"The mortality differences shown here were calculated by subtracting the death rate of the "no, no" group from the death rate of each of the four groups. The mortality ratios were calculated by dividing the death rate of each group by the death rate of the "no, no" group.
The mortality ratios are 1.00 for "no, no" (asbestos, no; cigarette smoking, no); 5.17 for "yes, no" (asbestos, yes; cigarette smoking, no); 10.85 for "no, yes" (asbestos, no; cigarette smoking, yes) and 53.24 for "yes, yes" (asbestos, yes, cigarette smoking, yes).
Now, suppose that occupational exposure to asbestos dust and cigarette smoking acted independently in respect to the production of lung cancer. In that event, the lung cancer death rate of asbestos workers with a history of cigarette smoking should be very close to the sum of the following three numbers: 11.3 (the rate for the "no, no" group), 47.1 (the mortality difference for the "yes, no" group), and 111.3 (the mortality difference for the "no, yes" group). The sum comes to 169.7 lung cancer deaths per 100,000 man-years which is a reasonable estimate of what the lung cancer death rate of the asbestos workers with a history of cigarette smoking would have been if there had been no synergistic effect of the combined exposure. In contrast, the observed lung cancer death rate of the "yes, yes" group was 601.6 per 100,000 man-years. The difference (601.6 – 169.7) = 431.9 lung cancer deaths per 100,000 man-years, was presumably due to a synergistic effect in men with both of the two types of exposure (asbestos dust and cigarette smoking)." (Hammond et al., 1979).

The mortality difference of asbestos workers who smoked (relative to blue-collar workers unexposed to asbestos and non-smokers) was expected to be 158.4 /100,000/yr, which corresponds to the sum of the individual effects of smoking and asbestos. But it was 590.3, that is, much larger than expected. The authors therefore concluded that there was synergy because smoking amplified the mortality difference (i.e., absolute causality) due to asbestos. But they would have come to a very different conclusion if their reasoning had been based on the mortality ratio (i.e., relative causality). The mortality ratios are [58.4 ÷ 11.3 =] 5.17 for asbestos alone, [122.6 ÷ 11.3 =] 10.85 for smoking alone. In the absence of interaction between asbestos and smoking we would expect the mortality ratio for those exposed to both asbestos and smoking to be [5.17 × 10.85 =] 56.09, which is very similar to the observed mortality ratio (53.24). What was then the correct interpretation?

Table 24, or similar findings observed in other studies, provoked a controversy about the definition and interpretation of interaction that took place, mostly in the American Journal of Epidemiology between 1976 and 1980. Three of the contenders coauthored a paper which they hoped would "lay to rest" the concept of interaction:

"We believe that the controversy surrounding the concept of interaction can be laid to rest with specification of the context in which the interaction is being evaluated. Four broad contexts can be distinguished: statistical, biological, public health, and individual decision-making. Each has different implications for the evaluation of interaction." (Rothman et al., 1980).

They distinguished four types of interactions according to the purpose or the context: statistical, biological, public health and individual decision-making.

1) The evaluation of *statistical* interaction depended on the model chosen, whether additive (modeling risk differences) or multiplicative (modeling relative risks). It served to describe the relation between the two factors and the outcome irrespective of the nature of their biological links.

Checking in Table 24 for smoking, asbestos and lung cancer, there is *additive interaction* as the observed attributable risk (AR, referred to in the table as mortality difference) is greater than the AR expected if the AR for smoking and the AR for asbestos were independent:

Observed AR for smoking & asbestos = 590.3
Expected AR for smoking & asbestos if no interaction = 47.1 + 111.3 = 158.4

In contrast, Table 24 does not suggest *multiplicative interaction* as the observed relative risk (RR, referred to in the table as mortality ratio) is not substantially different from the RR expected if the RR for smoking and the RR for asbestos were independent:

Observed RR for smoking & asbestos = 53.24
Expected RR for smoking & asbestos if no interaction = 5.17 × 10.85 = 56.09

2) In *biological* interaction, the choice of the additive or multiplicative model was based on some speculation about the underlying biologic model, whether the two factors were believed to act additively or multiplicatively.

3) *Public health* interaction had to be evaluated using *additive* models, as an additive interaction implied that the preventive yield of a public health intervention would differ according to the target population. Let's turn again to the example of smoking, asbestos and lung cancer. The AR associated with preventing smoking among asbestos-exposed workers is:

AR (smoking & asbestos) – AR (asbestos alone) = 590.3 – 47.1 = 543.2

The corresponding absolute risk reduction of lung cancer associated with removing asbestos exposure among smoking workers is:

AR (smoking & asbestos) – AR (smoking alone) = 590.3 – 111.3 = 479.0

The attributable risk for removing smoking among asbestos workers appears therefore greater (543.2 per 100,000 per year) than that of removing asbestos among smoking workers (479.0 per 100,000 per year). Hammond et al. (1979) had chosen the right model. Public health interaction can lead to key strategic choices, even if in practice things are not that simple and the absolute number of cases prevented by each of the interventions would require considering the prevalence of smoking and of asbestos exposure.

4) The *individual decision-making* interaction is similar to the public health interaction but in the context of medical practice. The presence of additive interaction between a specific drug (e.g., oral contraceptive), a risk factor (e.g., hypertension) and a disease (e.g., stroke) may imply that the drug is contraindicated (or particularly beneficial) in subgroups of patients.

Interaction is the most recent of the epidemiologic concepts. It has not been "laid to rest" yet.

3.9. Causal inference

Causal inference is another long-lasting conceptual development fostered by the smoking-lung cancer controversy. The criteria used by epidemiologists today to establish a plausible causal connection are primarily associated with the name of, once again, Bradford Hill (Hill, 1965). Hill's work summarized a generation of thought by several eminent epidemiologists including Jacob Yerushalmy (1904– 1973), Carroll

E. Palmer (1909–1969), Abraham Lilienfeld (1920–1985), Philip Sartwell (1908–1999) and Mervyn Susser.

Hill's 1965 paper entitled: *"Environment and disease: Association or causation"* has been so influential that it is worth citing some parts at length. Hill starts by stating the question underlying causal inference:

> *"In what circumstances can we pass from this observed association to a verdict of causation? Upon what basis should we proceed to do so? (...) The decisive question is whether the frequency of the undesirable event B will be influenced by a change in the environmental feature."* (Hill, 1965, p. 295).

Causal inference comes after we have ruled out the role of chance or bias in the interpretation of the data:

> *"Our observations reveal an association between two variables, perfectly clear-cut and beyond what we would care to attribute to the play of chance. What aspects of that association should we especially consider before deciding that the most likely interpretation of it is causation?"* (Hill, 1965, p. 295).

Then comes the list of nine aspects that tend to characterize causal relations, in the order given by Hill and, when relevant, accompanied by an example.

1. Strength: *"...prospective inquiries into smoking have shown that the death rate from cancer of the lung in cigarette smokers is nine to ten times the rate in non-smokers and the rate in heavy cigarette smokers is twenty to thirty times as great. But to explain the pronounced excess in cancer of the lung in any other environmental terms requires some feature of life so intimately linked with cigarette smoking and with the amount of smoking that such a feature should be easily detectable"*. [However] *"We must not be too ready to dismiss a cause-and-hypothesis merely on the grounds that the observed association appears to be slight."* (Hill, 1965, pp. 295–296).

2. Consistency: *"...the consistency of the observed association. Has it been repeatedly observed by different persons, in different places, circumstances and times ?(...) The Advisory Committee to the Surgeon-General of the United States Public Health Service found the association of smoking with cancer of the lung in 29 retrospective and 7 prospective inquiries (US Department of Health, Education & Welfare 1964). The lesson here is that broadly the same answer has been reached in quite a wide variety of situations and techniques. In other words we can justifiably infer that the association is not due to some constant error or fallacy that permeates every inquiry. (...)I would myself put a good deal of weight upon similar results reached in quite different ways, e.g. prospectively and retrospectively."* (Hill, 1965, pp. 296–297).

3. Specificity: *"If, as here, the association is limited to specific workers and to particular sites and types of disease and there is no association between the work and other modes of dying, then clearly that is a strong argument in favor of causation. (...) If other causes of death are raised 10, 20 or even 50% in smokers whereas cancer of the lung is raised 900–1,000% we have specificity - a specificity in the magnitude of the association."* (Hill, 1965, p. 297).

4. Temporality: *"...which is the cart and which the horse? Does a particular diet lead to disease or do the early stages of the disease lead to those peculiar dietetic habits?"* (Hill, 1965, pp. 297–298).

5. Biological gradient: *"For instance, the fact that the death rate from cancer of the lung rises linearly, with the number of cigarettes smoked daily, adds a very great deal to the simpler evidence that cigarettes smokers have a higher death rate than non-smokers. (...)The clear dose-response curve admits of a simple explanation and obviously puts the case in a clearer light."* (Hill, 1965, p. 298).

6. Plausibility: *"It will be helpful if the causation we suspect is biologically plausible. But this is a feature I am convinced we cannot demand. What is biologically plausible depends upon the biological knowledge of the day."* (Hill, 1965, p. 298).

7. Coherence: *"On the other hand the cause-and-effect interpretation of our data should not seriously conflict with the generally known facts of the natural history and biology of the disease - in the expression of the Advisory Committee to the Surgeon-General it should have coherence. Thus in the discussion of lung cancer the Committee finds its association with cigarette smoking coherent with the temporal rise that has taken place in the two variables over the last generation and with the sex difference in mortality - features that might well apply in an occupational problem. The known urban/rural ratio of lung cancer mortality does not detract from coherence, nor the restriction of the effect to the lung."* (Hill, 1965, p. 298).

8. Experiment: *"Occasionally it is possible to appeal to experimental, or semi-experimental, evidence. For example, because of an observed association some preventive actions are taken."* (Hill, 1965, pp. 298–299).

9. Analogy: *"In some circumstances it would be fair to judge by analogy. With the effects of thalidomide and rubella before us we would surely be ready to accept slighter but similar evidence with another drug or another viral disease in pregnancy."* (Hill, 1965, p. 299).

Then comes the crucial caveat that the aspects of causal relations should not be summed as a causality score:

"Here then are nine different viewpoints from all of which we should study association before we cry causation. What I do not believe – and this has been suggested – is that we can usefully lay down some hard-and-fast rules of evidence that must be obeyed before we accept cause and effect. None of my nine viewpoints can bring indisputable evidence for or against the cause-and-effect hypothesis and none can be required as a sine qua non. What they can do, with greater or less strength, is to help us to make up our minds on the fundamental question – is there any other way of explaining the set of facts before us, is there any other answer equally, or more, likely than cause and effect?" (Hill, 1965, p. 299).

Followed by the often forgotten reminder that there is no statistical test for causal inference:

"No formal tests of significance can answer those questions. Such tests can, and should, remind us of the effects that the play of chance can create, and they will instruct us in the likely magnitude of those effects. Beyond that they contribute nothing to the "proof" of our hypothesis. (....) Fortunately I believe we have not yet gone so far as our friends in the USA where, I am told, some editors of journals will return an article because tests of significance have not been applied. Yet there are innumerable situations in which they are totally unnecessary – because the difference is grotesquely obvious, because it is negligible, or because, whether it be formally significant or not, it is too small to be of any practical importance." (Hill, 1965, p. 299).

The elaboration of a structured approach to causal inference accompanied the preparation of the historical 1964 Surgeon General report stating that cigarette smoking caused lung cancer (US Department of Health, 1964). The unrelenting rise in cigarette sales in the US and in Europe from the 1920s was finally curbed in the early 1980s, at least among men.

3.10. The rare disease assumption

Superficially, cohort and case-control studies may appear to be two designs with opposite logic. Jerome Cornfield (1912–1979) has been, among many other prestigious positions, Chairman of the Department of Biostatistics at The Johns Hopkins University and Director of Biostatistics Center at The George Washington University. It is of historical interest to note that Cornfield was President successively of the American Epidemiologic Society (in 1972) and of the American Statistical Association (in 1974). Cornfield played a decisive role in demonstrating the close link between cohort and case-control study designs and therefore creating the basis for the modern understanding of case-control studies.

Table 25 – Results of the case-control study of cigarette smoking and lung cancer among white males of aged 40–49 used as an example by Cornfield (Cornfield, 1951). Source: (Schrek et al., 1950).

Cigarette per day	Lung cancer cases	Controls with tumors of other sites
10 or more	$p_1 = 77\%$	$p_2 = 58\%$
Else	$1-p_1 = 23\%$	$1-p_2 = 42\%$
N	35	171

P = proportion of cigarette smoking.
[Odds Ratio = $[p_1 \div (1-p_1)] \div [p_2 \div (1-p_2)]$ = (0.77 ÷ 0.23) ÷ (0.58 ÷ 0.42) = 2.42]*.
* Cornfield does not use the term odds ratio.

In 1951, Cornfield showed that it was possible to estimate a relative risk (in principle, only computable in a cohort study) from case-control study data. The procedure assumed that the cases and the controls were representative of the same groups in the general population. Cornfield's procedure is explained in Tables 25 and 26. Table 25 gives the case-control data and notation that Cornfield used as an example. They came from a paper by Schrek et al. (Schrek et al., 1950; Paneth et al., Part II).

The primary result of the study was that smoking 10 cigarettes or more per day was more common in cases ($p_1 = 77\%$) than in controls ($p_2 = 58\%$). Intuitively, it is logical to expect that if more cases of lung cancer smoked, the risk of lung cancer was greater in smokers. But, mathematically, there was apparently no relationship between the proportions of exposed in cases and controls and the smokers/non-smokers risks of lung cancer.

Going beyond simple proportions, p1 and p2 could be re-expressed as the odds of smoking in cases [$(p_1 \div 1-p_1)$ = (0.77 ÷ 0.23)] and the odds of smoking in controls [$(p_2 \div 1-p_2)$ = (0.58 ÷ 0.42)]. Dividing the odds of smoking in cases by the odds of smoking in controls yields the *odds ratio*, that is, 2.42. This odds ratio means that cases have 2.42 times the odds of smoking 10 or more cigarettes per day than controls. Still there is no apparent connection with risks of lung cancer in smokers and non-smokers.

Table 26 gives the formula proposed by Cornfield to compute the incidence rates based on the proportions of smokers, p_1 and p_2. For the purpose of the demonstration, Cornfield needed an additional piece of external information, that is, an "annual prevalence rate" of lung cancer in the population, which he estimated was 15.5 per 100,000 people per year. Cornfield was alluding to new cases of lung cancer diagnosed over a year and he must have meant annual *incidence* rate.

Table 26 shows that by some conjuring trick Cornfield had been able to transform proportions of smokers into incidence rates. This transformation allowed him to compute a relative risk from a case-control study. The trick depended on a simple

Table 26 – Formula used by Cornfield to transform smoking proportions (p_1 and p_2, see Table 25) into incidence rates. APR = "annual prevalence rate" of lung cancer in the population of = 15.5 /100,000. Source: (Cornfield, 1951).

Cigarette per day	Formula	Computations	Incidence rates (/100,000/yr)
10 or more	(p_1 × APR) ÷ [p_2 + APR × ($p_1 - p_2$)]	(0.77 × 0.000155) ÷ [0.58 + 0.000155 × (0.77−0.58)]	20.6*
Else	(1-p_1) × APR ÷ [(1-p_2) − APR × ($p_1 - p_2$)]	(0.23 × 0.000155) ÷ [0.42 − 0.000155 × (0.77−0.58)]	8.5**

Relative Risk = [incidence rate in '10 or more' ÷ incidence rate in 'else'] = [20.6 ÷ 8.5] = 2.40.
* 20.5 in Cornfield's paper.
** 8.6 in Cornfield's paper.

condition. If the proportion of the general population developing cancer of the lung, the "annual prevalence rate", is small relative to both p_2 and 1-p_2, the contribution of the term APR × (p_1-p_2) is trivial and can be neglected. In Table 26, this term is equal to [0.000155 × (0.77−0.58) =] 0.00003.

Table 26 also shows that once the APR × (p_1-p_2) term is deleted, we are left with a formula for the relative risk, which is:

$$RR \cong [p_1 \times (APR \div p_2)] \div [(1-p_1) \times (APR \div (1-p_2))]$$

The equality is not exact because the term APR × (p_1-p_2) was added to p_2 and subtracted from 1-p_2. But we need four digits to show the inequality. The relative risk = 2.4240 before simplification and 2.4243 afterwards. We can again simplify APR from the numerator and the denominator of the new equation. We are left with the relative risk being almost equal to the odds ratio:

$$RR \cong [p_1 \div (1-p_1)] \div [p_2 \div (1-p_2)] = odds\ ratio = 2.42$$

The great news was therefore that knowledge of the population incidence rate (i.e., Cornfield's APR) was not needed to approximate the relative risk by the odds ratios. The connection between the odds ratio and the relative risk was now obvious and confirmed the intuition:

> "...whenever a greater proportion of the diseased than of the control group possess a characteristic, the incidence of disease is always higher among those possessing the characteristic. This is the intuition on which the procedures used in

such clinical studies [i.e., case-control studies] is based. Although it has frequently been questioned, it can now be seen as correct." (Cornfield, 1951, p. 1270).

In 1960 Cornfield and William M. Haenszel (1910–1998), biostatistician at the National Institutes of Health (1960, pp. 525–526) re-expressed the derivation of what we now call the approximation of the relative risk by the odds ratio under the rare disease assumption. The relation between the odds ratio and the relative risk had become the relation between cohort and case-control studies, which they still referred to with the old terminology of prospective (= cohort) and retrospective (= case-control) studies:

"Studies which start with populations grouped initially into subclasses, for each of which one counts the number of new cases of a disease which develop during some subsequent period of time, are ordinarily referred to as "prospective" or "population-based" studies. The annual incidence of most diseases is sufficiently small, so that prospective studies designed to supply estimates of the incidence rate for different classes of the population, or of their ratios, must cover large numbers of persons. Thus, in a prospective study of lung cancer in a population of 100,000 males over age 40, one might at the end of 1 year of study expect to find 50 to 75 new cases. This is a small return for a large effort. The "retrospective" or "case-control" study provides a more economical way of estimating the relative risk than the prospective method because it does not require devotion of a large part of the study resources to those who did not develop the disease. In such a study one identifies all, or a well-defined sample, of the new cases of a disease as they occur during some period of time, and only after the occurrence of the disease does one classify them by the presence or absence of the characteristic (hence the name "retrospective"). The remainder of the population, i.e., those who did not develop the disease during the period, is also sampled and similarly classified by presence or absence of the characteristic. Thus, a retrospective study of lung cancer of the same population of 100,000 males over age 40 would (in principle) uncover exactly the same 50 to 75 newly developed cases but would be free to study the characteristics of only a fraction of the remaining 99,925 to 99,950 males who did not develop lung cancer. Retrospective studies might on the surface appear to supply only estimates of the proportion of persons with and without the disease who possess the characteristic and not to estimate relative risk. Such an estimate can easily be derived, however." (Cornfield and Haenszel, 1960).

3.11. Refinements of the theory of case-control studies

Two factors have stimulated the refinement of the theory of case-control studies. First, before the 1980s, the computational problems associated with the analysis of (moderately, e.g., n = 4,000) large cohort studies required computational alternatives that facilitated the sound treatment of the data. Nathan Mantel, statistician at the National Cancer Institute, proposed in 1973 that cohort studies could be analyzed as case-control studies without loss of validity in estimating the odds ratio:

> *"The prospective study can be converted into a synthetic retrospective study by selecting a random sample of the cases and a random sample of the non-cases, the sampling proportion being small for the non-cases, but essentially unity for the cases."* (Mantel, 1973).

Mantel called this new design "synthetic retrospective studies". We know it today as "nested case-control studies" (Doll, Part II). The computational burden is reduced by sampling a small fraction of the non-cases.

The second stimulus stemmed from the work of Cornfield (section 3.10) following which all case-control studies were now viewed as variants of cohort studies in which *cases* were a sample of all cases, and *controls* a sample of all the subjects who did not develop the disease during follow-up. In this context, did the way controls were sampled matter? In Cornfield's paper (Cornfield, 1951), controls were non-cases, that is, sampled among people who had not developed the disease at the end of the follow-up period. Miettinen (Miettinen, 1976a) had noted that waiting until all the cases had been recruited to sample the controls was an uncommon way of performing case-control studies of chronic diseases. Usually, the sampling of controls ran parallel to that of cases. Controls were free of disease at the time of their recruitment, but the investigator could not always rule out that they did not develop the disease later within the same risk period. There could therefore exist two different schemes of sampling controls. This distinction proved to be very fruitful for the evolution of the theory relating cohort to case-control study designs as well as odds ratios to relative risks or relative incidence rates.

3.11.1. Sampling schemes of controls

A series of papers in the seventies and eighties, including (Miettinen, 1976a; Greenland and Thomas, 1982; Hogue et al., 1983; Smith et al., 1984; Greenland et al., 1986) led to the conceptualization of three types of case-control studies according to the mode in which controls were sampled within the underlying cohorts.

To understand the theoretical reasoning we have to *imagine* that the cases and controls are sampled within fully enumerated cohorts of exposed and unexposed subjects, as if we were conducting *nested* case-control studies. If we define the "risk period" as the time interval during which cases are ascertained in the exposed and unexposed cohorts, controls could be sampled either: a) at the end of the risk period; b) from the population at risk during the risk period; or c) from the base. Building on Miettinen's work, Sander Greenland, from the Division of Epidemiology, UCLA School of Public Health and Duncan C. Thomas, then at the Department of Epidemiology and Health, McGill University in Canada, referred to these three sampling schemes as a) traditional b) incidence-density and c) case-base sampling (Greenland and Thomas, 1982; Greenland et al., 1986).

Figure 6 is an attempt to present graphically the differences between these three types of sampling schemes and modes of calculating odds ratios (Morabia et al., 1995).

a) In the *traditional* case-control study, controls are sampled among subjects remaining at risk at the end of the risk period. Thus, none of the controls has had the disease at some point during the risk period: controls are "non-cases" as in Cornfield's example. This is "cumulative incidence" sampling of controls (Greenland and Thomas, 1982). The traditional odds ratio is computed as:

$$\text{Odds ratio}_{traditional} = [cases_{exposed} \div cases_{unexposed}] \times [non\text{-}cases_{unexposed} \div non\text{-}cases_{exposed}]$$

Where "cases" and "non-cases" stand, respectively, for the number of cases and controls.

b) In the *incidence-density* case-control study, subjects in the population-at-risk are eligible as controls at multiple points in time within the risk period given that they are disease-free at the time of selection. However, they may also be sampled later as *cases* if they develop the disease. Controls are selected from all subjects still free of disease at the time of occurrence of the "index case", that is, the particular new case occurring at that time. Thus, the number of available controls for each index case is a function of the duration of follow-up. It is obtained by multiplying the number of subjects at risk times the average duration of follow-up (T), which is equivalent to computing person-times. Thus, it is as if controls were counted as person-times rather than individuals. This is "incidence density" sampling (Greenland and Thomas, 1982). The incidence density odds ratio is computed as:

$$\text{Odds ratio}_{incidence\ density} = (cases_{exposed} \div cases_{unexposed}) \\ \times (person\text{-}times_{unexposed} \div person\text{-}times_{exposed})$$

The "person-times" are the total number of person-times accrued in, respectively, the exposed and the non-exposed subset of the cohorts included in the case-control study. The OR$_{incidence\ density}$ is, strictly speaking, the ratio of two incidence rates. The formula above can be re-written as:

$$\text{Odds ratio}_{incidence\ density} = (cases_{exposed} \div person\text{-}times_{exposed}) \\ \div (cases_{unexposed} \div person\text{-}times_{unexposed})$$

$$= \text{Incidence Rate}_{exposed} \div \text{Incidence Rate}_{unexposed}$$

c) In the *case-base* (or case-cohort) study, controls are sampled from the baseline cohorts (i.e., the base), regardless of whether they become cases or not during the sub-

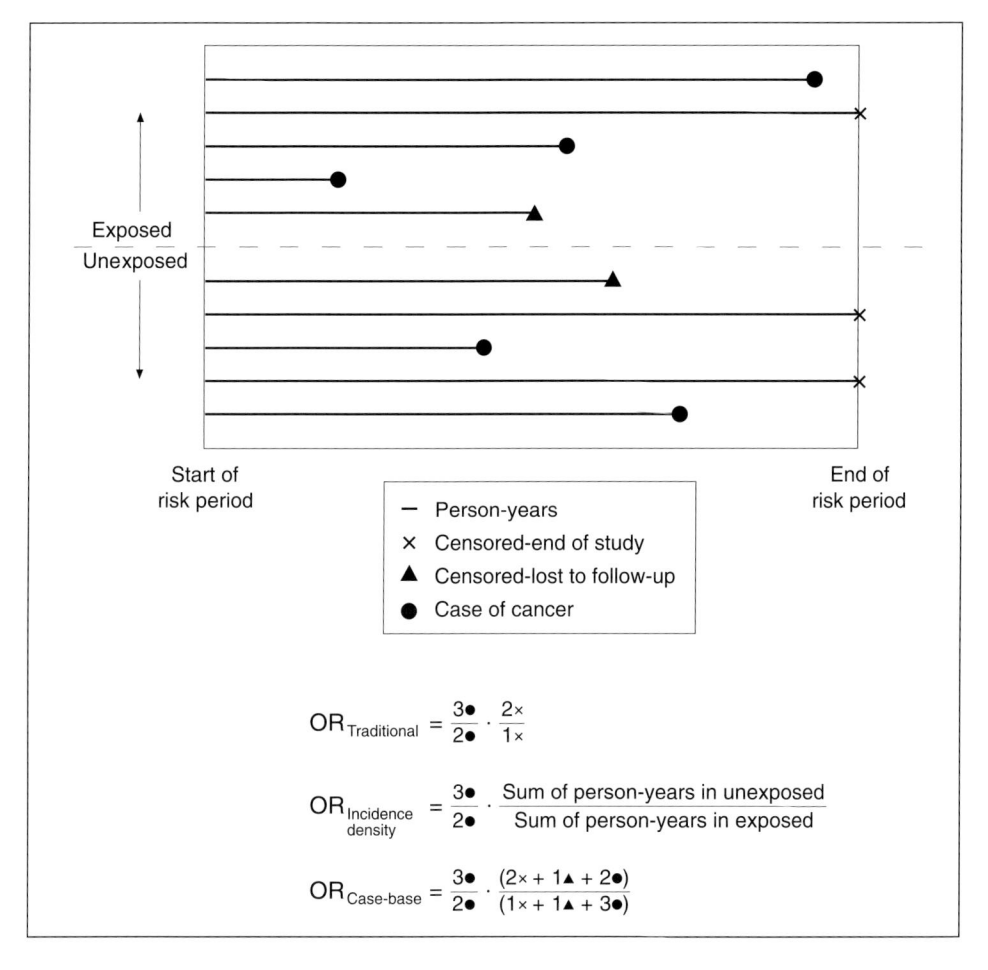

Figure 6
Methods for calculating traditional, incidence density and case-base odds ratios (adapted from Morabia et al., 1995).

$$OR_{Traditional} = \frac{3\bullet}{2\bullet} \cdot \frac{2\times}{1\times}$$

$$OR_{Incidence\ density} = \frac{3\bullet}{2\bullet} \cdot \frac{\text{Sum of person-years in unexposed}}{\text{Sum of person-years in exposed}}$$

$$OR_{Case\text{-}base} = \frac{3\bullet}{2\bullet} \cdot \frac{(2\times + 1\blacktriangle + 2\bullet)}{(1\times + 1\blacktriangle + 3\bullet)}$$

sequent follow-up (Greenland et al., 1986). Thus, some individuals count both as cases and controls. The "case-base" odds ratio is computed as follows:

$$\text{Odds ratio}_{case\text{-}base} = (cases_{exposed} \div cases_{unexposed}) \times (cohort_{unexposed} \div cohort_{exposed})$$

The "cohorts" are the total number of people in the exposed and the non-exposed subset of the baseline cohorts, respectively, who were included in the case-control study. The $OR_{case\text{-}base}$ is strictly speaking a ratio of two risks:

$$Odds\ ratio_{case\text{-}base} = (cases_{exposed} \div cohort_{exposed}) \div (cases_{unexposed} \div cohort_{unexposed})$$
$$= Risk_{exposed} \div Risk_{unexposed}$$

The important consequence of this theory was that the relation of the odds ratio to measures of relative risks, either as ratio of incidence rates, or of risks, was *independent* of whether the studied disease was rare in the population. For example, no "rare-disease assumption" was needed to interpret the incidence-density odds ratio as the ratio of two incidence rates. The complete theory is more complex than its simplified version presented above and takes into account the stability of incidence and exposure during the risk period (Miettinen, 1976a; Greenland and Thomas, 1982; Greenland et al., 1986). I also chose one terminology for the measures described in this section, but the latter varies according to the authors (Rothman and Greenland, 1998).

At the end of this theoretical big bang, Cornfield's "rare disease assumption" had become a special case of a case-control study design. Nevertheless, when the disease is "rare" – that is, when the risk of disease is lower than about 10% over the risk period – the values of all risk ratios and odds ratios are very similar. In these situations, Jerome Cornfield's contribution is valid and the theory of control sampling schemes has less practical relevance.

3.11.2. Sampling controls independent of exposure

Kenneth Rothman has summarized the new concept of the case-control study resulting from the evolution described above in his 1986 textbook "*Modern Epidemiology*" (Rothman, 1986). Imagine a case-control study in which h cases are individuals who became ill during an average duration of time t, some being exposed (a) and other unexposed (b) to the studied cause. The controls are exposed (c) and unexposed (d) individuals, representing a proportion, k, of the combined exposed and unexposed cohorts that gave rise to the cases. The total number of exposed in the underlying cohorts is, therefore, c ÷ k for the exposed and d ÷ k for the unexposed. The total person-times in the underlying cohorts is (c ÷ k) × t or (c × t) ÷ k for the exposed and (d × t) ÷ k for the unexposed. Thus, the cohort incidence rates among exposed and unexposed could be estimated as

$$I_{exposed} = k\frac{a}{c \cdot t} \quad \text{and} \quad I_{unexposed} = k\frac{b}{d \cdot t}$$

The relative risk is the ratio of the incidence rates in the exposed over the incidence rate in the unexposed. In a case-control study, k, the sampling fraction for controls, is usually not known. We cannot therefore estimate the disease incidence rates based on the known a, b, c, d and t. However, both k and t are in principle similar for exposed and unexposed and can be cancelled when we compute the *ratio* of the incidence rates. The relative risk can therefore be obtained as:

$$RR = \frac{I_{exposed}}{I_{unexposed}} = \frac{a \cdot d}{b \cdot c}$$

In Rothman's words:

> "Since the sampling fraction, k, is identical for both exposed and unexposed, it divides out, as does t. The resulting quantity, ad ÷ bc, is the exposure odds ratio (ratio of exposure odds among cases to exposure odds among controls), often referred to simply as the odds ratio. This cancellation of the sampling fraction for controls in the odds ratio thus provides an unbiased estimate of the incidence rate ratio from case-control data (Sheehe, 1962; Miettinen, 1976). The central condition for conducting valid case-control studies is that controls be selected independently of exposure status to guarantee that the sampling fraction can be removed from the status ratio calculation.
> The case-control design can be conceptualized as a follow-up design [follow-up = cohort] in which the person-time experience of the denominators of the incidence rates is sampled rather than measured outright. The sampling must be independent of exposure; by revealing the relative size of the person-time denominators for the exposed and unexposed incidence rates, the sampling process allows the calculation of the relative magnitude of incidence rates. Viewed in this way, the case-control study design can be considered a more efficient form of the follow-up study, in which the cases are the same as those that would be included in a follow-up study and the controls provide a fast and inexpensive means of inferring the distribution of person-time experience according to exposure in the population that gave rise to the cases." (Rothman, 1986, pp. 63–64).

3.12. Evolution of group comparisons in epidemiology

When do we find the first group comparison? Is it already present in Graunt? Graunt compared the mortality of plague across calendar years. In a mysterious sentence, he explains that the proportion of plague deaths in 1625, that is, 68.4% ([35,417 ÷ 51,758], or about 7 to 10) was three times larger than the corresponding proportion in 1592, that is, 44.4% ([11,503 ÷ 325,886], or about 2 to 5):

> "In the year 1625, we find the Plague to bear unto the whole in proportion as 35 to 51. or 7 to 10. that is almost the triplicate of the former proportion [2 to 5 or 40% in 1592], for the Cube of 7.being 343. and the Cube of 10. being 1000. the said 343. is not 2/5 of 1000." (Graunt, 1662, p. 34).

Why does Graunt conclude that 70% can be the "triplicate" of 40%? The exact relative mortality is [68.4% ÷ 44.4% =] 1.6. The puzzling aspect is that the odds of deaths from plague in the year of 1625 ([0.684 ÷ 0.316 =] 2.16) is about three times larger than the odds of death in 1592 ([0.444 ÷ 0.556 =] 0.80): odds ratio = [2.16 ÷ 0.80 =] 2.7. Graunt's conclusion seems meaningless except if we use our modern odds ratio. This important variation of plague mortality across times suggested to Graunt that the plague was more related to environmental than to human constitutional factors.

Around 1720, both John Arbuthnot (1665–1735), London physician, and James Jurin (1684–1750), physician and natural philosopher of Cambridge, tried to establish the mortality from natural smallpox and compare it with the mortality due to inoculation. They used the London Bills of mortality, other evidence when available, and a good deal of reasoning: Arbuthnot found 1 death out of 10 exposed to smallpox, and 1 death out of 100 inoculated. Jurin got 1 of 7 or 8, and 1 of 91, respectively (Rusnock, 2002). A fascinating example of population thinking and group comparison in the early 18th century.

3.12.1. Comparing like with like

The principle of comparing like with like already guides group comparisons in the 18th century. In his investigation of treatments for scurvy, the Scottish naval physician, James Lind (section 3.2) was very cautious to compare six pairs of seamen under similar conditions. He laid them together in one place and fed them with the same diet. One pair served as non-treated controls. Other examples from the 18th century can be found in the James Lind Library and in (Troehler, 2004).

About a century later, in his book about the effects of bleeding as a treatment of pneumonia and other illnesses, Pierre Louis (section 3.3.1) described the principle of valid comparisons:

> "...what was to be done in order to know whether bloodletting had any favorable influence on pneumonitis, and the extent of that influence? Evidently to ascertain whether, other things being equal, the patients who were bled on the first, second, third or fourth day, recovered more readily than those bled at a later period. In the same manner it was necessary to estimate the influence of age, or any other circumstance, on the appreciable effects of bloodletting." (Louis, 1836, p. 55).

For Louis, the experiment had to compare recoveries in groups of patients bled at different times. Louis was expecting that one group would recover "more readily" than the other. This was not an all-or-none response to treatment. The comparison had to be done "other things being equal". The potential influence of things that were not equally distributed had to be evaluated. In another section of the book, Louis mentioned diet before bleedings, age, severity of symptoms at the beginning of the disease and treatments other than bloodletting as

> "causes which, independently of the period of the first bleeding, must have affected some difference in the mean duration of the disease" (Louis, 1836, p. 6).

John Snow insisted in his description of the 1854 natural experiment that the clients of the different water companies were alike in many aspects (section 3.3.2). He was responding to the criteria that William Farr had expressed six months earlier, on November 19, 1853, in relation to Snow's hypothesis:

> "To measure the effect of bad or good water supply, it is requisite to find two classes of inhabitants living at the same level [elevation], moving in equal space, enjoying an equal share of the means of subsistence, engaged in the same pursuits, but differing in this respect, – that one drinks water from Battersea [supposedly polluted water], the other from Kew .... But of such experimenta crucis the circumstances of London do not admit ...." (cited by Vinten-Johansen et al., 2003, p. 260).

Basically, the proof required a study design that would minimize the confounding effects of those factors that were viewed as causes of cholera under different theories.

3.12.2. Fallacies resulting from group incomparability

The first half of the 20th century saw the first theories on potential fallacies that may have resulted from comparing incomparable groups. In 1903, Yule had published his *"Notes on the theory of association of attributes in statistics"* (Yule, 1903), which put in evidence, using a hypothetical example, "fallacies that may be caused by the mixing of records" (section 3.4.1). Yule's fallacy has been transmitted to us as Simpson's paradox and described the fundamental mechanism underlying what we now term "confounding".

In their 1916 investigation of the causes of pellagra, Goldberger and Sydenstricker used different forms of stratification and restriction in the data analysis to separate the effects of diet from those of income, age or gender and presented age-standardized risks (section 3.4.2).

In 1939, Wade Hampton Frost described a fallacy resulting from comparing the mortality from tuberculosis between people of different ages but born at different times (section 3.4.3). The mortality at different ages may in reality reflect different life exposures to the tuberculosis bacillus. We would say today that the effect of age on tuberculosis mortality was confounded by differences in exposure across cohorts.

3.12.3. Treatment allocation

The concern of comparing like with like rapidly led to the idea that allocating treatment could help. Louis had already written that:

> *"In any epidemics, for instance, let us suppose five hundred of the sick, taken indiscriminately, to be subjected to one kind of treatment, and five hundred others,*

taken in the same manner, to be treated in a different mode; if the mortality is greater among the first than among the second, must we not conclude that the treatment was less appropriate, or less efficacious in the first class than in the second? It is unavoidable; for among so large a collection, similarities of conditions will necessarily be met with, and all things being equal, the conclusion will be rigorous." (Louis, 1836, p. 59).

The notion of taking the patients "indiscriminately", taking the two groups between which the treatment is compared "in the same manner" and the large sample size (1,000 patients being "such a large collection") indicate that Louis had a theory of group comparisons, and even of random allocation of treatment, whereby all other factors would have been distributed equally between the compared groups.

There is plenty of evidence that the use of alternate allocation to constitute comparable groups was a common idea by the end of the 19th century. In his now classic public controversy with the British bacteriologist Almroth Wright (1861–1947) about the efficacy of anti-typhoid inoculation, the statistician Karl Pearson proposed:

"only to inoculate every second volunteer. In this way spurious effect really resulting from a correlation between immunity and caution [to avoid exposure] would be got rid of" (Pearson, 1904).

In 1898, the Danish Nobel laureate, Johannes Fibiger (1867–1928), published the apparently first clinical trial with alternate allocation of treatment (Hrobjartsson et al., 1998; Lilienfeld, 1982). In 1930, serotherapy was alternatively allocated to the patients of some the centers participating in the British Medical Research Council trial (section 3.4.4).

3.12.4. The name of the game

However, before 1945, it would be an anachronism to baptize the methods and concepts that were used with the names we use today. Take Louis's and Snow's analyses. Clearly, none of them consciously chose one study design or the other because its properties were more adapted to the questions they wanted to address. They could not rely on any existing theory of study designs. There were no epidemiology textbooks to which they could refer. Louis and Snow had to *invent* their way through the group comparisons. Indeed, there is little consensus among contemporary epidemiologists about how to categorize *a posteriori* Snow's 1854 "natural experiment". It has been viewed as a cohort study (Rothman, 1986; Sartwell, 1965), a survey (Doll, Part II), and a combination of ecologic and retrospective cohort studies (Winkelstein, Jr., 1995).

The same is true for Goldberger and Sydenstricker who performed exposed/unexposed (e.g., comparing incidence rates of pellagra in subgroups differing by diet or income) and affected/unaffected (e.g., comparing dietary habits in subgroups differing by pellagra) comparisons (section 3.4.2). Their methodological contribution is mentioned both in histories of "cross sectional field surveys" (Susser, 1985), cohort studies (Liddell, 1988) and of case-control studies (Paneth et al., Part II).

It would be decades before "investigations" or "analyses" would become "studies" and the logic of exposed/non-exposed or affected/unaffected comparisons would become formal study designs, with their measures of effect, biases, and ability to disentangle the effects of multiple causes. We can only find the unspoken premises of these methods and concepts in these early works.

3.12.5. Case-control and cohort studies

The study of chronic traits, such as lung cancer and cardiovascular diseases, would have to address complex problems: risk factors (e.g., cigarette smoking) could not be randomly allocated, diseases lasted long, had multiple causes, and those exposed to one of the causes tended to be exposed to many others. Typically, smokers were more likely to drink, eat more meat and less fruits and vegetables, and engage less in physical activity. When studying the effect of any of these factors, it was important to treat the effects of the other factors appropriately. In this context, a theory of observational study designs comparing exposed/non exposed (i.e., cohort study) or affected/non affected (i.e., case-control study) became indispensable (sections 3.5 and 3.6).

The elements of theory accrued before 1945 were eventually fused into a theory of study designs after World War II. This process was driven by the quest for the causes of a huge epidemic of lung cancer among Western men that became recognized around 1950. The data showing that exposure to tobacco was the cause triggered an enormous controversy, which contributed importantly to the refinement and formalization of case-control studies, prospective studies and concepts such as confounding, interaction and bias.

The story begins more or less in 1940 (White, 1990). According to Ernst L. Wynder, the medical profession in the forties and fifties did not seriously think about smoking as a potential cause of major diseases (Wynder, 1997). In contrast, physicians interested in public health were astonished when, after World War II, vital statistics were showing a dramatic increase of lung cancer mortality in men. Around 1900, lung cancer was extremely rare (White, 1990, p. 30). Its incidence seemed to grow at a fast pace but the evidence did not convince everyone. It was argued that better diagnosis and aging of the population could explain the trends. An editorial in the British Medical Journal in 1942 stated:

"It is doubtful whether the higher incidence of cancer of the lung observed in recent years is real or only apparent." (Editorial, 1942).

The Medical Research Council of Great Britain in 1950 still used the same expression as the British Medical Journal, that is,

"the increase [in lung cancer incidence] may, of course, be only apparent" (cited by White, 1990).

The opinion had clearly changed in 1952, when the other major British medical journal, The Lancet, wrote:

"Few trends are more dramatic than the rise during the last 30 years in the notified death rates from cancer of the lung. There is little doubt that the increase is both real and numerically important." (Editorial, 1952).

The population-based registries in Denmark and Connecticut reported marked increases in incidence in the forties and fifties. The Connecticut annual, age-adjusted incidence rates per hundred thousand were 9.7, 13, 20.6, 31.1 for 1935–39, 1940–44, 1945–49 and 1950–54 (White, 1990).

The smoking-lung cancer controversy epitomizes this new phase of methodological development, but the causes of many complex traits were discovered. In this process the theory of case-control studies (section 3.5), of cohort studies (section 3.6), concepts of confounding (section 3.4.5), bias (section 3.7), interaction (section 3.8) and causal inference (section 3.9) were further formalized. The relation of case-control to cohort studies was understood (sections 3.10 and 3.11).

Finally, the demonstration that a case-control study could be viewed as a way of sampling subjects within cohorts has unified concepts across study designs (section 3.10). It was also understood that the most usual way of sampling controls, that is, concurrently to case occurrence, yielded the relative incidence rates, without the rare-disease assumption (section 3.11.1). This led to the confinement of the need for the rare disease assumption to relatively uncommon ways of sampling controls (section 3.11.2).

There is a meaningful aspect of the smoking-lung cancer controversy for the history of epidemiologic methods and concepts: the arguments that were used to oppose the smoking-lung cancer connection finally contributed to strengthening epidemiologic methods. In trying to demonstrate that lung cancer was *not* related to smoking but to some genetic factor, the statistician of the University of Cambridge, Fisher contributed to the formalization of the concept of confounding (section 3.4.5). In his criticism of hospital-based case-control studies, another statistician of the Mayo Clinic, Joseph Berkson, laid the foundations for a theory of selection bias (section 3.7). Instead of derailing epidemiologists, these criticisms proved useful and were further elaborated and integrated into the emerging discipline by several epidemiologists.

4. Epistemology

4.1. Tribute to Piaget

The work of the epistemologist Jean Piaget (1896–1980) has inspired me to present the genesis of epidemiology as an evolving process from very intuitive to more theoretical and abstract concepts (Piaget, 1970). During the last phase of his career (1940 to 1971), Piaget was Professor of experimental psychology at the University of Geneva, Switzerland. He had created in 1955 and directed the International Centre of Genetic Epistemology. His description of the genesis of scientific disciplines offered an attractive model for explaining the development of epidemiologic methods, a model that fitted well my perception of the evolution of epidemiologic principles, population thinking, and group comparisons reviewed in this essay.

Before I present *my* understanding of Piaget's genetic epistemology, I want to stress that I do not pretend to be a Piagetian. I do not know if this essay reflects his views, first because he never dealt with epidemiology but, even more importantly, because of his intellectual style. Piaget was a fascinating thinker. He wrote thousands of pages of epistemology, which read as a continuous flow of ideas. His thinking was in perpetual construction (Piaget, 1967). Piaget constantly polished ideas, and debated against other schools of thought. But unlike manuals, his books neither really start nor end. Indeed, one can hardly find a synthesis in Piaget's writing. Syntheses written by his students and scholars are often less accessible than Piaget's original contributions. Of course, these scholars probably deeply disagree with what I just wrote.

Thus, I am hesitant to relate this essay to Piaget's ideas. But at the same time I want to acknowledge that his writings inspired me. In Piaget's terms:

"Genetic epistemology attempts to explain knowledge, and in particular scientific knowledge, on the basis of its history, its sociogenesis, and especially the psychological origins of the notions and operations upon which it is based."
(Piaget, 1970, p. 1).

There are in my view two key elements in Piaget's epistemology. The first is that humans actively gather knowledge. Human knowledge is derived from actions:

"I think that human knowledge is essentially active. To know is to assimilate reality into systems of transformations. To know is to transform reality in order to understand how a certain state is brought about." (Piaget, 1970, p. 15).

This may seem self-evident to most readers of this book, but Piaget was among the first to express it in a qualified way. The world does not reveal its truth passively. It resists and we must therefore act upon it and learn from these actions. We assimilate reality by developing systems that transform it in order to reveal how certain states are produced. We can learn *by acting* on a physical object using *simple* actions, such as throwing, pushing, touching. For example, we can lift different objects and realize that they have different weights. This is how sciences like physics accumulate knowledge, but what about mathematics? In abstract sciences, knowledge is derived from *coordinated* actions and it is the coordination of actions rather than the transformation of reality that generates knowledge. For example, I can count ten lined pebbles from left to right and then from right to left and find out that their sum is independent of their order. This concept is known in mathematics as commutativity. It was not acquired by changes in the pebbles but by the action of counting them in different orders. Actions can be concrete or abstract.

For Piaget, thoughts being invariably related to actions, they need to evolve. Knowledge consists of established causal relations, which he refers to as laws, "modes of production", explanations. Identified causal relations open the way to more action, and therefore more and increasingly elaborated knowledge.

This leads to the second key element in Piaget's idea: scientific knowledge and discipline are in perpetual evolution. Science is a process. It is in continual construction and organization. Other epistemologists may have defended similar ideas, but Piaget's thinking is characterized by the importance of psychological and sociological factors in this construction process. Piaget postulates that there is a parallelism between the progress made in the logical and rational organization of scientific knowledge and the development of human psychology during an individual's life.

> *"The fundamental hypothesis of genetic epistemology is that there is a parallelism between the progress made in the logical and rational organization of knowledge and the corresponding formative psychological processes. Well, now, if that is our hypothesis, what will be our field of study? Of course, the most fruitful, most obvious field of study would be reconstituting human history – the history of human thinking in prehistoric man. Unfortunately, we are not very well informed about the psychology of Neanderthal man or about the psychology of Homo siniensis of Teilhard de Chardin* [1881–1955, paleontologist]. *Since this field of biogenesis is not available to us, we shall do as biologists do and turn to ontogenesis. Nothing could be more accessible to study than the ontogenesis of these notions. There are children all around us. It is with children that we have the best chance of studying the development of logical knowledge, mathematical knowledge, physical knowledge, and so forth."* (Piaget, 1970, pp. 13–14).

As a psychologist, Piaget studied the development of intelligence in children and observed that it is a progressive but structured process that starts with the acquisition of very simple skills, which become in turn the bases for acquisition of more complex ones. Steps are added to the ladder and each step up offers a wider perspective on the world. In Piaget's view, the genesis of a scientific discipline follows an analogous process. Scientific disciplines evolve from very intuitive concepts based on primitive notions to always more abstract and formalized concepts, which are intellectual constructions, made possible by the previous steps. Each level of formalization is a precondition for reaching higher levels because simple theories become tools that allow us to construct theories that are more complex. Without the simple theories, we cannot achieve the more complex and abstract ones. In the process of transforming intuitive or naive notions into universal concepts and theories, scientific disciplines progressively became more abstract, theoretical and mathematical.

4.2. Evolution of physics

Before applying this interpretation scheme to epidemiology, let us see how it applies to physics, as this is the science on which common epistemological models are based. Physics is a very old science that can be viewed as an extension of the sensory and muscular systems of the human body (vision, muscle power, audition, touch, temperature, etc). Physics is related to the essential activities of social life: creation of utensils (flint) or weapons, control of fire, wind (navigation) and water, etc. (Bernal, 1972 chapter 2). Every craftsman develops an intuitive (empirical) knowledge. Seamen have their own theory about sailing, the pitcher about throwing the ball, the cook about the use of the fireplace. Their mode of acquiring knowledge is from a psychological perspective a very primitive one, based on action and reaction, trials and errors. Knowledge comes from repeating the same action and eventually modifying it until one gets what is expected or discovers something new. The first physical experiments were very intuitive. The law of buoyancy of the Greek mathematician Archimedes (BC 287-BC 212) is taught in high school. It is quite intuitive to understand that

> 1. A completely submerged body displaces a volume of liquid equal to its own volume. The buoyant force equals the weight of the fluid displaced.
> 2. When an object weighs less than the total volume of fluid it can displace, it will settle down until the buoyant force equals the weight and it floats partially submerged.

The law is easy to remember and the anecdote of Archimedes exclaiming Eureka! (which means: "I found" in Greek) while immersing himself in his bathtub belongs to popular wisdom. But intuition is insufficient to understand more subtle physical phenomena. The Greek philosopher Aristotle (BC 384-BC 322), founder of the Lyceum of Athens, stated, for example, a law of motion according to which

> *"the moving body comes to a standstill when the force which pushes it along can no longer so act as to push it"* (Einstein and Imfeld, 1966, p. 6).

This "law" reflects our intuitive perception of movement (in the presence of friction and air resistance) but it is false. You can compare it with the Newtonian definition of a force given above (section 2.4.1). Eventually, repeated and organized actions on nature reveal invariant phenomena, observations and laws. In the 16th century, mathematics would become the indispensable complement of experiments in physics. The Italian scientist Galileo Galilei (1564– 1642) claimed that he repeated his experiments a hundred times and always observed the *exact* same results (Bernal, 1972, p. 27). Galileo apparently ignored measurement errors but his experiments allowed him to state a law according to which falling bodies of different weights and sizes took the same time to reach the ground. Galileo's discovery of gravity required a more elaborated mode of reasoning to obtain a result that was, and still is, counter-intuitive (intuitively, most of us expect bodies of different weight to accelerate differently in their fall). After Galileo, the process of formalization went on. Newton built on Galileo's work and predicted the behavior of even less intuitive phenomena (planets), and needed advanced algebra to understand the nature of forces.

Physics finally moved to a form of population thinking, but in terms of particles. Classical physics defined the position and velocity of a single particle (or of one planet). The world of mechanical physics was three-dimensional. It was made of particles whose interactions were governed by a specific law depending on distance and fields. But this mechanical view did not explain why matter appeared to have a granular structure. Hence,

"quantum physics formulates laws governing crowds and not individuals ..." (Einstein and Imfeld, 1966, p. 297).

Quantum physics defined the probability of finding one particle of a certain velocity and a certain position, based on many observations. Thus, physics became statistical in the 20th century. Ultimately, from the 20th century on, physics became so abstract and theoretical that it went beyond intuition and only "geniuses" such as the mathematicians and physicists Albert Einstein (1879–1955) or Niels Bohr (1885–1962) could carry it on to new levels of knowledge.

Epidemiology, at least when defined as a set of methods and concepts, is a much younger discipline than physics. Physics has existed for more than 2500 years considering that its first levels of formalization occurred in ancient Greece. Or 400 years considering, as Einstein did, that scientific reasoning in physics began with Galileo. When did epidemiology first appear?

4.3. Was Hippocrates an epidemiologist?

In this review of the scientific work that has been referred to at one moment or another as "epidemiologic", I systematically searched for the simultaneous presence of population thinking and group comparisons. I started, of course, with the texts of Hippocrates (BC 460-BC 377), who is described in many epidemiology texts as the "father of epidemiology" (MacMahon et al., 1960; Lilienfeld and Lilienfeld, 1980; Pan American Health Organization, 1988, p. 3). These texts do not mention, however, who the "mother" was!

Hippocrates, we believe, was an independent and ambulatory physician, born on the Island of Cos, between current Greece and Turkey. He and others after him described their activity and thinking in medical texts that occupy an undoubtedly important place in medicine. At the time when most medicine, treatment, and cures relied on magical or divine phenomena, the Hippocratic texts used rational thinking, attributing diseases to environmental or other natural causes and proposing empirical treatments such as surgery, diet, herbal remedies, etc. They did not consider divine or magical causes in the etiology or treatment of diseases. Causes were to be found in nature. The quality of the description of diseases and symptoms in Hippocratic texts may explain their influence in the centuries that followed. They expressed 2,500 years ago the kind of materialism that still drives Western medicine today. Hippocratic theories are often easier to understand for a modern reader than the theoretical constructs of physicians who followed him. For example, the theory of reproduction based on the mixing/blending of male and female seminal fluids remain a perfectly satisfactory explanation for what most people observe with their own eyes, much more so than the homunculus theory of Aristotle (Sykes, 2002, p. 41).

A remarkable feature of Hippocratic thinking, which struck those defending the cause of public health in the 19th century and later, is its appraisal of environmental and lifestyle factors as health determinants. In his book "*On Airs, Waters and Places*" (Hippocrates, 400a BCE), we read that the traveling physician arriving to a foreign place had to examine its geographical position, winds, sun, quality of water and yearlong climatic variation:

"Whoever wishes to investigate medicine properly, should proceed thus: in the first place to consider the seasons of the year, and what effects each of them produces for they are not at all alike, but differ much from themselves in regard to their changes. Then the winds, the hot and the cold, especially such as are common to all countries, and then such as are peculiar to each locality. We must also consider the qualities of the waters, for as they differ from one another in taste and weight, so also do they differ much in their qualities. In the same manner, when one comes into a city to which he is a stranger, he ought to consider its situation, how it lies as to the winds and the rising of the sun; for its influence is not the same whether it lies to the north or the south, to the rising or to the setting sun." (Hippocrates, 400a BCE).

The second part of "*On Airs, Water and Places*" is less often quoted but reveals the speculative side of Hippocrates's thinking:

"The other races in Europe differ from one another, both as to stature and shape, owing to the changes of the seasons, which are very great and frequent, and because the heat is strong, the winters severe, and there are frequent rains, and again protracted droughts, and winds, from which many and diversified changes are induced." (Hippocrates, 400a BCE, Part 23).

Hippocratic texts indicate that there was a time when physicians included environmental factors in their diagnostic approach. The role of the environment may have been downplayed later until rediscovered in the 19th century. Hence the fascination of public health practitioners and early epidemiologists towards this major figure of antiquity who seemed to have shared their vision of the role of environment in disease causation. However, the gap between the Hippocratic treatises and modern preventive medicine has lasted so many centuries that it is not clear to me whether Hippocrates can be viewed as a pioneer of modern medicine.

But was Hippocrates an epidemiologist in the sense that he combined population thinking and group comparisons? Can we really trace the roots of epidemiology in antiquity? Here is Major Greenwood's opinion:

"Although Hippocrates was before all else a clinician, he was also a student of preventive medicine and epidemiology, of the doctrine of disease as a mass phenomenon, the units not individuals but groups." (Greenwood, 1935, p. 18).

Is it true that the Hippocratic texts considered diseases as mass phenomena? In *"On Airs, Waters and Places"* we find the distinction between "endemic" diseases, that are always present in a population and "epidemic" diseases, which can become excessively frequent and then disappear. Moreover, the following description of an epidemic (probably of mumps) shows that there is some qualitative description of the frequency of symptoms (e.g., "in many", "in all cases") and their distributions in the population (e.g., in children and adults but seldom attacked women):

"1. In Thasus, about the autumn equinox, and under the Pleiades, the rains were abundant, constant, and soft, with southerly winds; the winter southerly, the northerly winds faint, droughts; on the whole, the winter having the character of spring. The spring was southerly, cool, rains small in quantity. Summer, for the most part, cloudy, no rain, the Etesian winds, rare and small, blew in an irregular manner. The whole constitution of the season being thus inclined to the southerly, and with droughts early in the spring, from the preceding opposite and northerly state, ardent fevers occurred in a few instances, and these very mild, being rarely attended with hemorrhage, and never proving fatal. Swellings appeared about the ears, in many on either side, and in the greatest number on both sides, being unaccompanied by fever so as not to confine the patient to bed; in all cases they disappeared without giving trouble, neither did any of them come to suppuration, as is common in swellings

from other causes. They were of a lax, large, diffused character, without inflammation or pain, and they went away without any critical sign. They seized children, adults, and mostly those who were engaged in the exercises of the palestra and gymnasium, but seldom attacked women. Many had dry coughs without expectoration, and accompanied with hoarseness of voice. In some instances earlier, and in others later, inflammations with pain seized sometimes one of the testicles, and sometimes both; some of these cases were accompanied with fever and some not; the greater part of these were attended with much suffering. In other respects they were free of disease, so as not to require medical assistance." (Hippocrates, 400c BCE).

But the purpose of these concepts was to help clinicians better understand the reasons why individuals (their patients or clients) in some populations were more likely to be affected by some diseases than others:

"It appears to me a most excellent thing for the physician to cultivate Prognosis; for by foreseeing and foretelling, in the presence of the sick, the present, the past, and the future, and explaining the omissions which patients have been guilty of, he will be the more readily believed to be acquainted with the circumstances of the sick; so that men will have confidence to entrust themselves to such a physician. (...) Thus a man will be the more esteemed to be a good physician, for he will be the better able to treat those aright who can be saved, having long anticipated everything; and by seeing and announcing beforehand those who will live and those who will die, he will thus escape censure." (Hippocrates, 400b, BCE).

To the best of my knowledge, Hippocratic texts do not use the group as a unit of thinking. They describe patients one at a time and do not derive knowledge from looking at aggregated cases. There is no formal attempt to group the symptoms under the same disease entity or suggest that they occur in a well-defined combination.

The Hippocratic central preoccupation is to predict what will happen to an individual patient, a question that lies at the heart of medicine. And clearly, the environment was, in Hippocratic texts, an important predictor. But there are no traces of formal population thinking and practically no simple, controlled observations in Hippocrates's treatises. It is mostly, from the 17th century on, when population thinking became philosophically and mathematically founded, that disease entities started to be defined by a set of common symptoms in a population of patients. Before that, there could be no epidemiology.

4.4. Traces of epidemiology in the Bible?

This last statement seems to be contradicted by an example of a supposed group comparison reported in the Book of Daniel, which belongs to the Old Testament of the Bible. The Book of Daniel probably reflects attitudes from the 2nd – 1st centuries before our era (Weingarten, 2004).The episode belongs to the attempt of the King of Babylon to familiarize a group of noble Israelite prisoners, including Daniel, captured after the fall of Jerusalem with the customs of the Chaldeans. The text reports the following episode:

> *"Then Daniel said to the guard whom the master of the eunuchs had put in charge of Hananiah, Mishael and Azariah and himself 'Submit us to this test for ten days. Give us only vegetables to eat and water to drink; then compare our looks with those of the young men who have lived on the food assigned by the king and be guided in your treatment of us by what you see.' The guard listened to what they said and tested them for ten days. At the end of ten days they looked healthier and were better nourished than all the young men who had lived on the food assigned them by the king. So the guard took away the assignment of food and the wine they were to drink and gave them only the vegetables."* (Weingarten, 2004).

Apparently, this story suggests that a controlled experiment took place. Hananiah, Mishael, Azariah and Daniel received a vegetarian diet and water and their looks were compared after 10 days to those of "all the young men" who ate the meat and wine assigned by the king. This example is exceptional in many aspects. The principle of comparing two groups to assess the benefit of some diet appears as a crafty tactic of the prisoners to keep their dietary practice. The comparison must have appealed to the king's sense of logic, which may not have been culture-specific. The results of the experiment were absolutely convincing, almost miraculous: the *four* Jewish men looked healthier and were better nourished than *all* the young men who had lived on the food assigned by the king. But here stops the analogy with group comparisons as we mean it today. It did not come to anybody's mind that the better look of Daniel and his friends could be attributable to something else than their diet. Daniel did not expect his friends and him to look *on average* healthier and better nourished than the other young men. There is no population thinking in Daniel's ruse: each of the Jewish men looked healthier than each of the king's men. The tale is therefore not eligible as a first epidemiologic trial. Epidemiologic group comparisons go along with population thinking, and population thinking did not exist before the 17th century. Such an innovation could not have skipped centuries.

4.5. The impossible comparison

The propensity to trust non-controlled observations is a striking feature of human populations. Consider a patient complaining about flu-like symptoms, who is given antibiotics and feels rapidly better thereafter. The improvement will be attributed to the antibiotics. Similarly, the person who drinks herbal tea after each meal and does not catch the flu for the whole winter will tend to causally relate the herbal tea and his/her resistance to the flu. These are examples of *"post hoc, ergo propter hoc"* ("after it, therefore because of it") reasoning. Conclusions may have been radically different if controlled observations were available, that is, had there been an instance to compare what happened with the antibiotics or with the herbal tea to what would have happened without them.

It seems impossible that brilliant thinkers and clinicians such as Hippocrates, Galen, Thomas Sydenham (1624–1689), also called the "English Hippocrates", Jean-Nicholas Corvisart (1722–1809), etc., in addition to generations of shamans and other primitive therapists had not reflected about this issue. There must be some deep, essential reason for which no therapist integrated controls in their approaches. A simple explanation is that a controlled observation with oneself is *logically impossible*. Once the antibiotic has been prescribed and eventually taken, the situation of the patient has irreversibly changed. We cannot go back in time to the situation where the patient was suffering from flu-like symptoms and had not been treated yet. There is a logical impossibility to get the "counter fact" that would be needed to perform a perfect controlled observation.

The principle of a controlled experiment is therefore logically impossible when we are dealing with an individual human, and more generally with an individual living, complex organisms. Once an action has occurred, we cannot go back to square one and act as if that action had never occurred. Both the subject (e.g., the clinician) and the object (e.g., the disease of the patient) of the action have been modified by the action itself.

To make a cautious step in the direction of Piaget, we can ask whether this logical impossibility of the counterfactual action explains why children do not develop an intuition for controlled experiment. Children develop their psychology by experimenting with the world around them. They compare all the times. They compare what they expect to what they observe. They do this repeatedly. They learn by repeated trials and errors, but they *cannot* compare what happened after their specific action to what would have happened if they had not acted like that.

We are therefore facing a dilemma: there is no scientific knowledge without comparison or controlled experiment, but comparing or controlling medical intervention on a specific patient is impossible. It is actually more than a dilemma. Physicians develop the art of predicting outcomes in individuals and are reluctant to see any relationship between their art and the techniques of mass or crowd prediction.

4.6. Why did epidemiology appear so late in human history?

The logical impossibility of experiments in which the same individual serves *simultaneously* as her own control can only be overcome if the problem is posed at the population level, in probabilistic terms. While individuals are unique, unpredictable and incomparable, the average behavior of groups is predictable and comparable.

Often paradoxes have a solution only if we radically change our perspective on the problem.

Consider one of Zeno's paradoxes. Anyone who wants to move from one point to another (say, 100 meters) must first reach half the distance (i.e., 50 m), and thereafter half of half distance (i.e., 25 m), etc. Since space is infinitely divisible, one has to reach an infinite number of mid-distances in a finite time. This being impossible, we cannot go anywhere and motion is illusory. This seems logically correct but intuitively absurd. To formally perceive the logical error, we have to change perspective. We stop viewing ourselves as being unable to make a first step across the first mid-distance of our journey. We consider each mid-distance as belonging to a geometric series (e.g., 1 + 1/2 + 1/4 + 1/8 + 1/16 + 1/32 + ...), which luckily for us does converge when the multiplicative factor (in our example, 1/2) is less than one. Thus, 1 + 1/2 + 1/4 + 1/8 + 1/16 + 1/32 + ... is equal to 2. Here we go.

Similarly, the controlled observation has no solution at the individual level but, paradoxically, it has one at the population level. As Sherlock Holmes told Dr Watson who was once more amazed by the sagacity of his friend:

"Winwood Reade [novelist, William Winwood Reade, 1838–1875] is good upon the subject," said Holmes. *"He remarks that, while the individual man is an insoluble puzzle, in the aggregate he becomes a mathematical certainty. You can, for example, never foretell what any one man will do, but you can say with precision what an average number will be up to. Individuals vary, but percentages remain constant. So says the statistician."* (Doyle, 1890a, chapter 10).

Population thinking implies that one can establish what would happen on average in the presence (or the absence) of the cause, and use this as the *best guess* to make predictions at the *individual* level. A controlled experiment is possible, but only at the population level.

Glimmerings of population thinking in epidemiology appear in the work of William Farr 175 years ago. In *On Prognosis*, which is reproduced in this volume (Farr, Part II), Farr begins by discussing the Greek etymology of the word "prognosis":

"Fore-telling presupposes fore-knowledge; and prognosis is employed, in medicine, to designate the art of fore-seeing and foretelling the course and issue of diseases." (Farr, Part II).

He then explains how the probabilities have different interpretations when applied to populations or to predict the occurrence of an event in an individual "case":

"In prognosis patients may be considered in two lights: in collective masses, when general results can be predicted with certainty; or separately, when the question be-

comes one of probability. If 7,000 of 10,000 cases of fever terminate fatally, it may be predicted that the same proportion will die in another series of cases; and experience has proved that the prediction will be verified, or so nearly verified as to leave no room for cavil or skepticism. The recovery or death of one of the cases is a mere matter of probability. (...). The rate of mortality determined for 10,000 cases applies, as a general standard, to each patient; and the probability of death is 0.07, of recovery is 0.93; the probability that the fever patient will recover is 93 to 7, raised or lowered by particular circumstances." (Farr, Part II).

The concepts expressed in this paragraph are radically different from those found in Hippocrates's treatises. Farr was much more clearly a population thinker. Population thinking allows Farr to make an observation which would have certainly fascinated Hippocrates, and which is probably valid for medicine at large:

"It is, nevertheless, rare that the physician has to perform this mournful function, and to prophesy death. There is almost always a chance, and generally a strong probability of recovery. Nine times in ten he is the messenger of glad tiding; and it is seldom that he cannot point out some dawn of hope – some streak of light – when the horizon is darkest." (Farr, Part II).

In other words, around 90% of the patients will live regardless of the physician's intervention. Physicians should first avoid aggravating the death risk by their intervention.

A radical change occurred between antiquity and the 19th century, between Hippocrates and Farr. Population thinking emerged as a mode of conceptualization, observing, and approaching problems. It made the development of group comparisons as a methodological tool possible. Group comparisons could from then on belong to a formal scientific activity, because probabilistic statements and probabilities had become part of "high sciences" thinking. Epidemiology came late in human history because it had to wait for the emergence of probability.

4.7. Emergence of probability

According to the Professor of History of Philosophy Ian Hacking,

"the decade around 1660 is the birth time of probability" (Hacking, 1975, p. 11).

The reasons for the late emergence of probabilistic thinking in philosophy and mathematics are not clear. A vulgar version of probability had been present for hundreds of years in "low sciences" such as alchemy, astrology, geology, or in games. The first textbook of probability was written by Huygens in 1657 (Hacking, 1975). It is of major interest for epidemiology that the application of probabilities to human health-related issues also occurs during this decade, around 1660. Graunt's opus *"Natural and Political Observations upon the Bills of Mortality"* appeared in 1662.

Hacking notes that there are immediately two usages of probability: a) for producing frequencies that have "law-like" regularity on the basis of statistical data, b) for assessing reasonable degrees of belief in propositions, even if they are guesses not based on statistical evidence (Hacking, 1975, p. 44). The second point would represent a major revolution in science because it opened the way to the existence of scientific knowledge that was not necessarily "demonstrated" by irrefutable and reproducible experiments. Before probability, and more specifically according to Hacking, before the publication in 1739 of the English philosopher David Hume (1711–1776) *"A Treatise of Human Nature"* (Hume, 1739), knowledge was the privilege of the sciences such as mechanics or optics, which could demonstrate the existence of natural laws. Sciences that could not achieve demonstrations could not produce knowledge either, only opinions.

Hume explained that past observations did not necessarily determine what would happen in the future. The fact that by custom and habit we come to associate two qualities does not legitimize the belief that the association will hold in the future. Bread nourishes me but this is no demonstration that the next piece of bread will also prove nourishing. Nevertheless, most of us would bet that it would still be nourishing. Why? Because we do believe that we can generalize on the basis of what we have repeatedly observed in the past and make reasonable predictions. The work of Hume has lent support to the view that in addition to the knowledge of *what has been demonstrated* there is a knowledge of *what is probable*, based on sound generalizations (Hacking, 1975, p. 176 and 183).

Both aspects of probability were to be used in epidemiology. Population thinking in epidemiology may correspond to the statistical usage of probability described by Hacking. We have seen that the word statistics itself means the systematic collection of data about the state. The City of London began in 1603, a bad year of plague, to keep a weekly tally of births and deaths. This activity provided Graunt with "statistical", population data, which he used as evidence to compute the frequencies of different causes of deaths.

4.8. A theory of group comparison

John Stuart Mill (1806–1873) is one of the most famous British philosophers of the 19th century. He wrote extensively on epistemology. In *"A System of Logic"*, first published in 1843, he described four methods (which he calls "canons") of experimental enquiry: the canons of agreement, difference, residues, and concomitant variations, which are all based on the principle of comparison.

The method of difference, Mill's second canon, states the fundamental principle of group comparisons:

"In an instance in which the phenomenon under investigation occurs, and an instance in which it does not occur have every circumstance in common save one, that one occurring only in the former; the circumstance in which alone the two instances differ, is the effect, or the cause, or an indispensable part of the cause, of the phenomenon". (Mill, 1950, pp. 215–216).

This is typically the rationale for epidemiologic designs, either cohort or case-control studies, aiming to compare like with like. In epidemiology, however, the method has to be reformulated in probabilistic terms.

The method of agreement, Mill's first canon, is the counterpart of the method of difference. It searches for "the only one circumstance in common". The method of residues has become Holmes's maxim:

"Eliminate all other factors, and the one which remains must be the truth." (Doyle, 1890b).

The method of concomitant variation is needed when the objects of the experiment cannot be manipulated in full, such as the moon or the earth. We cannot remove the moon, but we can correlate the position of the moon with water levels.

There is an aspect in Mill's canons that is particularly appealing to epidemiologists: the causes that the methods of difference, agreement, etc., contribute to discover are single invariable antecedents of the studied phenomenon. This is the type of cause that epidemiologists usually seek: a single preventable risk factor, such as smoking, polluted water, alcohol, saturated fat, physical activity, etc. (Vineis, Part IIb). It is therefore not surprising that Mill's canons of causality are often referenced in the writing of epidemiologists (Susser, 1973; MacMahon et al., 1960). Mervyn Susser, former director of the Department of epidemiology at Columbia University School of Public Health (Susser, 1973) has cited and illustrated the canons with modern examples. Rothman's theory of sufficient causes comprising multiple component causes (Section 2.6) evokes Mill's concept of a cause (Rothman, 1976):

"The cause, then, philosophically speaking, is the sum total of the conditions, positive and negative taken together; the whole of the contingencies of every description, which being realized, the consequent invariably follows..." (Mill, 1950, pp. 197–198).

In summarizing the modes of coordinating actions that can contribute to the discovery of causes, Mill has established a theory of comparison. The examples he gives indicate that these methods apply primarily to experimental sciences: "the planetary path" as an example of the method of agreement, the law of "falling bodies" as an example of both the methods of agreement and difference, the "cosmical motions" as an example of the methods of agreement and of concomitant variations (Mill,

1950, p. 236). But for Mill these methods could be successfully applied in the social sciences, where by definition population thinking is the rule. Thus, Mill can also be viewed as having formalized a theory of *group* comparisons. From Mill on, group comparisons combined with population thinking became a philosophically valid principle of knowledge acquisition.

4.9. Causal inference

The second aspect of probability identified by Hacking, that is, its usage to generate *degrees of belief* associated with specific statements not (directly) based on data were to permeate epidemiology much later. This apparently occurred as part of the tobacco-lung cancer controversy, when the question of the causal nature of the association was posed. A theory of causal inference would then be built in successive steps.

In 1959, Yerushalmy and Palmer, from the Division of Biostatistics of the University of California at Berkeley and the Division of Special Health Services in Washington, published a paper entitled "*On the methodology of investigation of etiologic factors in chronic diseases*" (Yerushalmy and Palmer, 1959). They first summarized the criteria of causal inference proposed in textbooks of bacteriology, putatively attributed to the German bacteriologist Robert Koch (1843–1910) and known as "Koch's postulates". Causality required

> "A. The simultaneous presence of organism and disease and their appearance in the correct sequence, and
> B. The specificity of effect of the organism on the development of the disease."
> (Yerushalmy and Palmer, 1959, p. 31).

These two types of evidence were incompatible with the multiplicity of causes for chronic diseases. Yerushalmy and Palmer therefore restated Koch's postulates in terms of population thinking and group comparisons:

> "1. The suspected characteristic must be found more frequently [population thinking] in persons with the disease in question than in persons without the disease [group comparisons], or
> 2. Persons possessing the characteristic must develop the disease more frequently [population thinking] than do persons not possessing the characteristic [group comparisons]." (Yerushalmy and Palmer, 1959, p. 32).

But that did not suffice. For example, concluding that smoking was a cause of lung cancer could not be based strictly on data. Yerushalmy and Palmer (Yerushalmy and Palmer, 1959) contributed, along with many epidemiologists, to a lively debate. Austin Bradford Hill, the British epidemiologist and perhaps the most creative methodologist of the 20th century, authored the consensual paper. The question addressed by Hill was:

"In what circumstances can we pass from this observed association to a verdict of causation? Upon what basis should we proceed to do so?" (Hill, 1965, p. 295).

Epidemiologic studies were what they were and no more. Their results could be indicative of statistical associations but it became clear that causal statements had to be based on a synthesis of all available information, epidemiologic, biological, toxicological, etc. Hill described nine "aspects" or "viewpoints" that could help the causal inference process by precisely increasing or decreasing our degree of belief in the causal statement (Section 3.14).

Hill, in contrast to Yerushalmy and Palmer, did not mention some philosophical or scientific origin to the causal viewpoints. There are, however, striking similarities between them and the "rules by which to judge of causes and effects" (Hume, 1739, pp. 173–6) given by David Hume in his 1739 *"A Treatise of Human Nature"* (Morabia, 1991).

Table 27 matches Hill's and Hume's aspects of causality as they are expressed in their two publications (Hume, 1739; Hill, 1965). Because Hume's treatise was published 225 years before Hill's report, it is obviously impossible to get a perfect match. For example, Hume presented his rules as universal statements, whereas Hill's viewpoints are worded specifically for preventive medicine. The comparison suggests nevertheless a potential philosophical kinship between Hume and Hill.

The identity is striking for the aspects of causal relations Hill has identified as "temporality," "biologic gradient" and "consistency". Strength of the association, as a measure of relative effect, does not have an exact complement in Hume's rules. Nevertheless, Hume's constant-conjunction formula is, just like the relative risk, a measure of association. There is some resemblance between Hill's concept of analogy and Hume's fifth rule. It is possible to find in Hume's writing formulas that correspond to Hill's concepts of specificity and coherence. For historical reasons, Hume could not have expressed two aspects of causality mentioned by Hill. The concept of "biological plausibility", as biology is a 19th century science, and that of experimental or semi-experimental evidence. Again, the key element is the similarity of the intellectual approaches rather than the exact formulations.

I do not know whether Yerushalmy or Hill were familiar with Hume's rules. However, independently of whether Hume's Rules were known to Hill or Hill's predecessors, Hume had a concept of causality assessment that was very similar to that of most contemporary epidemiologists. Hume's rules sound reasonable to us, and most likely Hill's ideas would have sounded reasonable to Hume. Actually, both Hume and Hill say essentially the same thing: when deterministic demonstration is not available, it is imperative to screen the causal statement for illogicalities or gross contradictions between what has been found and what we think we know. Hume and Hill's com-

Table 27 – Hill's criteria and corresponding Hume's "Rules by which to judge of causes and effects".

Hill's criteria (see section 3.9 for more details)	Hume's rules
1. Temporality: "The temporal relationship of the association – which is the cart and which is the horse?"	1. "The cause must be prior to the effect" (Rules 1 and 2)
2. Dose-response: "If the association is one which can reveal a biological gradient, or dose-response curve, then we should look most carefully for such evidence. (…) The clear dose-response curve admits of a simple explanation and obviously puts the case in a clearer light."	2. "When any object encreases or diminishes with the encrease or diminution of its cause, 'tis to be regarded as a compounded effect, deriv'd from the union of the several different effects, which arise from the several different parts of the cause. The absence or presence of one part of the cause is here suppos'd to be always attended with the absence or presence of a proportionable part of the effect. This constant conjunction sufficiently proves, that the one part is the cause of the other" (Rule 7).
3. Consistency: "Has it [the association] been repeatedly observed by different persons, in different places, circumstances and time?"	3. "…multiplicity of resembling instances, therefore, constitutes the very essence of power or connexion" (not a specific rule but in the premises of the catalog, p. 163)
4. Strength of association	4. "There must be a constant union betwitxt the cause and effect" (Rule 3)
5. Analogy: "In some circumstances it would be fair to judge by analogy. With the effects of thalidomide and rubella before us we should surely be ready to accept slighter but similar evidence with another drug or another viral disease in pregnancy."	5. "…where several different objects produce the same effect, it must be by means of some quality, which we discover to be common amongst them" (Rule 5). "Like effects imply like causes" (Rule 5).
6. Specificity	6. "The same cause always produces the same effect, and the same effect never arises but from the same cause" (Rule 4)
7. Biological possibility	7. Not applicable
8. Experiment	8. Not applicable
9. Coherence	9. Not a rule

plicity may thus have a historical ground. Hume provided the philosophical bases of the 17th century "probabilistic" revolution, which gave birth to the two fundamental epidemiologic principles, population thinking and group comparisons.

Thus, the logic of causal inference described by Hill and generally regarded as the appropriate approach by today's epidemiologists finds its origin in the intellectual changes that occurred in Western philosophy in the 17th and 18th centuries.

4.10. Principles of knowledge acquisition in epidemiology

According to Piaget, the genesis of a scientific discipline is based on a principle of knowledge acquisition. Direct action on an object has been traditionally the principle of knowledge acquisition in physics. What is then the corresponding knowledge-generating tool in epidemiology? Group comparisons combined with population thinking appear as good candidates. Indeed, group comparisons consist of coordinated actions. The process is very similar to that of the mathematical example described previously in which we were able to discover the law of commutativity by counting the same pebbles in different orders. In group comparisons, people are sampled from a population and rearranged (e.g., grouped into exposed and unexposed categories and simultaneously followed) in such a way that the perspective offered by the reorganization of the population in groups differing by exposure or affection can reveal potential causal links. The mode of knowledge acquisition in epidemiology is therefore closer to logic and mathematics than to physics.

Group comparisons and population thinking started to contributing to knowledge as soon as they merged, in the 18th century. The physician "experimenting" with treatments from one scurvy patient to the other was not able to derive universal knowledge that would still be valid today. But when Lind showed that, *other things being equal*, the sailors who ate the oranges and lemons were cured from scurvy while those in the other groups were not, some knowledge had been acquired that is still valid today. Lind and his successors did not know why citrus fruits could treat scurvy. But it did not really matter. They had a cause, on which they could act to modify a health outcome. Lind succeeded with an n = 12 experiment where centuries of trials and errors by physicians had failed. This shows how powerful the group comparison approach was. It is likely that physicians had had many opportunities to observe the beneficial effect of citrus fruits, but it is only when the observation was made within a given experimental design with coordinated actions that it generated knowledge, exportable to other places and valid for other populations than the sailors of the Salisbury.

In the 18th and 19th centuries, it suddenly became obvious that group comparison was the only strategy available if the outcome was to be observed only in a fraction of subjects exposed to the postulated cause. Consider Snow's London experiment in the summer of 1854. There had been an average of about 9 cholera deaths per thousand households. There was no way the role of the water supply could be put in evidence without grouping the households based on a clear definition of exposure. Snow and Farr knew that a controlled experiment was needed to demonstrate the effect of polluted water but such an experiment obviously could not be conducted. This may explain why Snow immediately recognized the "Grand Experiment" in the data produced by Farr's administration when the 1854 epidemic took place. And indeed, after grouping the households by water providers, there were about 30 cholera deaths per 1,000 households supplied by the Southwark and Vauxhall Company *vs.* 4 per 1,000 households supplied by the Lambeth Company and 6 per 1,000 households in the other districts of London.

Human thinking, philosophy, and mathematics became mature enough to embrace group comparison in the 19th century. Once the principles of knowledge acquisition existed, the evolution of epidemiology could be traced as the progressive refinement or enrichment of these principles by methods and concepts. At the beginning, these were very intuitive forms of counts and comparisons of like with like. With time, they became more abstract and formalized. We saw how ratios led to proportions, and then risks and rates, and how intuitive group comparisons paved the way towards a theory of epidemiologic study designs. The work of Lind, Louis or Snow consisted of simple forms of comparisons and frequency measures. When Einstein discovered relativity, there was not a single methodological textbook of epidemiology. As theory developed, methods became less intuitive and served for designing experiments suitable for solving complex problems. Still, the understanding of epidemiologic methods did not require any mathematical skills. In its latest phase, the methods and concepts have become much more abstract and are virtually out of reach for people who do not have some mathematical background.

5. Phases of epidemiology

On the basis of the evidence available today to a non-historian, it is reasonable to conclude that before the 18th century there was no research based on population thinking or group comparisons and that there could therefore be no epidemiology as the discipline we know today. In the 18th century, group comparisons and population thinking merged in the activities of physicians such as James Lind or the English proponents of the "medical arithmetik", that is, the usage of mass observations collected on patients as an additional source of knowledge for medical practice beyond the teaching of the great clinicians (Troehler, 2000). Since then, epidemiology has emerged as a set of research methods, which have contributed to elucidating important questions related to human health. Over about 150 years, epidemiologists have developed and refined the designs of cohort and case-control studies, the concepts of confounding and interaction, the categorizations of types of bias, and the process of causal inference.

In this continuous genesis of epidemiologic methods and concepts, I propose to distinguish four phases, characterized by qualitative changes in the level of formalization and abstraction of the concepts and methods: preformal, early, classic and modern epidemiology. "Preformal" means that none of the concepts and methods had been *formally* defined.

The point of this section is to show that this categorization in four phases is meaningful and that each phase had unique features of its own, mostly using material that has been already presented in the previous sections. An exhaustive historical review has still to be written.

5.1. Preformal epidemiology

Until the end of the 19th century, there was no specific theory of population thinking and group comparisons backing the activity of epidemiologists. The mathematical and philosophical bases existed but no formal theory. Let us call this first phase, *Preformal epidemiology*, during which scientists used population thinking and group comparisons, spontaneously, without referring to some theory. People such as Lind, Snow or Farr *invented* their way into epidemiologic research and therefore set the bases for the future development and formalization of methods and concepts.

5.1.1. Preformal epidemiologists

Preformal epidemiologists were mainly physicians but with diversified interests. For example, Farr was a physician, a public health professional and a statistician. Snow was an anesthesiologist, a clinician and a public health scientist. These people had different objectives. Some searched for ways to act on the environment to improve public health, other assessed the efficacy of treatments to improve patient care, and probably all aimed to develop human knowledge with respect to the determinants of health and disease. But their common denominator is the fact that they strived for their objectives using the same two principles: population thinking and group comparisons. Eventually, the use of these two principles was to characterize epidemiology, and differentiate it from medicine, statistics, economics, etc. with its own conceptual and methodological corpus.

5.1.2. Population thinking and group comparisons

We have seen that the use of different measures of disease occurrence, such as risks and rates, can be traced back to Graunt. William Farr established a clear conceptual difference between risks and rates. This first theory of risks and rates shows that the distinction of phases in the evolution of epidemiologic methods and concepts is somewhat arbitrary, and that the evolution has really been a continuous process. It is also true however that people like Farr were exceptional. Population thinking and group comparisons found a lot of resistance, especially in medicine, hampering their use by medical doctors.

For physicians, population thinking appeared to conflict with the fundamental principles of medicine. How can we generate information from a group of patients that is relevant for the single patient? Isn't the patient unique? How can medical knowledge rely on probabilities? The controversy that surrounded Louis's numerical method illustrates the types of criticism that were expressed by physicians.

A first group of physicians rejected Louis' numerical method because they believed medicine was an art of individual prediction and could not rely on group-based probabilities. A professor of pathology and general therapy from Montpellier, in the south of France, Benigno Juan Isidoro Risueño d'Amador (1802–1849) represented the category of opponents for whom medicine was the art of healing individual patients. He requested an audience at the April 25, 1837 session of the French Royal Academy of Medicine. His point was that the role of the physician was care for individual patients, and that no statistics could predict what would happen to a specific patient. If on average 10% of the patients died from a given intervention, the physician could not forecast which patients these would be. The information was therefore useless to the physician whose primary concern is to determine which individual would become sick or die. Thus, the uniqueness of each patient made it impossible to generalize from past patients to future patients, and made the calculus of probabilities "completely useless in medicine" (cited by Matthews, 1995a, p. 27).

Claude Bernard (1813–1878), one of the most esteemed and influential medical physiologists of his century, is emblematic of another category of opponents to Louis's methods. Bernard agreed that group comparisons were needed to evaluate therapies. But he also professed that medical knowledge could not be based on probability. For Bernard, averages did not exist in nature. Physiology, in contrast to statistics, described medical phenomena as they were repeatedly and constantly observed across experiments. Physiology discovered facts and laws. In the presence of variation across experiments, the physiologist would search for the determinants of such variation and certainly not hide it by making average descriptions of experiments.

Joseph Lister (1827–1912), the English founder of modern antiseptic surgery, expressed ideas similar to those of Bernard. Lister had actually compared the mortality related to surgical procedures some years before (1864 & 1866) the introduction of antiseptic methods and during the three following years (1867– 1869). Mortality had been cut by three, from 1 death every 2.17 cases to 1 every 6.66 cases (Lister, 1870a). For some reason Lister did not include the data for 1865. He and many of his contemporary colleagues interpreted these results as strong evidence in favor of anti-sepsis. But much fewer were those who recognized that the effect of antiseptics was due to their capacity to kill germs. Antiseptics prevented infections, which were the real causes of death, but still physicians were inclined to attribute their striking effect to "some specific virtue" of the antiseptic:

"... the striking results which were recorded were too often attributed to some specific virtue of the agent. The antiseptic system does not owe its efficacy to any such cause, nor can it be taught by any rule of thumb. One rule, indeed, there is of universal application – namely this: whatever be the antiseptic means employed (and they may be very various), use them so as to render impossible the existence of a living septic organism in the part concerned." (Lister, 1870b, p. 288).

Thus, for Lister, group comparisons were too superficial. They could not reveal that the true scientific foundation of the antiseptic effect was the presence of germs responsible of infection, that is, the "germ theory of putrefaction" (Lister, 1870b, p. 288).

Finally Auguste Comte (1798–1857), the leader of the French school of positivism, relied some biological arguments to oppose Louis's principles, arguing that comparing the statistical effects of two treatments was "impossible" because a sick human organism reacted differently than a healthy one.

These episodes indicate how isolated population thinkers, and therefore epidemiologists, were in the 19th century scientific, and especially medical, environments.

It is of note that preformal epidemiologists were at ease with exposed/non-exposed or affected/non-affected group comparisons. John Snow's 1854 Grand Experiment compared households exposed to polluted water and households that were not. But in another investigation performed during the same epidemic around the Broad Street pump, frequencies of exposure to the water pump were compared in people affected *vs.* non-affected by cholera (Paneth et al., Part II). Pierre Louis describes his work on the use of bleeding in the treatment of pneumonia in terms of exposed/unexposed comparison, but he also used affected/unaffected comparisons in other circumstances, as for example, to assess the potential hereditary origin of emphysema, a chronic lung disease leading to respiratory insufficiency:

"Of 28 patients with emphysema, 18 had their mother or father affected by that same disease", while *"of 50 individuals free of emphysema, only three had affected relatives."* (Louis, 1837, p. 255).

The conjunction of population thinking and group comparisons was necessary for the emergence of the new discipline of epidemiology. There was no progress in the understanding of the causes of infectious diseases when public health data were not ordered and analyzed according to the principles of group comparisons. A recent re-analysis of a report of the City Council of Ferrara, Italy, on the cholera epidemic of 1855 illustrates the limitations of public health without epidemiology (Scapoli et al., 2003; Morabia, 2003; Vandenbroucke, 2003). The cholera epidemic in Ferrara occurred a year after the London cholera epidemics during which Snow's Grand Experiment took place. Why is it that the determinants of the Ferrara epidemic are barely understandable, even using modern statistical techniques to analyze them, whereas in London, John Snow was able to successfully demonstrate that the cause of cholera was related to polluted water? The dominant model in public health was that air pestilence, poverty, overcrowding, and lack of hygiene were responsible for the epidemic of cholera. The data from Ferrara showed that more people tended to be diagnosed and die from cholera when they lived in dirtier streets, smaller and less hygienic houses, etc. This corroborated the model, even though the data also indicated higher case fatality rates in large and more hygienic houses, which did not fit the poverty model too well. The Ferrara City Council may not have been pursuing the correct hypothesis, but, more important, it was not using the right methodological approach either. For an 1855 observer in Ferrara, ecological correlations indicated that socio-demographic and urbanistic factors had weak and sometimes paradoxical effects on mortality from cholera. Its records did not lend themselves to non-ambiguous group comparisons. What was missing was the conceptual leap that gave birth to the corpus of epidemiologic methods and concepts, that is, collecting data in such a way that *comparing groups* on specific exposure and outcome could shed light on potential causal associations.

5.1.3. More examples

In the first part of this essay, we have glimpsed the work of Lind, Snow, Farr and Louis. These were not the sole pre-formal epidemiologists who combined population thinking and group comparisons. In his investigation of the epidemic of measles on the Faroe Islands in 1846, the Danish physiologist Peter Ludwig Panum (1820–1885) used an early form of relative risk to compare the age-specific number of deaths during the first 8 months of 1846 with the average number of annual deaths from 1835 to 1845. For example, there had been 50 deaths under age 1 in 1846 vs. "18 1/11th" in 1835–45, yielding a relative risk of about 2.8. Panum wrote that:

> "Number of times mortality in first two-thirds of 1846 was greater than the usual in an ordinary whole year: about 2 9/11." (Pan American Health Organization, 1988, p. 38).

Ignaz Philipp Semmelweis (1818–1865), a Hungarian physician teaching medicine in Vienna, observed that the mortality from puerperal fever was two to four times higher among women delivered by physicians compared to women delivered by midwives. In 1846, mortality had been about 11.4% in medical deliveries ("First clinic") *versus* 2.7% in midwife deliveries ("Second clinic") (Carter, 1983). Semmelweis speculated that these differences were caused by the fact that examining physicians went from pathological dissections and contact with dead bodies to deliveries without thorough cleansing between the two activities. At the end of May, 1847, Semmelweis introduced the practice of washing the hands with a solution of chloride of lime before the examination of lying-in women. Subsequently, the mortality from puerperal fever stabilized around 2% or less for both midwives and physicians (Carter, 1983).

In his report on the mortality of Cornwall miners, 1860–1862, William Farr presented annual mortality rates by ten-year age groups, which were, for metal miners, 3.77, 4.15, 7.89, 19.75, 43.29 and 45.04, and, for "males exclusive of metal miners", 3.30, 3.83, 4.24, 4.34, 5.19 and 10.48. He used these rates to compute relative risks of mortality from pulmonary disease comparing metal miners to males who were not miners:

> "...assuming as before that the rate of mortality among the males exclusive of miners is represented at each period of life by 100, then that among the miners would be represented by 114 between the ages of 15 and 25 years, by 108 between 25 and 35, by 186 between 35 and 45, by 455 between 45 and 55, by 834 between 55 and 65, and by 430 between 65 and 75 years. It is therefore evident that pulmonary diseases are the chief cause of the excess mortality among the Cornish miners." (Pan American Health Organization, 1988, pp. 68–69).

William Augustus Guy (1810–1885), Professor of Forensic medicine and Hygiene at King's College Hospital in London, compared the occurrence of "pulmonary consumption" across a variety of occupations. Guy used odds, that is, the ratio of the number of cases with pulmonary consumption to the number of other diseases, as a measure of risk (Lilienfeld and Lilienfeld, 1979). Guy, in 1843, had also considered (and ruled out) the possibility that the relation of job and health could reflect the self-selection of jobs by workers according to their health status rather than to the effect of the job on health (Vineis, Part II).

Christiaan Eijkman (1858–1930), a Dutch physician, received the Novel Prize for having established that beriberi was a nutritional disease. Beriberi was a fatigue disease, involving weight loss, muscle weakness, loss of feeling and eventually death in up to 80% of the cases. In the local idiom, the word beri means weak, and doubling it intensifies its meaning. The contribution of epidemiology to this discovery came from Adolphe Vordermann (1857–1902). Between May and September of 1896, this supervisor of the Civil Health Department of Java compared the occurrence of beriberi among the 280,000 inmates of 100 Java prisons. According to local customs, prisoners were fed either polished rice, half-polished rice, or a mixture of both. Beriberi was found in 2.7% of the prisons feeding half-polished rice (corresponding to 1 in 10,000 prisoners), in 46.1% of the prisons preparing a mixture of polished and half-polished rice (1 in 416 prisoners), and in 70.6% of the prisons serving exclusively polished rice (1 in 39 prisoners) (Allchin, 2000; Carpenter, 2000). On the other hand, beriberi was not associated with hygienic conditions of the prisons such as the age of the building, the permeability of the floor, ventilation, or population density. It was later established that it was the polished rice deficiency in thiamine (vitamin B1) that was causing beriberi.

5.1.4. Definition of epidemiology

Overall, the balance between successes and failure is positive for epidemiology during this preformal phase. There was no discipline called epidemiology, and defined as such, but the fight against infectious disease was a domain of activity that acquired a name. The first scientific society of epidemiology, the London Epidemiology Society, was created in 1850. Some of its members were epidemiologists, but none had an academic appointment and extremely few (e.g., Farr) wrote theoretical/methodological work. The situation changed dramatically in the 20th century.

5.2. Early epidemiology

Let us call *early epidemiology* the development phase in which some epidemiologic concepts and methods were assembled for the first time into a theory of population thinking and group comparisons.

5.2.1. Early epidemiologists

Before 1880, epidemiologists were essentially amateurs (general practitioners like Snow, Semmelweis, military and naval physicians and surgeons). After 1880, public health professionals were hired in England to practice "epidemiology" (e.g., John Simon, William Frederick Barry, Theodore Thompson, H. Timbrell Bulstrode, Edward Ballard, William G. Savage) (Hardy, Part II).

A salient trait of this second phase is the creation of university positions of professors of epidemiology and the publication of the first textbooks. Almost simultaneously in the US and the UK, epidemiology became an academic field. After World War I, Major Greenwood was appointed lecturer and in 1930 professor of epidemiology in the Department of Epidemiology and Vital Statistics created in 1927 at the London School of Hygiene and Tropical Medicine, where he remained until he retired in 1945 (Hardy and Magnello, Part II). In the United States, Frost was appointed in 1922 as Professor and Chairman in the Department of Epidemiology and Public Health Administration at The School of Hygiene and Public Health of the Johns Hopkins University in Baltimore (Comstock, Part II).

The line of demarcation between epidemiology and statistics remained fuzzy. Major Greenwood considered himself a "professed statistician" (Greenwood, 1935, p. 21) and wrote one of the first textbooks of epidemiology (Winkelstein, Jr., 2002; Winkelstein, Jr., 2003; Lilienfeld, 2003; Bracken, 2003). Greenwood and Bradford Hill had strong connections with statistics, and were disciples of the Cambridge statistician Karl Pearson. Bradford Hill entitled his textbook "*Principles of medical statistics*", but the text contained very little mathematics and could perfectly have been called "*Principles of clinical epidemiology*". Even though the title of Hill's book referred to medical statistics, it had a lot to do with epidemiology and group comparisons. For Hill

"The essence of the statistical method lies in the elucidation of the effects of these multiple causes." (Hill, 1939, p. 3).

And by statistical method he understood:

"methods specially adapted to the elucidation of quantitative data affected by a multiplicity of causes" (Hill, 1939, p. 3).

We may consider the scientific duet between Snow and Farr as a preformal collaboration between epidemiology and statistics. Other duets of this type existed in this early phase. Edgar Sydenstricker was the "first national public health statistician" (Wiehl, 1974). He played a key role in the methodological developments of the early phase of epidemiology. He worked closely with Goldberger on the pellagra investigations and developed a life-long collaboration with Frost, whom he provided with the Massachusetts data used for the cohort analysis paper (Section 3.4.3).

5.2.2. Population thinking

Preformal epidemiology had paved the way for population thinking by early epidemiologists. The latter further refined the description of disease occurrence in population by separating prevalence from incidence. In a lecture given on December 15, 1931 at the Johns Hopkins University School of Hygiene and Public Health in Baltimore, Sydenstricker distinguished the "prevalence of illness" based on surveys, which are affected by "cases of long duration and of chronic type" from the "incidence of illness", based on continuous recording of an illness in a population. According to Sydenstricker, incidence of illness was first measured on a large scale in the studies he had conducted with Goldberger on the causes of pellagra (Pan American Health Organization, 1988, pp. 168–169).

Somewhat related to the distinction between prevalence and incidence, the study of chronic diseases also called for new methods of surveillance and of group comparisons. In 1935, the Connecticut State Legislature authorized a population-based cancer registry. In Denmark, a cancer registry covering the whole population was set up in 1942. These registries played an important role in revealing the rising trends of lung cancer incidence, which motivated the following generation of epidemiologists (Terracini and Zanetti, Part II).

5.2.3. Group comparisons

In 1927, Frost published an article entitled "*Epidemiology*" in the Nelson Loose Leaf Encyclopedia (Frost, 1941), which, according to his successor as Chair of epidemiology at The Johns Hopkins School of Public Health, Abraham M. Lilienfeld, was "the first systematic exposition of epidemiology as a scientific discipline" (Lilienfeld, 1983). The paper can be viewed as the module of a textbook. Two citations from "*Epidemiology*" show that for Frost, epidemiology consisted in the conjunction of population thinking and group comparisons. Population thinking:

> "*For the clinical description of a disease the unit is an individual, and the phenomena of the clinical reaction may be described in terms of the character and distribution of the anatomic lesions and the nature and sequence of symptoms. For epidemiologic description the unit is the aggregation of individuals making up a population, and description of mass-phenomena of a disease consists of a statement of its types and frequency of occurrence in the population as a whole and in its different component groups.*" (Frost, 1941, p. 494).

And group comparisons:

> "*In every epidemiologic investigation, whether its immediate purpose be to explain a localized epidemic or to elucidate the general spread of an obscure disease, the first step is to investigate the association between the occurrence of the disease and some special condition or set of conditions. This is primarily a statistical process of ascertaining the frequency of the disease in two or more populations separated with respect to the particular condition.*" (Frost, 1941, p. 540).

Frost referred to the work of Snow as being a model of group comparisons. It is of note that Frost also gave one of the earliest descriptions of the cohort study design. Frost wrote that:

> "*The simplest and most direct method of determining whether or not such an association exists* [that is, "*that the occurrence of the disease is in some way associated with the use of sewage polluted drinking water*"], *is the method used by Dr. Snow, namely, that of ascertaining what different water supplies are used within the area of investigation, and how those supplies differ with respect to sewage pollution; then classifying (1) the persons who have died from cholera, and (2) the entire population, according to their sources of water supply. It remains to ascertain the frequency of deaths from cholera in each of the two groups of the population, which differ with respect to the sources and sewage pollution of their water supplies, that is, to ascertain the ratio of deaths to total of persons in each group. If the difference of incidence in the two groups is found, as in this instance, to be entirely outside the range of such differences as may be expected in two*

groups of such size drawn at random from the population, it may reasonably be inferred that in this area the use of sewage polluted water is positively associated with the liability to death from cholera. It is further found, by still another independent inquiry, that the two groups are, so far as can be ascertained, quite similar in all other conditions of composition and environment, hence the association of cholera mortality with character of water supply is a rather direct one. It is, of course, equally necessary to show that the two water supplies actually differ materially with respect to the degree of sewage pollution." (Frost, 1941, pp. 537–538).

The oral history of epidemiology says that Frost taught the "techniques of prospective and retrospective studies" already in 1933–34 (Susser, 1985, p. 152). Thus, early epidemiologists built on the experience accrued in the 19th century to strengthen the foundations of group comparisons. Frost "made John Snow a hero" (Vandenbroucke et al., 1991) because, in retrospect, Snow was *the* historical example of the successful combination of group comparisons and population thinking.

Distinct improvements also occurred for the affected/non-affected comparisons. Clinicians started to compare groups of patients suffering from disease believed to have different etiology on a larger scale than ever before. In 1926, the British physician and former Dean of the London School of Medicine for Women Janet Lane-Claypon (1877–1967) compared 500 hospitalized breast cancer cases and 500 controls with non-cancerous illnesses from both inpatient and outpatient settings in London and Glasgow (Lane-Claypon, 1926). This early case-control study, which had Major Greenwood as statistician, indicated that cases were more likely to be single or to have lower fertility when married. In 1928, a New England Journal of Medicine's paper (Lombard and Doering, 1928) compared the habits, characteristics and environment of individuals with and without cancer in Massachusetts and showed that cancer patients had smoked more pipes and cigarettes than non-cancer controls. These were first experiences with a new type of study design, eventually termed the case-control study.

In the first half of the 20th century, epidemiologists also contributed to improving the design, analysis and interpretation of therapeutic trials. The James Lind Library (http://www.jameslindlibrary.org) has already assembled the documentation of a substantial collection of therapeutic trials performed during that time.

5.2.4. Concepts

During this second phase, epidemiologic methods and concepts acquired some theoretical foundations. These were somewhat less intuitive than in the previous phase but remained quite basic. A major theoretical contribution of this phase consisted in identifying sources of fallacious interpretations of group comparisons, and in proposing solutions to minimize them.

The idea that an observed association may in reality be indirect or spurious because the compared groups differ in some important way has always been present in the epidemiologic thinking. Preformal epidemiologists intuitively understood the concept of "confounding". Lind, Louis, Snow were always preoccupied with comparing like with like. The examples that we reviewed in this essay speak for themselves of the evolution of the concept of confounding during the following phase.

In 1904, Yule gave the first formal description of the mechanism of confounding. He referred to it as a fallacy associated with the mixing of records. The mechanism of confounding described by Yule was also reported in their textbooks by Greenwood in 1935 and by Hill in 1937. Hill did not cite Greenwood, who did not cite Yule. They must have thought that this was an exercise of simple logic and not a meaningful discovery. Indeed, Greenwood mentions that this type of fallacy has "vitiated many published reports" (Greenwood, 1935).

In 1920, Goldberger and Sydenstricker performed stratified analysis and computed standardized rates to separate the effects of diet, age, gender and income, which were correlated causes of pellagra. In 1930 Hill applied the alternate allocation of treatment in the British Medical Research Council therapeutic trial as a form of study design that could increase the comparability of groups and allow the researcher to compare "like with like". In a posthumous paper published in 1939, Frost explained the use of cohort analysis as a way to prevent fallacious interpretations of cross-sectional data, especially when looking at diseases with a prolonged survival such as tuberculosis. The formalization of the mechanism and modes of control of confounding had clearly progressed.

5.2.5. Definitions of epidemiology

It is also during this period that epidemiology got its first definitions as a discipline. The evolution of the definitions of epidemiology reflects its process of differentiation from other scientific disciplines. "Epidemiologists" themselves were still unclear about what epidemiology was. In 1919, Frost defined epidemiology as the study of the determinants of infectious diseases (Comstock, Part II). This definition implied that people studying non-infectious diseases were not epidemiologists. The case of Goldberger around the time of Frost's first definition is an interesting one. He studied the causes of pellagra, a disease people believed to be infectious, but which he believed was produced by diet and poverty.

The epoch of early epidemiology was characterized by the transition from the dominance of acute infectious diseases to that of chronic diseases in the "global" burden of disease. Epidemiologists became increasingly involved with the study of chronic conditions and the definitions of epidemiology changed accordingly. In 1927, Frost expanded his definition to include some but not all non-infectious diseases. In 1935 Greenwood defined epidemiology as

> *"the study of disease, any disease, as a mass phenomenon"* (Greenwood, 1935, p. 15).

or as

> *"a science of group etiology"* (Greenwood, 1935, p. 21).

In 1937 Frost finally generalized his definition to all aspects of human health (Comstock, 2001).

5.3. Classic epidemiology

The years after 1945 were particularly fruitful for the development of epidemiology. The discipline of epidemiology, in contrast to all other human and social sciences, has been uniquely able to perform vast community-based studies to investigate the causes of heart disease, cancer and other chronic conditions, which characteristically have a long incubation and require long-term follow-up. Millions of people have been involved in epidemiologic studies. As a result, new epidemiologic methods were developed and older ones were refined, in particular in the context of the controversy about the health effects of tobacco smoke. The process occurred almost in parallel in the US and in Great Britain.

5.3.1. Classic epidemiologists

Most classic epidemiologists who authored textbooks were medical doctors (e.g., Jerry Morris, Brian MacMahon, Mervyn Susser, Abraham Lilienfeld). Few had formal training in epidemiology or statistics. The close collaboration with statisticians persisted in this phase. The case of Jerome Cornfield is an interesting one. Cornfield, who played a decisive role in creating the bases for the modern understanding of case-control studies, graduated from New York University in 1933 with a B.A. in history but later became President successively of the American Epidemiologic Society (in 1972) and of the American Statistical Association (in 1974).

5.3.2. Population thinking

We have reviewed in previous sections the considerable development of population thinking during this phase, related to a better understanding of the relation of prevalence to risk. On the one hand, the prevalence of a *disease* could be viewed as the product of its incidence and of its duration (i.e., $P = I \times D$). On the other hand, large fractions of disease cases in a population could be produced by small risks applied to large fractions of the population with low levels of exposure (i.e., Rose's prevention paradox).

A special note must be made here about ecologic correlations, a form of population thinking which had been used in the past but which received a strong impetus in classic epidemiology. Ecologic correlations consist of relating exposure and outcome data, which are only available as group averages and not as individual observations. Typically, the 1964 Surgeon General Report included a graph showing that countries with higher per capita cigarette consumption in 1932 tended also to have higher mortality rates from lung cancer in 1970 (US Public Health Service, ed, 1964, p. 176). Ecologic correlations were common in other fields, such as sociology, in which it had been established that they could not be used as substitutes for individual correlations (Robinson, 1950).

The very influential article by Doll and Richard Peto, also epidemiologist at Oxford University, entitled "*The causes of cancer*" (Doll and Peto, 1981) was essentially an ecologic study. The Office of Technology Assessment of the US Congress had commissioned it:

> "*If the foregoing is accepted as justifying that much human cancer is avoidable, then a crude estimate of the proportion of cases that might be avoided in any one community can be obtained by comparing for each separate type of cancer the incidence in that community with the lowest reliable incidence recorded elsewhere.*" (Doll and Peto, 1981, p. 1205).

That is, the lowest incidence observed was considered inevitable, while the entire excess incidence beyond the lowest level could be attributed to external factors and, in theory, be prevented. Doll and Peto concluded that:

> "*75 or 80% of the cases of cancer in both sexes might have been avoidable.*" (Doll and Peto, 1981, p. 1205).

In particular, they estimated that 30% of U.S. cancer deaths were due to tobacco, 35% to diet, and 4% by occupational exposures (Doll and Peto, 1981, pp. 1256). The section of the article entitled "*4.3. Use of epidemiological information*" (pp. 1217–1219) reflects the level of self-assurance reached by classic epidemiology:

> "*... to make estimate of the proportion of today's cancers that are attributable to avoidable causes (...) epidemiology, influenced by laboratory investigation, is by far superior to the latter alone. Epidemiology has at present an undeservedly low reputation among people who have first artificially limited themselves to wondering which environmental pollutants to restrict and who then find that almost none of the few thousand chemicals they are worried about have been adequately studied by epidemiologists. This is, however, to condemn epidemiology for failing to achieve ends that it does not have.*" (Doll and Peto, 1981, p. 1219).

In his 1973 textbook (Susser, 1973), Susser stressed that individuals and the group represented different "levels of organization". This second feature of ecologic correlations provided qualitatively distinct insights into exposure-disease associations. Elucidating the source of discrepancy between individual and ecological correlations could illuminate causal links. The debate on the interpretation of ecologic correlations and their role in the armamentarium of epidemiologists is still ongoing (Schwartz, 1994).

5.3.3. Study designs

Large cohort studies are one of the major features of classic epidemiology. In October 1951, Doll and Hill launched the British Doctors prospective study (Doll and Hill, 1954; Doll, Part II).

> *"Bradford Hill suggested that doctors would make a suitable population to study as they might be more interested in responding to a questionnaire about smoking habits than most other people, that having had a scientific training they might be more accurate in the description of their smoking habits, and, most importantly, that they would be relatively easy to follow up, because of the need to keep their names on the Medical Register for legal reasons."* (Doll, Part II).

In October 1951, Doll and Hill sent a short questionnaire (seven questions) to 59,600 members of the medical profession in the United Kingdom eliciting their smoking habits. Of the 41,024 replies, 40,564 were sufficiently complete to be utilized. Initially, the Office of the Registrar General of births and deaths (the national bureau of vital statistics which Farr had directed 100 years before) provided the death certificates from all doctors. Hammond and Horn began the first American Cancer Society Cancer Prevention Study sending questionnaires to 188,000 white males, aged 50 to 59 (Hammond and Horn, 1958). The causal nature of the association of smoking and lung cancer was finally fully recognized in both countries in the early sixties.

Several cohort studies were performed on the basis of historical records, that is, "retrospective cohort studies", especially to study occupational exposures (Stellman, Part II). In this volume, Doll describes the Framingham Heart Study, whose results have had an enormous impact on clinical medicine (Doll, Part II).

During this phase, case-control studies acquired a theoretical basis as a study design. It was three case-control studies, two in the United States (Levin et al., 1950; Wynder and Graham, 1950) and one in Great Britain (Doll and Hill, 1950) that firmly launched the debate on the association between smoking and lung cancer. Cornfield established that the odds ratio computed in the case-control study was, under certain assumptions, a close approximation to the relative risk. From then on, case-control studies became the most common study design in epidemiologic research (Paneth et al., Part II).

The theory of study designs made its appearance progressively in the literature (Cornfield et al., 1959; Cornfield, 1951; Cornfield and Haenszel, 1960; Dorn, 1959), but especially in textbooks, which flourished during this phase (Zhang et al., Part II).

5.3.4. Concepts

Classic epidemiology brought the concepts of confounding, bias and interaction to a higher level of generalization. In previous sections we have reviewed the developments that occurred during this phase around the concepts of interaction and causal inference.

In this essay, I only discussed the evolution of selection bias (section 3.7). The history of bias is of course much richer. The concept evolved from a list of dozens of biases to types of based on their mechanism, the two main ones being information (i.e., misclassification) and selection bias (Vineis, Part IIa). The history of misclassification bias is relatively recent as it is closely related to that of screening. The new availability of simple diagnostic devices (e.g., blood or urinary sugar concentration, Papanicolaou smear tests) created the conditions for the development of population-wide screening, especially for diabetes, cervical and breast cancer (Morabia and Zhang, 2004). The screening tests were not dangerous but had imperfect validity. A whole theory of test interpretation, involving the concepts of sensitivity, specificity and predictive values, was developed (Morabia and Zhang, 2004). Applied to group comparisons, these new concepts contributed to the development of a theory of misclassification bias (Newell, 1962; MacMahon et al., 1960).

5.3.5. Definition of epidemiology

The "*Dictionary of Epidemiology*" sponsored by the International Epidemiology Association provides the following definition of epidemiology:

> "*The study of the distribution and determinants of health-related states of events in specified populations, and the application of this study to control of health problems.*" (Last, 2001).

This "classic" definition of epidemiology integrates population thinking ("study of distributions") and group comparisons ("study of health determinants"). The second part of the definition specifies that the usage of these principles is oriented towards the improvement of the public health. Indeed, in classic epidemiology, the theory cannot be separated from its medical and social applications. "Classic" textbooks read like essays on the determinants of human health and the methods to assess them (Zhang et al., Part II).

Not only did classic epidemiology develop epidemiologic theory, but it had some distinct achievements, the most salient being the establishment of a causal link between exposure to tobacco smoke and risk of lung cancer synthesized in the classic *"US Surgeon General Report"* of 1964. Classic epidemiology created the foundations for further theoretical developments.

5.4. Modern epidemiology

Let us call this latest phase of the genesis of epidemiology *modern epidemiology*, in reference to the most influential textbook presenting these new theoretical developments (Rothman, 1986; Rothman and Greenland, 1998).

5.4.1. Modern epidemiologists

There is a strong contrast in the professional backgrounds and profiles between the generation of epidemiologists who contributed to this new phase and the classic epidemiologists. Many have PhDs but not MDs. This is the case for many authors of the textbooks of this new phase (Rothman and Greenland, 1998; Kelsey et al., 1986; Kleinbaum et al., 1982). Most if not all have a strong background in mathematics or statistics. This generation of epidemiologists went further in the formalization of methods and concepts. As a result the discipline became much more mathematical. Where classic epidemiology expressed concepts that had no necessary mathematical translations, almost all concepts (e.g., bias, confounding, interaction, etc.) in modern epidemiology can be written either in words or equations.

The methodological and conceptual core of modern epidemiology can be found in a textbook entitled *"Theoretical Epidemiology"* (Miettinen, 1985). Its author, Olli Miettinen, expressed the watershed between classic and modern epidemiology by saying that epidemiology was previously

> *"widely regarded as commonsense activity, a line of research that any physician – even one without statistical education – is prepared to engage in"* (Miettinen, 1985, p. VIII).

Modern epidemiology went beyond common sense. The novelty of the approach proposed was first only understood by a small circle of students, who re-expressed the new concepts and made them accessible to a wider audience.

Let us make a short digression here and consider again the analogy with physics. There is a point at which theoretical progress becomes irrelevant for our everyday life. As far as physics is concerned, we can comprehend most of the phenomena in our daily life if we don't go beyond the Newtonian, mechanical vision of the world. Few people are versed in relativity, even less in quantum physics.

It is the same in epidemiology. At a given moment, the theoretical developments become irrelevant for the bread and butter activity of the epidemiologist. A

Cornfieldian vision of epidemiology suffices. For example, the algebraic relationship between cumulative incidence and incidence density, the impact of control sampling schemes on effect estimation, are usually pointless when the phenomenon studied is rare. This is why classic epidemiology remains for many active epidemiologists the phase of reference. But the developments of modern epidemiology are crucial for our understanding of what we do, for the identification of the exceptional situations in which the choices of study design and of measure of disease occurrence matter, and for our ability to carry the discipline forward. They are progressively becoming part of the intermediate epidemiology curriculum.

5.4.2. Population thinking

We have seen in the earlier sections that the concepts of risks and rates underwent a profound transformation during this phase, with new names (e.g., cumulative incidence and incidence density), and new formal, mathematical links (e.g., cumulative incidence can be viewed as a function of incidence densities).

5.4.3. Study designs

Classic epidemiology had established a theory of cohort and case-control studies, and discovered that the relative risk could be estimated from both designs. Still, there remained many doubts about the validity of case-control studies. In an influential paper published in 1959 by the New England Journal of Medicine (Dorn, 1959), Harold Dorn (?–1963), chief of the Biometrics Branch at the Division of Research Services of the National Institutes of Health, wrote:

> *"I do not wish to give the impression that I reject retrospective studies as a method of investigating the etiology of chronic diseases. The retrospective method, in theory, can provide data of reliability and validity comparable to that obtained from prospective studies. But, as usually applied, it does not do this. The fundamental defect of many retrospective studies is that they are based on an unspecified sample of persons chosen by an unknown method of sampling from an unidentified population"* (Dorn, 1959, p. 577).

The paper was rather favorable to case-control designs but it set very high standards for a valid design. Modern epidemiology has clarified which were these standards.

It became clear that the key criterion for the validity of the case-control study was that the cases and controls originate from the same source population. All case-control studies became viewed as being nested within cohorts, whether the cohort has been actually enumerated and characterized as a cohort study (i.e., nested case-control studies) (Doll, Part II; Doll, 1998), or whether the cohorts are hypothetical. This led to a new conceptualization of the different ways of sampling controls and to the decline of the "rare disease assumption" formulated by Cornfield to equate the case-control study odds ratio with the cohort study relative risk.

5.4.4. Concepts

Modern epidemiology is the first phase comprising a coherent set of methods and concepts spanning the different circumstances that the researcher faces when trying to establish the causal nature of an association: methods for comparing groups, sources of biases, presence of multiple independent causes (i.e., confounding), presence of multiple interrelated causes (i.e., interaction), and causal inference.

Without going into details, the theory of confounding became enriched by: a) a more rigorous formulation of the conditions under which confounding occurs; b) a theory of matching in cohort and case-control studies; c) the simultaneous treatment of multiple confounders.

The theory of biases was further developed with a better understanding of the effects of losses to follow-up in cohort studies and selection in case-control studies, the implications of misclassification of exposure, disease and confounders, whether differential or not, across the compared groups.

The concept of interaction became, as we also saw, much more refined, with a distinction between interaction of attributable risks (i.e., additive interaction or public health interaction), and interaction of relative risks (i.e., multiplicative interaction).

Causal inference did not evolve much in this new phase even though it was intensively debated. The debate turned in particular around the question of the relevance of the "falsification of hypotheses" approach proposed by the epistemologist Karl Popper (1902–1994) for the design and interpretation of epidemiologic studies (Greenland, 1987a; Rothman (ed), 1988). The Popperian approach did not succeed in replacing the traditional Humean approach formalized by classic epidemiologists.

5.4.5. Definition of epidemiology

What is the definition of modern epidemiology? The second edition of "Modern Epidemiology" states that:

> *"the ultimate goal of most epidemiologic research is the elaboration of causes that can explain patterns of disease occurrence"* (Rothman and Greenland, 1998, p. 29).

This definition is a good reflection of the state of the discipline, because it relates its methods (elaboration of causes or "etiology") to its subject matter (disease occurrence). The evolution of epidemiologic methods and concepts has been driven by the search for causes of human diseases. It is likely that this will remain the driving force of epidemiologists and of epidemiology. Nevertheless, it is important to note that at that stage of abstraction, concepts and methods become independent of specific issues, such as public health or simply health-related problems. They can be applied in any field in which combining group comparisons and population thinking can be an appropriate mode of knowledge acquisition.

5.5. What will come next?

If the scheme of analysis used to describe the genesis of epidemiology is correct, modern epidemiology is a transitory phase, just like the early and classic epidemiology phases were. The new theoretical tools allow us to address problems of increasing complexity both in the biological and the social dimensions. These will require further theoretical developments and lead to a new phase, the nature of which can probably be perceived in the latest theoretical work of epidemiologists.

6. Conclusion

In this essay, I have attempted to show that:

1) epidemiology is characterized by the combination of population thinking and group comparisons aiming to discover the determinants of human health;
2) the set of methods (study design) and concepts (measures of disease occurrence, confounding, interaction, bias) have evolved since the 17th century. This evolution is consistent with Piaget's theory of genetic epistemology.
3) In this evolution, we can identify four phases characterized by qualitative leaps in formalization and abstraction of the methods and concepts. After a preformal phase, in which epidemiology was discovered intuitively by scientists, most of all physicians, epidemiology has gone through an early, a classic and a modern period.

History and epistemiology are not a type of a general culture, a knowledge that it is nice to have but that is not essential for the active life of the epidemiologists. On the contrary, I argue that they are an integral part of the background of epidemiologists. Understanding the origin and evolution of epidemiologic methods and concepts can stimulate Scientific creativity. Methods and concepts are tools. These tools improve with time. Each epidemiologist should be ready to contribute to this improvement by adapting the methods and concepts to the solution of new or more complex problems than those which the available methods have contributed to solving in the past.

What will be the next phase in the evolution of epidemiologic methods and concepts? I am not sure we can tell yet. But the discipline is certainly undergoing a period of uneasiness. Our current methods have been successful for the discovery of major, relatively independent determinants of health in the environment (e.g., germs, tobacco smoke, radiation, asbestos, or social inequalities), in our behaviors (e.g., physical activity, vitamins, alcohol, drugs) and in our biology (e.g., genes, lipids, blood pressure, obesity). They are not that well adapted to assess the more complex manifestations of many (e.g., genetic, social, infectious) health determinants. These contradictions between old methods and new problems should induce theoretical developments, and make epidemiology enter into a new qualitative phase in order to continue to improve human health.

Part II
Collection of papers on the history of epidemiological methods and concepts

The changing assessments of John Snow's and William Farr's cholera studies

John M. Eyler

University of Minnesota, Program in the History of Medicine, 511 Diehl Hall, Minneapolis, MN 55455, USA

Summary

This article describes the epidemiological studies of cholera by two major British investigators of the mid-nineteenth century, John Snow and William Farr, and it asks why the assessments of their results by contemporaries was the reverse of our assessment today. In the 1840s and 1850s Farr's work was considered definitive, while Snow's was regarded as ingenious but flawed. Although Snow's conclusions ran contrary to the expectations of his contemporaries, the major reservations about his cholera studies concerned his bold use of analogy, his thoroughgoing reductionism, and his willingness to ignore what seemed to be contrary evidence. Farr's electic use of current theories, his reliance on multiple causation, and his discovery of a mathematical law to describe the outbreak in London in 1849 was much more convincing to his contemporaries. A major change in thinking about disease causation was needed before Snow's work could be widely accepted. William Farr's later studies contributed to that acceptance.

The judgment of posterity is certainly unpredictable. Witness the changing acclaim for the cholera studies of John Snow and William Farr. Today John Snow is celebrated as the one who solved the mystery of cholera's transmission and as a founder of modern epidemiology. His work is held in the highest regard, and he is one of few nineteenth century medical figures whose name is likely to be known to most members of the health professions. William Farr, on the other hand, seems to be known today only to those very few in these professions who have well-developed historical interests. But in 1855, the year when the second and more famous edition of John Snow's "*On the Mode of Communication of Cholera*" (Snow, 1855) was published, the situation was reversed. Farr was then the recognised authority on vital statistics and epidemiology and the one whose report on the 1848–49 cholera epidemic was considered authoritative (Farr, 1852; Review, 1852). Snow's publications on cholera, on the other hand, were regarded as ingenious but seriously flawed (Pelling, 1978, pp. 218, 221–36; Brown, 1961, pp. 525, 527; Brown, 1964, pp. 651–652). My purpose here is to suggest why the assessments of both men's work on cholera have changed so fundamentally since they wrote.

John Snow formulated his basic theory early in the 1848 outbreak by analogical reasoning on the pathology and therapeutics of the disease (Snow, 1849a; Snow, 1849b; Snow, 1855, pp. 10–15; Shepard, 1995, pp. 1643–1644, 173–174; Brown, 1961, pp. 519–520, 523–524; Brown, 1964, pp. 649–650; Pelling, 1978, pp. 204–205). Unlike other epidemic diseases which begin with general symptoms, such as fever, and whose morbid material was believed by most medical men to be present in the blood, cholera, Snow explained, began with local abdominal symptoms. This fact suggested to Snow that the disease was caused by a morbid material or poison which acted locally as an irritant on the surface of the stomach and intestines producing the pain, vomiting, diarrhoea, and dehydration that were the hallmarks of cholera. The fact that in its early stages cholera responded to treatments such as opium, chalk or catechu, which acted locally, seemed to confirm that cholera was a local disease of the gut. If the cholera poison acted solely on the surface of the alimentary canal, it seemed to follow that it must enter the body by being swallowed. It also suggested that the cholera poison ought to be present in the intestinal discharges of the sick. By his second edition Snow boldly drew on the examples of smallpox, cowpox and syphilis, inoculable diseases universally acknowledged to be contagious, to suggest that during an attack of cholera its morbid material was also multiplied in the body of the sick. If this were the case, as Snow clearly believed it was, then the cholera poison must be present in abundance in the intestinal discharge of cholera victims. Cholera, it followed, must be a communicable disease which spread when humans swallowed food or water contaminated with the dejecta of previous cholera victims.

Snow was not the only one to arrive at this conclusion in 1848–49. William Budd, later famous for demonstrating that typhoid fever was waterborne, reached a similar conclusion also by reasoning on pathological evidence. In a book published a mere 29 days after Snow's, Budd announced that he and a group of other Bristol medical men had found the agent of cholera, a fungus they had observed consistently in the stools of patients (Budd, 1849). Snow never endorsed this theory, and the fact that it was soon discredited seems to have convinced him that his only hope of convincing others of his theory was to collect epidemiological evidence (Pelling, 1978, pp. 157–188, 216–8; Brown, 1961, pp. 521–523). Snow was a general practitioner who had developed a practice in anesthesia and had conducted research in respiratory physiology and anesthesia, but he had no prior experience with epidemiology (Shephard, 1995).

He relied on two types of evidence. The first was the result of outbreak investigations in which he could make the fecal-oral route of transmission plausible. Examples include his account of the cases at Albion Terrace in 1849 and the Broad Street outbreak in 1854 (Snow, 1855, pp. 25–31, 38–54). In the former, after inspecting the site, Snow reconstructed how the spring-fed water supply to this row of 17 houses could have become contaminated by leakage from the cesspools and surface water drains that served these same houses. Snow also examined a specimen of water from one of the domestic water tanks at Albion Terrace and found that it smelt like privy soil and contained bits of undigested food that had clearly passed through the alimentary canal. The Broad Street outbrak was much larger. In this instance Snow failed to find direct sensory evidence of fecal contamination of the water, although a subsequent investigation published by the parish suggested how the Broad Street pump may have been contaminated by the water used to wash the diapers of an infant who died of what may have been cholera (Chave, 1958). The bulk of Snow's evidence in the Broad Street incident was drawn from his investigation of the circumstances of those who died of cholera in the vicinity. He could show that most of these had, or most likely had, consumed water from the public pump in Broad Street. Remarkably he could also implicate two cholera deaths in an area otherwise free from cholera, a widow in Hampstead and her daughter, who drank the water from the Broad Street pump after it was brought to them. Snow's colleagues found the two Hampstead deaths linked to the Broad Street pump water highly suggestive, but they did not find the evidence from Broad Street itself at all convincing. As one reviewer pointed out, Snow had not eliminated other explanations or the role of coincidence. Wells were so common in London that wherever the outbreak had occurred there probably would have been a well near its center (Parkes, 1855; Brown, 1964, pp. 651–652).

Snow's second type of evidence was the comparison of cholera mortality among large populations who had water supplies of varying degrees of sewage contamination. Circumstances provided an unusual opportunity for such an investigation, because in South London there were several areas served by two competing water companies (Snow, 1855, pp. 68–69, 74–5; Simon, 1856, pp. 4–5). In these districts the companies competed for customers house by house, so that the patrons of the two companies seemed indistinguishable except for their source of water. In 1854 one of these, the Southwark and Vauxhall Company, took its water from the Thames in central London at Battersea, while its competitor, the Lambeth Waterworks Company, had recently moved its inlet upstream to Thames Ditton, above Teddington Lock and hence beyond reach of most of London's sewage. In 1849 both companies had drawn their water from the Thames in central London. In neither 1849 nor 1854 did either company filter or treat its water. The circumstances seemed to be an ideal natural experiment for Snow's purposes. By comparing the mortality from cholera among the patrons of the two companies in 1854 and by comparing the experience of each set of patrons in 1849 with that of 1854, Snow obtained impressive results (Snow, 1855, pp. 68–92). Analysing the results he obtained from the first four weeks of the outbreak in 1854 Snow concluded that cholera mortality was fourteen times higher among those served the more impure water (Snow, 1855, p. 80). During the epidemic the gap in mortality narrowed, but, as he figured it, the patrons of the Southwark and Vauxhall Company remained between eight and nine times as likely to die of cholera during the first seven weeks of the outbreak and five times as likely during the next seven weeks (Snow, 1855, pp. 86–88).

Unfortunately the study of the water supply in South London was not nearly as ideal as this brief description suggests. First of all, as Snow acknowledged, in the districts with the mixed supply it was difficult to learn the source of water for the houses in which cholera deaths had taken place. Tenants often did not know the name of the company that supplied water to their building. Attempting to surmount this difficulty Snow relied on a chemical test. He took apparently one sample of Lambeth Company water at Tharnes Ditton and one sample of Southwark and Vauxhall Company water and tested each for their common salt content using silver nitrate. He found a significant difference. The silver nitrate precipitated only 2.28 grains of silver chloride from a gallon of the Lambeth Company water but 91 grains from an equal quantity of the Southwark and Vauxhall Company water. This difference was so great that Snow felt he could distinguish the two water supplies at a glance by adding a little silver nitrate to the sample in question (Snow, 1855, pp. 78–79). Only later did he realise that the saline content of the river water varied widely over time, in the recent past by a factor of 20 for the Southwark and Vauxhall Company, which took its water from an area under tidal influence (Shephard, 1995, p. 211).

But much more important to contemporaries was the fact that Snow did not know the number of people at risk of cholera in his test case. In fact, when he composed the second edition of his book, he did not even know the number of households supplied by each company in the districts with the mixed water supply. It is not immediately obvious in reading this work that his estimates of relative risk of dying of cholera, such as those just quoted for the first four weeks of the epidemic, are based on houses not persons and are computed for all households supplied by the two companies and not on those households in the areas of mixed supply. In reviewing this work Snow's contemporary, E.A. Parkes, at first missed what Snow had done, but on rereading he discovered that Snow had ignored entirely the natural experiment offered by the mixed districts. A comparison of the experience of all patrons of the two companies was not convincing to Parkes, because the whole of the areas served by the two companies differed substantially in ways thought to be relevant to cholera's prevalence, in elevation, in family income, and in the quality of housing (Parkes, 1855; Brown, 1964, pp. 651–652).

The reserve with which Snow's contemporaries greeted his results stemmed in part from the technical defects of his evidence and argument, but there was more to this skepticism. Witness the fact that his conclusions remained unconvincing even after Snow remedied some of these methodological problems, when additional information came into his hands. As Margaret Pelling has ably pointed out, Snow's colleagues did not so much oppose his theory as they objected to his dismissing other explanations for cholera's occurrence (Pelling, 1978, pp. 205–206, 222–235). It was the exclusiveness of his views that gave them pause. As we have seen, Snow began with his theory nearly formed and worked as an epidemiologist to collect evidence in its favor. He was untroubled by negative evidence, and he was overtly unsympathetic to the multifactorial theorizing about epidemic disease that was the hallmark of mainstream medical thinking at the time. His approach seemed to ignore what the profession had already learned in its experience with the disease. A few years later E.A. Parkes recalled his initial skepticism of Snow.

> "There seemed at once an a priori argument adverse to this view, as, at that time, all evidence was against the idea of cholera evacuations being capable of causing the disease. They had been tasted and drunk (in 1832) by men, and been given to animals, without effect. Persons inoculated themselves in dissections constantly, and bathed their hands in the fluids of the intestines; in India, the pariahs who removed excreta, and everywhere the washerwomen who washed the clothes of the sick, did not especially suffer. And to these arguments must be added the undoubted fact, that there were serious deficiencies of evidence in Dr. Snow's early cases. Add to this the unfortunate circumstance, that Dr. Snow, with all the enthusiasm of a discoverer, adopted the view that cholera entered only by means of water, and not at all by air, an hypothesis which is quite irreconcilable with the history of cholera..." (Parkes, 1864; Brown, 1961, p. 527).

It is quite possible that some of them may have associated such determined unifactoral explanations with the glib explanations of quacks or the simplistic understanding of lay people.

The second edition of Snow's book was widely reviewed in the medical press, and it stimulated discussion and further investigation. But Snow's colleagues were more impressed with his evidence than with his conclusions, and true to form, they tried to accommodate this evidence into the multifactorial explanations of the time. The Committee of Scientific Inquiry of the General Board of Health, which investigated the 1853–54 outbreak, may serve as an example. The Committee was most impressed with the results of the cholera study in South London, and it was willing to concede that sewage-contaminated water was a contributing factor to the cholera tragedy. But it could not accept Snow's pathological theory of cholera or his contention of specific contamination or sufficient causation (Pelling, 1978, pp. 222–235). The Committee concluded that the exciting cause of cholera brews poison from air or water containing ample organic impurities (The Committee for Scientific Inquiries 1854). John Simon, one of the most influential members of the Committee, regarded Snow's demonstration as very significant but concluded that Snow had established that both fecalized air and water were to blame for cholera's incidence (Simon, 1856, p. 9).

No one in the profession took Snow's work more seriously than William Farr (Eyler, 1973; Eyler 1979, pp. 114–122). Farr, the Statistical Superintendent of the General Register Office and a member of the Committee of Scientific Inquiries in 1854, devoted much attention to cholera and published important studies of three of

England's cholera epidemics: monographs on the epidemics of 1848–49 and of 1866 and sections in his weekly and annual reports for the 1853–54 outbreak (Farr, 1852; Farr, 1867–68; Farr, 1856). If Snow was exclusive in his analysis, Farr was inclusive in the extreme. His much-acclaimed study of the 1848–49 epidemic consisted of 300 pages of tables, charts, and maps prepared in the General Register Office under his supervision and a 100 page introduction in which he analysed the outbreak. Using the mortality records at his disposal Farr traced the cholera in England over time and space, compared this epidemic to its predecessor in 1832 and to the plague epidemics of earlier centuries, and analysed the possible influence of a host of demographic, social and environmental factors: age, sex, temperature, rainfall, wind, day of the week, domestic crowding, or property value. What impressed Farr most was the fact the cholera mortality was geographically concentrated. He found that in 1849 80% of the registered cholera deaths occurred in only 137 of the nation's 623 registration districts among 40% of the population living on one-seventh of its territory (Farr, 1852, pp. I–III). Coastal districts had on average three times the cholera mortality of inland districts. Farr further analysed local influences in nine cholera fields, areas of intense cholera mortality, each centered on a large port town. One of these, the London cholera field, was subjected to the closest analysis.

It was in the London cholera field that Farr made his most prized discovery, that cholera mortality is inversely related to elevation of the soil. He found that, if he arranged the districts of London into terraces by mean elevations above the high water mark of the Thames, cholera mortality varied according to a simple formula $C = C'\ (e' + a)/(e + a)$ where C and C' are cholera mortality rates per 10,000 in two districts having mean elevations in feet of e and e', and a is a constant, (12.8) (Farr, 1852, pp. LXIII; Langmuir, 1961). He demonstrated his elevation law by calculating for elevations 0, 10, 30, 50, 70, 90, 100, 350 a theoretical series of mortalities 174, 99, 53, 34, 27, 22, 20, 6 that agreed remarkably well with the observed series 177, 102, 65, 34, 27, 22, 17, 7.

This was exactly the sort of result Farr was looking for, demonstrating as it did that human mortality was regular, predictable, and capable of description in mathematical terms (Farr, 1852a). It also was a result in keeping with the understanding of epidemic disease held by Farr and by many in the profession. Farr's statements of his disease theory are most explicit, when he was presenting or defending new versions of the official nosology he had prepared to bring order and usefulness to the national system of death registration and, when he discussed the uses to which the registration material could be put in the campaign to prevent disease (Eyler, 1979, pp. 53–60).

Of greatest interest to us here is the first Class of Farr's nosology, the Epidemic, Endemic, and Contagious Diseases. As I have explained in detail elsewhere, Farr, like Snow, used analogies to the inoculable diseases – smallpox, cowpox, syphilis – to insist that diseases of this class were specific, disease entities produced by specific material causes that were reproduced in the blood of the victim (Eyler, 1973, pp. 81–87; Eyler, 1979, pp. 97–108). But unlike Snow, in the 1840s, Farr was certain that these material causes, while organic, were non-living, and he drew heavily on the writings of the German organic chemist Justis Liebig to explain the processes of fermentation or putrefaction (Pelling, 1978, pp. 113–145). To emphasise the similarity between these chemical processes and disease processes, Farr called the epidemic, endemic and contagious diseases zymotic, and held that a specific, non-living zymotic material caused each one. Cholera, for example, was caused by the as yet unidentified zymotic material "cholerine".

While Farr recognised that a few zymotic materials were inoculable, he held that most entered the body through the lungs. A long medical tradition of miasmatic explanations allowed him to explain why the epidemic, endemic and contagious diseases were most prevalent in urban slums, in prisons, or in squalid tropical port towns. In such places the air was ladened with organic material from respiration, perspiration, decomposition, or putrefaction. Zymotic material was abundant in the air in such circumstances. Furthermore, under extreme conditions zymotic material might be produced from ordinary organic material by chemical means without the presence of a prior case of the disease (Farr, 1840c; Farr, 1866a). Farr's purpose throughout his mortality studies was to demonstrate that the prevalence of the epidemic, endemic and contagious diseases was dependent on local environmental conditions and to provide compelling evidence that environmental, particularly sanitary reform, was essential.

Farr's discussion of the zymotic theory demonstrates not only the eclectic and inclusive nature of his thought, a feature of his work that contemporaries found appealing, but it also suggests why he was so delighted with his elevation law for cholera (Farr, 1852, pp. LXXX–LXXXLII). The low, moist soil on margins of the Thames, the filth and debris on the banks of a tidal river in a large industrial city provided ample organic material for putrefaction and decay. The concentration of miasmata, the airborne organic particles, resulting from these processes was greatest at lower elevation, and it could be expected to decrease at a regular rate as one ascended the sides of the river basin. The elevation law he discovered in analysing the epidemic of 1848–49 was a result that was easy for Farr's contemporaries to accept, so consistent did it seem to be with the majority opinion on the nature and cause of the epidemic diseases. They soon affirmed his discovery. William Duncan, Medical Officer of Health for Liverpool, wrote that when he grouped the districts of his city by elevation as Farr had done, that cholera mortality in the last epidemic obeyed Farr's elevation law for Liverpool as well (Ducan, 1852).

In his report on the 1848–49 cholera Farr labeled Snow's the most important of the various cholera theories he reviewed, and he quoted from Snow's recent pamphlet and accurately summarised Snow's explanations (Farr, 1852, pp. LXXVI–LXXVIII). Farr acknowledged that river water was highly polluted, but he was unconvinced by Snow's conclusions (Farr, 1852, pp. LIII, LXIX–LXX, LVIII–LXII). He recognised that river towns inherited the sewage and other organic debris of the towns upstream and invariably had higher cholera mortalities than the towns upstream. When he analysed cholera mortality in London's water fields, the areas of the Metropolis served by water of different origins, he found that the water fields with the highest cholera mortalities were not only those at the lowest elevation but also those that drew their water from the Thames furthermost downstream. But in 1852 Farr viewed sewage-contaminated water as only another source of miasmata. Sewage contaminated river water, he emphasised, contained abundant organic material undergoing putrefaction and decomposition. Particularly telling is his use of the Royal Observatory's estimates of the quantity of vapor evaporated from the surface of the Thames in London and his emphasis on air and water temperatures during the weeks of the cholera epidemic in 1849 to demonstrate that "the wide simmering waters were breathing incessantly into the vast sleeping city tainted vapors, which the temperature of the air at night would not sustain" (Farr, 1852, pp. LIX).

While he could not accept Snow's conclusions in 1852, Farr had become intensely interested in his theory, and when cholera broke out in England again in 1853, he wasted no time investigating. On 13 October at his suggestion the General Register Office requested from each water company information on the source(s) of the water it supplied, on the methods of filtration or purification used, and any change in source since the last epicemic (Farr, 1856, p. 91). The responses alerted Farr to the change in the Lambeth Waterworks Company's source and hence to the importance of the mortality patterns in South London. He began publishing in his weekly reports data on cholera mortality by water field as he had done retrospectively for the previous outbreak (Farr, 1856, pp. 91–97). His weekly report for 26 November 1853 carried the table that probably alerted Snow to importance of the arrangements in the water supply in South London (Snow, 1855, p. 69; Farr, 1856, pp. 75–76). Farr fully co-operated with Snow's efforts to test his theory, giving Snow unpublished material from the death registers, and, when Snow's preliminary results appeared promising, ordered local registrars in South London to inquire into the source of water, when a cholera death was registered (Snow, 1855, pp. 76–77; Farr, 1856, p. 94).

It was Farr who suggested that the Committee for Scientific Inquiries of the General Board of Health pay particular attention to cholera in South London in its report on the 1853–54 epidemic (Simon, 1890).

Farr's own investigations of this outbreak appeared in his weekly reports and in a section of his letter in the Registrar-General's Seventeenth Annual Report (Farr, 1856). He repeated the sort of analysis of the outbreak that he had published for the previous epidemic, and again he found cholera mortality to depend on local conditions. What was new was his conviction that sewage-contaminated water had exercised a decisive influence. He ended his report by saying that the collective efforts of Snow, the G.R.O., and the Board of Health had proven that "cholera matter or cholerine, where it is most fatal, is largely diffused through water, as well as through other channels" (Farr, 1856, p. 99). This statement might be taken to mean that Farr now agreed with Snow. But the fact is that Farr simply added polluted water to contaminated air as a vehicle for morbid matter. He continued to believe that zymotic material entered the body primarily through the lungs. He pointed out that evaporation from cisterns, taps, drains, and local reservoirs took place constantly. Sewage-contaminated water "comes into contact with the body in many ways and it gives off incessantly at its temperature, ranging from the freezing point to summer heat, vapors and effluvia into the atmosphere that is breathed in every room" (Farr, 1856, p. 95). Thus the differences between Snow and most of the profession, including Farr, continued to be over Snow's pathological theory and his exclusiveness. Strictly speaking, what had been established in South London was only that patrons of a company supplying highly contaminated water were at greater risk of dying of cholera. No one had proved how that contaminated water acted.

By the time of the 1866 epidemic of cholera John Snow was dead, and William Farr had become one of the waterborne theory's few champions. Farr's sympathy for Snow's hypothesis can be properly gauged, when his views are contrasted with the skepticism of most Medical Officers of Health in the Metropolis when the 1866 epidemic began (Luckin, 1877). Farr had been deeply impressed by the analyses of cholera mortality in South London in 1853–54, but the next epidemic provided a case study that was decisive. Farr's analysis of the cholera returns pointed very early in the epidemic to excessive cholera mortality in the East London Waterworks Company's water field. Farr not only made this information public, but he lobbied to have the causes of the outbreak and the quality of the East London Company's water investigated. The series of official investigations that followed showed that the company had been illegally pumping water from its reservoir at Old Ford, which it claimed was no longer in use, and which had been contaminated from the new sewage system of West Ham (Farr, 1867, pp. XII, XVII–XX; Luckin, 1877).

Farr's monograph on the 1866 epidemic, like that on the 1848–49 eidemic, provided a comprehensive analysis of the epidemic, treating it as a complex social and medical phenomenon. But this time it passed quickly over the influence of age, sex, weather, income, occupation, and housing density in order to concentrate his analysis on water, particularly on the outbreak in East London. Farr demonstrated not only that cholera mortality was extremely high only in the East London water field, particularly among those people receiving water from the Old Ford reservoir, but he also showed that the law of the epidemic, the rates of the outbreak's rise and fall, for the East London water field in this epidemic was different from the law that prevailed in either previous London cholera outbreaks or in other water fields in 1866 (Farr, 1867, pp. XX–XXIV, XXX–XXXIII). One of the anomalies in the East London outbreak was its sudden decline. Farr attributed this peculiarity to changes the company made in its supply once the high mortality among its patrons was exposed.

Farr now concluded that cholera was spread by cholera flux, the intestinal discharges of cholera patients, and that it could be transmitted in four ways: by personal contact, by air, by sewer vapor, and by water. This list was familiar. What was new was how he ranked these means. The first three, Farr thought, may have exercised a slight influence over all of London, not exceeding five deaths per 10,000. But in a city like London the first three were insignificant in comparison to the fourth. The character of the outbreak was determined by waterborne contagion (Farr, 1867, pp. XV–XVLL, LXXX). Except for a vestige of miasmatic notions, represented by air and sewer vapor as media that were retained to explain a few exceptional cholera cases that seemed intelligible in no other way, Farr had accepted Snow's explanation of cholera's transmission (Farr, 1867, pp. XIV–XVI).

The intellectual climate in the mid-1860s was more congenial to Snow's pathological theory of cholera than the climate of the 1840s had been, and that change in theoretical context was instrumental in Farr's conversion to Snow's position. In Farr's discussion of disease in his monograph on the 1866 cholera epidemic we find that biological evidence replaced much of the former reliance on chemical authorities. Liebig, Dumas, and Thomas Graham are displaced by Pasteur on fermentation and by pathologists such as Filippo Paccini and Lionel S. Beal, who reported seeing corpuscles in the intestinal discharges of cholera patients and in the cases of the cattle plague, respectively. In this Farr was reflecting a heightened interest of the profession in elementary units in biology and a suspicion that they were particulate (Crellin, 1968). I have shown elsewhere that Farr began to hold that zymotic material consisted of elementary particles he called zymads. Thus the agent of cholera, cholerine, consisted of cholrads. Over the next few years he responded to contemporary biological research by endowing these zymads with additional properties of life, until they became nearly indistinguishable from living organisms (Eyler, 1979, pp. 105–107). What was true for Farr may have been true of others in the profession as well. The *Lancet* suggested that Farr had led the way by making the waterborne theory "irresistible" (Lancet, 1868).

The contrast of Farr's and Snow's approaches to the study of cholera highlights the importance of disease theory in epidemiological investigations. The studies of both men were predicated on their understanding of the nature and causation of disease, and their methodology reflected those theoretical differences. Snow was exclusive or reductionist in theory, and he focused his empirical investigation on finding collaborating evidence and ignored negative evidence or anomalous cases. For him epidemiology was a means of verification; for Farr it was also a means of discovery. Farr was eclectic and inclusive in his theory, and he approached his cholera studies by trying to weigh a large list of social, environmental, and biological factors in accounting for cholera's behaviour. These qualities of mind made Farr responsive to new ideas and adaptable, as we can see in both the changing emphasis and the conclusions in his investigations of three cholera epidemics. A recent biographer of Snow briefly compares Snow and Farr and praises Snow for his openmindedness (Shephard, 1995, pp. 179–180). By implication Farr was closed-minded. On the cholera question I would conclude just the opposite. Judged by the standards of his time Snow was the dogmatic contagionist and premature reductionist. Farr was the more cautious in weighing all evidence.

One final comment on Farr must be made. He may have been eclectic and flexible in his understanding of the mechanism of disease, and he might have been open to new hypotheses, but he was firmly committed to his conviction that disease, in fact all vital phenomena, were law-abiding. He was convinced that a statistical law with as much predictive value as his elevation law must reveal something fundamental about disease. He never accepted Snow's claim that the elevation law Farr discovered in the data for the 1848–49 epidemic was merely a "remarkable coincidence" (Snow, 1855, pp. 97–98). Farr's increased sympathy for Snow's theory did not mean that he abandoned the elevation law. In fact it appears, suitably modified, in his reports on both subsequent epidemics (Farr, 1856, pp. 88–90; Farr, 1867, pp. XIV–XVXX). The tenaciousness and the ingenuity with which Farr worked to salvage an elevation law in each of his later cholera reports speaks volumes for his faith in the power of statistical inquiry. This faith made numerically strong relationships that confirmed expectations irresistible to him. Today it is his results and not Snow's that are considered merely ingenious, and Snow's publications are read perhaps more sympathetically than they deserve, because the modern medical reader can "fill in the gaps in his reasoning with the comforting knowledge that Snow was, after all, right" (Brown, 1964, p. 652; Pelling, 1978, pp. 209–210).

Appendix

A Note on Sources

The second edition of Snow's "*On the mode of communication of cholera*" of 1855 is cited from the reprint in Snow on cholera: Being a reprint of two papers by John Snow, M.D. together with a biographical memoir by B.W. Richardson, M.D. and an introduction by Wade Hampton Frost, M.D. London and New York, 1936 and is cited as Snow, "*On the Mode of Communication (1855)*". Farr's annual letter in the "*Annual Report of the Registrar-General of Births, Deaths, and Marriages in England and Wales*" is cited as Farr, "*Letter, nth A.R.R.G*". This important source was reprinted in the British Parliamentary Papers, here abbreviated as "*B.P.P.*" In some years the pagination differed between the separately published version and the version in the Parliamentary Papers. The version in "*B.P.P.*" is cited, but when the pagination differs, the page number in the separately published version is given in parenthesis.

Changing images of John Snow in the history of epidemiology

Jan P. Vandenbroucke

Clinical Epidemiology, Leiden University Medical Center, PO Box 9600, NL-2300 RC Leiden, The Netherlands

Summary

Ever since the end of the 19th century, the story of John Snow and his investigations into the contagiousness of cholera has fascinated epidemiologists. Several different lessons have been extracted from the interpretation and reinterpretation of Snow's work – according to prevailing insights. The story of John Snow continues to evolve, even into the 21st century.

The purpose of this commentary is to ask, and try to answer, the questions: "Why did it take so long before people recognised the importance of John Snow's work?", and "Who was first responsible for this belated recognition?". I will first of all show how long a time it took before Snow was recognised as a "hero" of epidemiology. But in searching why and how it took such a long time, an even more intriguing idea developed. It seemed to me that the name of Snow was needed to replace a part of the history of epidemiology of which 20th century epidemiologists were a little bit ashamed: the period when epidemiology still believed in miasmata. In doing so, however, some of the sounder themes that epidemiology really inherited from miasmatic thinking (an inheritance which we prefer to forget), were suitably ascribed to John Snow. Somehow, the Snow which we know is a construct of several ideas from the history of epidemiology; some of which we are ashamed of, and others of which we are proud (Vandenbroucke et al., 1991).

The role of "preconceived ideas"

Before embarking on the main theme, let me indicate that I have two interests in John Snow. The query about the way in which he became a hero of epidemiology was only my second interest. My first interest had to do with the origin of his ideas (Vandenbroucke 1988a; Vandenbroucke, 1988b). When reading John Snow and some of the commentators about his work, I was struck by the amount of a priori reasoning in his book "*On the Mode of Communication of Cholera*". When you read it closely, you see that Snow was already a convinced contagionist and already believed that water was an important factor before he made his observations about the Broad Street Pump and about the water companies. Haven't philosophers already said for a long time that we only see what we know? Anyway, Snow already had ideas about small amounts of cellular and self-replicating matter that would propagate disease. He had developed and strengthened these ideas, among others by simple clinical observation: case histories of children who shared beds in hospital and subsequently caught cholera from each other, and many similar observations that seemed to fit very well with his preconceptions about "germs", contagion and disease. To the concept of "direct contagion" he added the idea that, when there is no immediate person-to-person contact, then water will carry the infection. And for that idea too, he already had "proofs" long before his epidemiologic observations.

If you want to see for yourself how much a priori reasoning there was in Snow's work, you only have to read the first edition of his work on the "*Communication of Cholera*". Few people realise that Snow's celebrated book of 1855, which we know because it was reprinted so successfully in 1936 by Wade Hampton Frost, is only the second edition (Snow, 1936a). When you read the first, much smaller edition of 1849 (Snow, 1849a), excerpts of which were also published in the London Medical Gazette (Snow, 1849b), you will find already essentially the same reasoning, the incrimination of drinking water. Then you understand that Snow made his observations with a very prepared mind. In the first edition, he makes already a first attempt, on very crude data borrowed from earlier epidemics of cholera, to point at differences between London districts and their water supply. He also has many anecdotes about pumps, overflowing cesspools etc. In retrospect, it was a "dress rehearsal" for the Broad Street Pump and the "water companies". But even to a very benevolent observer like myself, it is clear that he was bending his data, or I should say, his anecdotes in the "right" direction. His was a highly single minded affair – and perhaps all scientists need a little of this single-mindedness to cling to one's own theory, whatever the data and the objections of others. Even in his second edition, he "obliterates" part of the data: he only emphasises the first part of the epidemic that shows most clearly the association between drinking water and cholera; he avows that the second part of the epidemic is less clear in this respect, because by that time the spread of the cholera went on from person to person.

I am not the first to point to the role of preconceived ideas in Snow's work. In the 1936 reprint of the second edition of Snow's work (with the data that made Snow's reputation) there is an introduction by Wade Hampton Frost, as well as a short biography by Snow's contemporary and friend Richardson (Snow, 1936a). They wrote clearly that Snow had very specific ideas "in mind" before he made his observations. Therefore, I do oppose certain epidemiologic interpretations that say that Snow just observed an association between water and cholera without having any inkling of the bacterial cause of cholera – 30 years before Koch made the discovery of the cholera bacillus. Such interpretations of the history of epidemiology lead to the notion that somehow "observing associations" is "the superior science". This is to me a distortion of Snow's writings. Quite on the contrary, what he describes as the background theory from which he set up his observations, is firmly rooted in "germ theory" convictions about causes of disease. I am neither the first (Buck, 1975; Cameron and Jones, 1983), nor will I be the last to make this observation. In a recent commemorative issue of the American Journal of Epidemiology, Winkelstein made exactly the same observations, based on other writings of Snow (Winkelstein, 1995).

Enough on my first interest in the interpretation of John Snow's work. I related it with some purpose, however, as it will come back. This first interest drew me into the second, because I started wondering how the interpretation of Snow might have evolved over time. I already knew that in his time he was a clear contagionist, was in a minority position (perhaps because people thought that his observations were merely made to confirm his prejudices), and that the publication of his book was almost a financial loss to him.

The emergence of Snow in the medical literature of the Netherlands

To delineate my search, I started to study the influence of Snow in the Dutch medical literature. However much I was prepared for surprise, my findings were still unsettling. In the Dutch medical literature, Snow's work only grew into a "classic" between 1930 and 1950: some 80 to 100 years after the initial publication. During the first decades after his publication, his work was hardly mentioned. In the Dutch medical literature, i.e. in the contemporary issues of the leading medical journals in the Netherlands, there were occasional footnotes about a drinking water theory – mostly without mentioning Snow by name. On the whole, the leading paradigm of the 1850 to 1880s and even 1890s was Von Pettenkofer's "boden theory", a multicausal variant of miasma theory (von Pettenkofer, 1887). Von Pettenkofer's work about cholera was enthusiastically described and paraphrased in lengthy articles with a wealth of very supportive geographical data. His books and writings were abundantly translated and popularised. The greatness of Von Pettenkofer's work was sung in all modes and it was often said that it would almost be impossible to improve on his work. His ideas completely permeated Dutch medical society. A very lone critic in 1873 showed that there was only a poor correlation between the composition of the soil and mortality in different areas of Rotterdam, the Netherlands (Ballott, 1873). In the first decades after John Snow's initial publication, his drinking water theory only surfaced once in the Netherlands in a cautious 1868 report (some 15 years after the facts!). Mind, that this is about the same time that Simon in England started to give Snow some credit (Vandenbroucke et al., 1991).

The idolatry with Von Pettenkofer reached an absolute height at the time of his celebrated controversy with Robert Koch about the commaform bacillus that the latter had discovered in 1883 in Egypt and had designated as "the cause" of Cholera (Brock, 1988, p. 149). Von Pettenkofer, who initially might have made some room for bacteria in his theory, was by that time so entrenched that he devised his famous experiment in which he swallowed pure cholera broth and successfully proved that neither he nor his co-experimenters got sick (among his co-experimenters were famous people like Metchnikoff who later converted himself to work with Pasteur) (Altman, 1987). Ironically, this very successful experiment became Von Pettenkofer's Swan song. Strange if you think of it: that a successful experiment can be the beginning of scientific defeat.

From about 1900 onwards, when bacteriology emerged as the "stronger science", we find a gradual decline in the number of references to Von Pettenkofer, and a concomitant gradual increase in references to Snow. In a 1913 Dutch book of public health, we can read how refreshing it is to read the clear-headed work of John Snow as a rare treasure amidst the volumes of theoretical trash that hygienism had produced. Koch's discoveries were held to bring real understanding, and underscored Snows findings (Saltet, 1913). The same Dutch author goes as far as to scorn hygienists for their mistakes: for example, he describes how hygienists had so much zeal to clean the city that they ordered to dump the street dirt of the city of London (including human excreta at that time) into the Thames River (from where the drinking water was obtained). So, it was written in 1914 that those hygienists might have prolonged the epidemic! At the same time Snow is praised for the equanimity by which he supported miasmatic slandering (Saltet, 1914). Still in a 1935 new book on public health in The Netherlands, Snow is not mentioned (van Loghem, 1935). Von Pettenkofer is mentioned eight times, be it always in the negative. It is only in 1955, in the fifth edition of the same book on public health in the Netherlands that we read for the first time unequivocally that Snow's work is a "classic" (van Loghem, 1955)! In 1955, one hundred years after the original publication! At the same time, attention is drawn to the equally forgotten work of Budd on Typhoid Fever. In between, of course, there had been the reprint of Snow's work by Frost in the USA. The aim of the reprint was to make the work widely available. And it succeeded. The original work by Snow had almost been lost – for example in the Netherlands, there are still roughly 80 copies of books by Von Pettenkofer in libraries; but only one original, and two reprints of Snows 1855 second edition of the Mode of Communication of Cholera. Of the first edition of 1849, there must only be a few copies all over the world.

The motives to make John Snow a "hero"

The motives of 20th century epidemiologists for making Snow a hero to replace Von Pettenkofer, became clear to me when studying the opposition between bacteriology and miasma theory. The new "science of bacteriology" had swept some of the greatest heroes of public health off their feet. The only historical figure of the 19th century to which epidemiologists and public health officials of the early 20th century could still relate to was John Snow, because he had proved to be "right" in his application of the "germ theory". Ironically, in his own time, the position of Snow's theory was a marginal one.

Epidemiologists of the first half of the 20th century have succeeded very well, maybe too well, in screening off the heritage of Von Pettenkofer. In introductions to epidemiology only Snow is mentioned, giving young students the impression that he was an important leader of epidemiology and public health in the middle of the 19th century. Thereby, the greatest irony of it all is that Snow's work is almost always described as a triumph of a type of thinking that is quite miasmatic or hygienic in character. It is forgotten that Snow had very firm convictions about germ theory and contagionism. His work is almost described as a victory of "black box" epidemiology, looking for environmental causes, without having any inkling of the biologic background. Somehow, the spirit of miasma still succeeds in blurring our view of Snow. What is more, all the credit that should go to hygienic thinking is brought to Snow. All hygienic precepts in combating cholera, i.e., not only those about drinking water, but also those about personal cleanliness, sewage disposal, etc. are now ascribed to Snow because he proved the contagion.

Snow in the international literature

It might be argued that too much of the above is based on a study of Dutch medical literature only, and that the Dutch are too close to the Germans, hence the all-pervasive influence of Von Pettenkofer. The first historian who called attention to the fact that Snow's work was so slowly and erratically accepted was Garrison in his 1929 textbook in the USA (Garrison, 1929, pp. 661–662, 781). There we also learn that Britain was the country where Snow's work was most readily accepted. Already in 1866, only 11 years after the publication, Simon would have reported favourably about it to the Queen's council. Yet, we have Simon recognising in the 1890s how it took him 30 years to understand the "rightness" of Snow (Simon, 1897).

Nevertheless, even British epidemiology remained ambiguous. We have seen that in 1936 Frost secured the reprint of Snow's work, because he found it so important, and it proved an instant success. Yet, one year earlier, in 1935 Greenwood, the first professor of Epidemiology at the London School of Hygiene, published his magnum opus, "Epidemics and Crowd Diseases", about the history of epidemiology, partially written for the lay public and partially for professional audiences (Greenwood, 1935). In Greenwood's account of the epidemiology of cholera in this 1935 book, neither Snow, nor the drinking water theory are mentioned (Greenwood, 1935, pp. 165 et ss.)! To Greenwood the real epidemiologic hero of the past was Creighton –

Charles Creighton who in the 1890s had published extensively on the history of epidemics in Britain from the year 600 to the 1800s (Creighton, 1891; Creighton, 1894). Creighton was a staunch follower of Von Pettenkofer; he was not only one of the last anti-contagionists, but also much opposed to smallpox vaccination. In his great book on the history of epidemics, a book that is still readable, both for its style and for its scrupulously factual accounts, Creighton sneered at Snow in a footnote as "one who had seized upon the occasion of a pump" (Creighton, 1894, p. 854). And still in 1929 Garrison – who had somewhat more sympathy for Snow – continued to describe Creighton as the founder of modern British epidemiology (Garrison, 1929, p. 742).

In Germany, Virchow originally opposed the germ theory on cholera (Virchow, 1985, vol I, p. 124; vol II, pp. 259–260); he admitted defeat in 1884 (Brock, 1988, p. 168). But even worse: Robert Koch who gave the ultimate demonstration that the drinking water theory was right by the isolation of the Vibrio Cholera in a water tank in India, even Koch did not mention Snow in his early papers (Brock, 1988, p. 162). Either Koch did not know his writings, or Snow was thought to be irrelevant – we will never know. So much for the importance of epidemiology.

Wade Hampton Frost

It will have become clear that the person responsible for making John Snow a hero was W.H. Frost. I ended one of my papers about Snow by citing an anonymous reviewer, who really seemed to have personal background information (Vandenbroucke et al., 1991). The review was typed by old-fashioned type-writer. I have never known who the reviewer was, and I repeat the quote here:

"Snow's studies of cholera were introduced to America, and perhaps the rest of the world by Wade Hampton Frost, the first Professor of Epidemiology at the Johns Hopkins School of Hygiene and Public Health. Not only did Frost republish the papers, but he introduced the studies to his classes. This practice was continued by his successor, Dr. Kenneth F. Maxcy, who as editor of the eight edition of the Rosenau text on Preventive Medicine and Public Health described in detail the Broad Street pump study. Material from Frost's introduction and republication of Snow's paper was used as a class problem in the introductory course in epidemiology. This practice was continued by the third chairman, Sartwell, whose description of the case-control method used in comparing two London populations was described in the ninth edition (Sartwell, 1965a, p. 6). He also gave a lecture at the American Epidemiological Society praising the Snow studies (Sartwell, 1972).

The use of the "Snow exercise" has since that time spread over the world (Vandenbroucke, 1992). I was introduced to it by Hans Valkenburg, Professor of Epidemiology at Rotterdam, the Netherlands, when I became a member of his department, because it was used as a class exercise for medical students. I took it over to Leiden University, the Netherlands, but was forced to abandon it because medical students opposed it as "too lengthy, outdated and a mere exercise in reading".

All in all, 20th century epidemiology has accepted a strange mixture of ideas: the methodological example of John Snow was revived but it was intertwined by a continuation of the multicausal way of thinking by Von Pettenkofer. The basic reason for this attitude of 20th century epidemiologists might have been that deep in their hearts they preferred a multicausal miasmatic way of reasoning, but that they were nevertheless forced under the uni-causal umbrella of bacteriology. Snow was the best compromise.

The image of John Snow continues to change

Our view of our past is constantly changing, because of the discovery of new facts, the re-examination of existing material by new techniques, and, perhaps most importantly, because of the reinterpretation of known facts. The history of John Snow is not different. Since the lecture that I gave at Annecy, France, in 1996, and upon which the above text is largely based, the literature about John Snow has continued to grow, and has been enriched with many new insights, and even discoveries. In particular there was the paper by David Lilienfeld who discovered a transcript of a testimony that Snow gave before a British parliamentary committee (Lilienfeld, 2000); in that testimony, Snow adamantly refuses to take into consideration that "toxic fumes" could cause any disease whatsoever, and seems to take a political stand that sounds "reactionary" to modern readers. I tried to comment how we might interpret this episode (Vandenbroucke, 2000), which is so reminiscent of many of today's discussions in occupational health (Sandler, 2000).

Next, there was the paper by (Brody et al., 2000), which builds upon their earlier work (Paneth et al., Part II), to draw attention to the neglected role of map-making in the work of Snow. It resulted in a flurry of letters by different authors in the correspondence pages of *The Lancet*, pointing at diverse interpretations (Correspondence, 2000). Most recently, as to this writing, and as to my limited capacity to select and read the relevant literature, there was a new book completely devoted to Snow (Vinten-Johansen et al., 2003), which took a new approach. Up to now the history of John Snow consisted of two almost separate histories: the history of the anaesthesiologist and physiologist who helped Queen Victoria giving pain-free birth, and the history of the epidemiologist. The new book, written by several authors who have been writing on Snow before, tries to bring alive the "whole Snow", and his links with contemporary medical science. In doing so, it somewhat de-emphasises the idea that Snow's ideas on cholera found little support with his contemporaries, which has been up to now a constant theme in the history of Snow. As in the past, debates on the right interpretation of the work of John Snow will continue. He will continue to be cited in epidemiologic editorials, as a lesson for the future (Smith and Ebrahim, 2001). And finally, what else could one expect: a brief look at the internet shows that over the past years dozens of web pages have been devoted to Snow, so that the youngest generations of epidemiologists can quickly turn to history (see references, short list of web pages devoted to Snow)!

Acknowledgement

The text of this commentary is based on a talk given at the symposium "Measuring our scourges – the history of Epidemiology" at Annecy, France, July 1–10 1996, and on a previously published text (Vandenbroucke et al., 1991). A note covering a selection of papers since 1996 has been added in 2001.

Constructing vital statistics: Thomas Rowe Edmonds and William Farr, 1835–1845

John M. Eyler

Department of History of Medicine, University of Minnesota, Minneapolis

Summary

This paper describes the role of these two English statisticians in establishing mortality measurements as means of assessing the health of human populations. Key to their innovations was the uses for the law of mortality Edmonds claimed to have discovered in 1832. In reality he had merely rediscovered a relationship between aging and mortality first described mathematically by Benjamin Gompertz a decade earlier. During the 1830s Edmonds attempted to interest the medical profession in his discovery and to suggest how his discovery could be used to assess health of large communities and to study case fatality and therapy. Using the rich data of the General Register Office William Farr would develop Edmonds's suggestions to produce some of the most sophisticated uses of vital statistics in the 19th century. In understanding the motivation of these two statisticians, it is essential to recognise their reform sympathies in an age deeply troubled by the human costs of rapid industrialisation and urbanisation. The two set out to reform both their professions and society.

The work of two relatively unknown Victorians, Thomas Rowe Edmonds and William Farr, was key to the creation of the modern discipline of vital statistics and of the use of those statistics to assess health and welfare. My thesis is that their contributions originated in their reform aspirations in the politically troubled 1830s and drew heavily on life insurance practices. In 1835 both men were ambitious, young, provincial Englishmen living in Fitzroy Square, London, looking for the places in the professions to which they believed their geniuses entitled them. Edmonds had the advantages a middle class family could provide, including a Cambridge education (Eyler, 2002a; Driver, 1929; Walford, 1873). Farr, on the other hand, was born to impoverished farm labourers who abandoned him to the parish. He was able to obtain a piecemeal education and to enter the lowest rung of the medical profession through the largeness of a patron who recognised his intelligence and promise (Eyler, 1979; Humphreys, 1885b). Both Farr and Edmonds tried to make their way with their pens. By 1835 Edmonds had already published three books and had begun the series of articles for the *Lancet* that we will consider below. Frustrated with general practice, Farr turned to medical journalism; he helped edit the British Medical Almanack, and co-founded and edited the short-lived British Annals of Medicine, Pharmacy, Vital Statistics, and General Science.

Both men considered their professions in desperate need of reform. Farr made his journals a voice for the frustrations and complaints of ordinary practitioners about the privileges and power of the London medical establishment (Anonymous, 1837a; Anonymous, 1837b; Anonymous, 1837c). That establishment, according to its rank-in-file members, neither recognised merit founded on scientific training nor represented the interests of the whole profession. Farr identified himself with a group of radical medical reformers in London that included Thomas Wakely, the editor of the Lancet. It is no surprise to find that in these years Wakely gave space in his journal to both Farr and Edmonds. Edmonds had found a place as an actuary. In journals edited by Farr and by Wakely he also took aim at his seniors, subjecting John Rickman, the head of the English census, to scorn for gross errors and for letting great opportunities for gathering invaluable information slip by and accusing John Finlaison, the government's actuary, of costing the nation over £ 300000 through poor advice he gave about the government annuity scheme (Edmonds, 1835–36a, p. 369; Edmonds, 1835–36c, p. 357; Edmonds, 1835–36d, pp. 692–93; Edmonds, 1836–37).

The reform impulse of these two men ran deeper than their professional ambitions. Like the other middle-class professional and business men of radical or Whig sympathies who formed the statistical societies of the 1830s, they were preoccupied by the problems of urban poverty and the condition of the industrial working class, and they believed that these problems could be studied objectively and solved peacefully (Cullen, 1975; McGregor, 1957; Ashton, 1934). Unlike most members of the early statistical societies whose interests proved to be short-lived, Edmonds and Farr found places in the civil service and in the insurance industry where data collection and analysis had become critical functions and where they could function as professional statisticians.

Edmonds's response to the great social problems of his youth was economic and utopian. In 1828, two years out of university, he published his first book, "*Practical, moral and political economy: or, the government, religion, and institutions most conducive to individual happiness and to national power*" (Edmonds, 1828). This book offered a critique of early industrial capitalism in the tradition of Ricardian socialism. Edmonds accepted the labour theory of value and explained British poverty as the result of private property, or the expropriation of the value of the labour of the working class by the unproductive classes (Driver, 1929; King, 1983; Perelman, 1980). Edmonds estimated that one man and one horse could provide the necessities for 15 people. He also calculated that one-third of the population produced all the necessities of life for the entire nation and yet retained only one-third of the product. The remaining two-thirds went to capital and to arbitrary expenditures such as rent. He deplored the utter dependency of wage earners on their masters, observing that there was little difference between slaves and such labourers (Edmonds, 1828, p. 141). It was surplus labour, the excess of labourers over jobs, that drove wages down and made the wage earner's position so uncertain. Such notions anticipated Karl Marx by 15 years. Like Marx, Edmonds also explained capitalism, the "money system" he called it, as a passing stage in human history to be succeeded by a more communal stage he called the "social system." He provided a blue print for radical social reform by describing a utopian, communal society created on an island.

Farr's critique was more limited, and, perhaps because he was a medical man, it was centred on human health. Farr would devote his career to demonstrating that the growth of industrial cities created conditions that caused unnecessary human disease, shortened human life, and cost the nation enormous sums in lost labour (Eyler, 1979, pp. 90–96, 123–149). His reports from the General Register Office over a period of 40 years would do much to sustain interest in the long process of eliminating the worst hazards to human health in the urban environment. But that was in the future. In 1835 Farr was just formulating the ideas and the methods that served him later, and, as I argue below, Edmonds was important to him in this formative process. In 1835 Farr had just begun to publish. His first two articles were lectures on hygiene (Farr, 1835–36a; Farr, 1835–36b). Although these lectures broke no new ground, they mark him as a reformer. He was confident that disease could be prevented and health improved, and he called on his fellow practitioners to put the public interest before professional fees and to support public efforts to prevent disease.

Those who advocated social reform faced a formidable adversary in Thomas Malthus, who had argued that a genuine improvement in the condition of the people was impossible. Population increasing geometrically would always outpace the means of subsistence, which increased arithmetically. Therefore it seemed that laws of nature precluded any genuine improvement in the lot of the mass of the population. Farr and Edmonds felt obliged to respond. Here again Edmonds led in the 1830s. His second book, *"An enquiry into the principles of population"*, was his answer to Malthusian pessimism (Edmonds, 1832a). As we have seen, Edmonds accepted Malthus's analysis, up to a point. The economic condition of workers under capitalism was a reflection of the existence of surplus labour, and he believed that any improvement in the plight of the poor depended on encouraging the working class to forego or to delay marriage, so that its size would grow in proportion to that of the upper classes which provided much of the demand for its labour. But unlike Malthus, he was optimistic that such population restraint was possible. This second book also offered a utopian scheme. This time it was a system to replace the old Poor Law. Edmonds's scheme was vastly different from the system of institutional deterrents to relief that the New Poor Law would soon create. He proposed creating artificial wants and providing a modest improvement in the standard of living to give the working class an incentive to delay marriage. Workers would also be encouraged to become independent craftsmen, and the working class itself would be given a hand in policing abuses in relief.

Edmonds also criticised Malthus's analysis of human misery. His own study of history showed that at every stage of human existence misery depended not on population pressure but on ignorance and bad government. He pointed to examples of an advanced and a "barbarous" people occupying the same land. In every case the knowledge, technology, and institutions of the advanced people supported a large population with an abundance of food, while the people lacking these blessings of civilisation lived in misery in small numbers (Edmonds, 1832a, pp. 7–8, 16, 22–24, 33–37). Knowledge, Edmonds concluded, was more important than either capital or natural resources, and human knowledge was boundless. His faith in science and human progress made him confident that Malthus had seriously erred in assuming that the means of subsistence could only grow arithmetically. Edmonds was certain that science was an inexhaustible source of useful discoveries, and that with the application of such useful knowledge, the means of subsistence could grow faster than the population (Edmonds, 1832a, pp. 57–67).

This objection, that Malthus erred in assuming that the means of subsistence could grow only arithmetically, was raised frequently in these decades (Finer, 1952, pp. 23–24). Farr would raise it as well, most often in the 1850s and 1860s, pointing out that the plants and animals on which humans depend also multiply geometrically and that human ingenuity and art amplify this productivity still further (Farr, 1875a, pp. XV–XVI, XX; Farr, 1868–69, p. 210). Farr offered an additional objection, however, by challenging Malthus's assumption that humans, like rabbits, reproduce without regard to the consequences. In the Registrar-General's fourth annual report, which appeared in 1842, Farr used the early results of civil registration to demonstrate not only that was it possible for the mass of the population to limit their reproduction but that in England population growth was already under such human control; thus Malthusian positive checks were not necessary (Farr, 1842, pp. 133–142 [85–90]). Specifically using the marriage and birth registration for 1839 through 1841, Farr showed that although women were capable of producing children from at least the age of 16 or 17, the average age of first marriage in England was 24 for women and 25 for men. Moreover, the registration records showed that a full 21% of women and 22% of men who reach the mean age of marriage never marry, and that in the years 1839–41 only one in seven women of childbearing age produced a child annually.

My claims for Edmonds's seminal influence on vital statistics are based on a book he published in 1832 and on his series of 22 articles that appeared in the *Lancet*, 15 of these between 1835 and 1839. His book, "*Life tables founded upon the discovery of a numerical law regulating the existence of every human being*" (Edmonds, 1832b), demonstrated that according to the best available data human mortality varied in geometrical series in three periods of life which he call infancy; manhood, florescence, or the period of procreative power; and old age or senescence (Edmonds, 1834–35a, p. 6; Edmonds, 1855, p. 128). In the first period mortality fell each year of life by 32.4%; in the second it increased each year by 2.99%; and in the final period of life it increased annually by 7.97% (Edmonds, 1832b, pp. V–VII). Edmonds held that this was a universal law of human existence. The exact ages dividing the three periods of life and the absolute rate of mortality might vary from people to people or from one historic period to another, but the pattern of change was innate to the human constitution. Edmonds demonstrated how one could use this law of mortality to construct theoretical or model life tables. He assumed a minimum mortality and the age limits of his three periods of life, and computed for each year of life a mortality rate from which he could calculate the number remaining alive at each age. Using this technique he produced three tables, his *"Mean, village, and city mortality tables"* that agreed quite well with the best available tables compiled from observation (Edmonds, 1832b, pp. XVIII–XIX).

Edmonds was certainly not the first to recognise that human mortality varied regularly with age. He mentioned that Richard Price had observed this general pattern. He failed, however, to properly acknowledge that in 1825 Benjamin Gompertz had published a mathematically equivalent law of human mortality in the *Philosophical Transactions* (Gompertz, 1825). This overreaching did not go unnoticed, nor was it forgotten. Years later, when Edmonds was proposed for fellowship in the Royal Society of London, his claims for discovery were contested, and his failure to prove that his law was different from Gompertz's in the ensuing dispute cost him a fellowship (De Morgan, 1860–61a; De Morgan, 1860–61b; De Morgan, 1861–62; Edmonds, 1859; Edmonds, 1860; Edmonds, 1860–61a; Edmonds, 1860–61b; Edmonds, 1861–62; Sprague, 1861–62). The editor of the Assurance Magazine, who had presided over this personally bitter controversy probably got it about right, when he observed that Edmonds's law was merely Gompertz's in a slight different form but that Edmonds had applied the law with "great ingenuity, neatness, and effect" (Anonymous, 1861).

Edmonds's historic importance does in fact reside in the applications he found for the law of mortality and particularly in the efforts he made to interest the medical profession in the uses of vital statistics. His series of articles in the Lancet was occasioned by the publication of the 1831 census. Much to Edmonds's disgust this enumeration did not collect information on the ages of the living, but that information was available from the 1821 census. The enumeration of 1831 did elicit information from the parish registers on the ages of the dying for the years 1813–1830. Now for the first time life tables for the general population of the entire nation or for geographical regions could be computed with the requisite information, the ages of the dying and the number of individuals at risk at each age of life (Edmonds, 1835–36a, pp. 365–367, 368–369; Edmonds, 1835–36d, p. 690). Edmonds lost no time in demonstrating that his law of mortality applied to life tables computed from these national data, and he made the important discovery that infant mortality was actually much lower than had been previously assumed (Edmonds, 1834–35b).

In these early articles in the Lancet Edmonds presented the law of mortality as a fundamental tool of social and medical analysis. He not only repeated in less technical language the explanations he had offered in his book "*Life tables*" of how the law could be used to construct accurate life tables, but he argued that the collective vitality these tables reflected was the only accurate measure of public health and medical progress (Edmonds, 1834–35a, p. 5). Age-specific mortality was a test of general health and well-being. To demonstrate he constructed tables using his law of mortality for each county of England and for six large towns and displayed in tables age group mortality rates by gender for each locality (Edmonds, 1835–36a). He considered adult female mortality the best sanitary criterion, since it eliminated occupational hazards outside the home. There was great variation in this mortality. Some counties had double the rate experienced by others. When Edmonds arranged the counties of England in groups according to female mortality ages 15 to 30, he found that a line of high mortality extended from Brighton northwest to Liverpool and that the counties with the lowest mortality were furthest from this line (Edmonds, 1835–36a, p. 411). This sort of sanitary topography would be developed much further and with greater emphasis on urban mortality by William Farr at the General Register Office.

Using the very limited data available in the middle 1830s, Edmonds also applied his law to sickness. Using data published by the Highland Society of Scotland on its members and by the Society for the Diffusion of Useful Knowledge on the experience of English mutual benefit societies, Edmonds concluded that the law of mortality applied to human sickness as well (Edmonds, 1835–36b). Specifically he found that the number of persons constantly sick in a population changed with age in the same way that mortality did. This fact suggested that there should be a fixed ratio between morbidity and mortality, so that if one knew the mortality for an area, one should be able to compute the number constantly sick. Edmonds went even further. Employing data Thomas Southwood Smith had published on 6000 cases at the London Fever Hospital between 1824 and 1834 and returns for the London Hospital made to Parliament for 13000 cases during the six years ending in 1833, Edmonds demonstrated that in at least these instances the law of mortality also described case fatality (Edmonds, 1835–36b, pp. 857–858; Edmonds, 1835–36e). He was convinced that the law applied to other human disease as well. If this were the case, the methods used to assess the value of therapy must change. Since case fatality varied with age, claims for effectiveness of therapy based on the numbers of recoveries or deaths without regard to age of patients were invalid (Edmonds, 1835–36e, p. 778). Edmonds challenged medical men to take this investigation further.

Farr was impressed with Edmonds's papers and he made good use of Edmonds's findings. In 1836 and 1837 he published two articles by Edmonds in the British Medical Almanack, and in his own chapter in John Ramsay McCulloch's "Statistical account of the British Empire", a chapter that appeared in 1837 and helped establish Farr as an authority on vital statistics in his own right, Farr made good use of Edmonds's articles in the Lancet (Edmonds, 1836; Edmonds, 1837; Farr, 1837f, pp. 568–572, 585). Farr also took up Edmonds's challenge to study the law of sickness.

Using clinical records from the London Smallpox Hospital, Farr published three articles in 1837 and 1838 in the periodicals he edited on the law of sickness in smallpox (Farr, 1837a; Farr, 1837b, pp. 134–143; Farr, Part II). These not only confirmed that the law of mortality described the change in case fatality with age in smallpox as Edmonds had predicted, but they also displayed what Farr called sickness tables for smallpox which showed for an initial group of 100 000 cases the number sick, the number recovering, and the number dying in five-day periods during the disease. This sickness or survivorship table was analogous to a life table, and Farr showed how the rates of recovery or dying varied for separate periods of the disease in geometrical series. The exercise provided further demonstration that vital processes were law abiding, and it suggested to Farr that the construction of sickness tables, "nosometry" in his parlance, could be used to judge therapeutic effectiveness (Farr, 1837a, p. 73).

Although Farr repeated the latter claim as late as 1862 before the British Medical Association (1962), it was in matters of public health that his debt to Edmonds is most obvious. In this work Farr had great advantages over Edmonds. In 1839 he became compiler of abstracts at the newly-created General Register Office, a minor clerical post that he would turn into a much more important position than its creators could possibly have imagined. He suddenly had at his disposal an unprecedented quantity of vital data in a continuous series for the entire population created by the system of vital registration that had gone into effect in 1837, and he had the unique opportunity of establishing the system in which it would be organised and used.

Edmonds's intellectual legacy can best be seen in three aspects of Farr's work. First and most explicit is Farr's use of life tables. Like Edmonds he constructed life tables for the entire population from public vital data. During his career Farr would compile three national life tables. The first of these is the only one we can consider here. It appeared in the Registrar-General's fifth and sixth annual reports and was based on the deaths registered in 1841 and on the 1841 census (Farr, 1844; Farr, 1839). Farr could have computed the entries for this table at each age directly from census and registration records, but such a procedure would have required enormous labour and been subject to all the inaccuracies and omissions of the raw data at his disposal. He instead used a method of interpolation which he acknowledged was suggested by the law of mortality first described by Gompertz and independently discovered by Edmonds (Farr, 1843b, pp. 345–346). Farr proceeded by calculating mortality at selected ages, and assuming that mortality varied with age in three geometric series as the law of mortality suggested, found the probability of living one more year at each age, and then the number living at each age (Eyler, 1979, pp. 77–80). Farr saw the life table as a tool of the widest possible application, and he computed life tables using similar techniques for local areas and for different occupational groups. Life table analysis suggested other techniques to Farr was well: the sickness tables that we have already noticed, a fertility table for English women, a table to describe the life time of English government ministries, and a table to describe promotions in the army and civil service (Eyler, 1979, pp. 80–84, 133–135).

The second way in which Farr followed Edmonds was in his use of mortality as a measure of health. Edmonds first measured the healthiness of places by comparing age group mortality rates for entire English counties and began to construct a topography of health for the nation. Over the course of his career, Farr would carry this goal to a high level of development. But let us here consider how he dealt with the problem at the beginning of his career, in his reports to the Registrar-General which appeared between 1839 and 1843 (Farr, 1839; Farr, 1840a; Farr, 1841a). Much more than Edmonds, Farr had the particular goal of demonstrating how conditions in large towns undermined human health, and he proposed to do that by comparing the mortality of urban with rural areas. In the first three reports he merely compared total mortality and mortality rates for particular causes of death for two pairs of districts, one composed of urban areas and the other of rural. The districts in each pair had approximately equal population. The comparison demonstrated a dramatic increase in the burden of mortality in towns, and it suggested that the epidemic, endemic, and contagious diseases, the diseases Farr labelled "zymotic", were largely responsible. But this comparison was subject to the objection that the age structures of the urban and rural populations were not the same, and since mortality varied with age, a direct comparison of mortality was subject to error. With the 1841 census enumeration and the preparation of his first national life table Farr was prepared to tackle this problem. He did so in the fifth annual report where he presented not only life tables for the nation, but local tables chosen to represent the spectrum of national mortality experience: the rural areas of Surrey, the Metropolis, and Liverpool. Using these four life tables he could compare age-specific mortality rates and life expectancies, and he drew survivorship diagrams which dramatically illustrated how a population cohort dwindled with the passage of years in each place (Farr, 1843c; Eyler, 1979, pp. 131–136). This analysis suggests the direction Farr's investigations would take him. By the middle 1850s Farr had a model healthy population to serve as a standard, his Healthy Districts, the districts having crude annual death rates of 17 per 1000 or fewer. He would eventually publish a life table for the Healthy Districts, but even before he did so, he had begun to compute age-specific mortality rates for the healthy districts and to use those rates to calculate the excess mortality in other districts (Farr, 1859a; Farr, 1859b). Such mortality comparisons form the basis of Farr's famous decennial supplements to the Registrar-General's 25th and 35th annual reports which were published in 1865 and 1875 (Farr, 1865; Farr, 1875a). In these magnificent reports he made ample use of life tables for standard populations and of age-standardised mortality rates. The analysis in these reports is a long way from the simple comparisons Edmonds had offered, but the trajectory leading to these sophisticated studies of Farr begins in Edmonds's articles in the Lancet in the 1830s.

Third and finally we can find the origins of Farr's idea of a statistical law in these publications of Edmonds. The law of mortality provided confirmation for these two young men that vital phenomena could be described in mathematical terms and that the discovery of mathematical regularities in sickness and death would have great utility. Such a law also defined for Farr the goal of statistical analysis. Farr constantly tried to demonstrate mathematical regularities in the data he collected, and over the course of his career he announced statistical laws of several sorts. Some described the changes in the probability of recovery or death during illness. We have noticed that his first statistical law, the law of recovery and death in smallpox, was of this sort. About the same time he announced another such law for recoveries and deaths among the institutionalised insane (Farr, 1837c; Farr, 1837e; Farr, 1841b). Others described the course of an epidemic over time. An early one allowed him to describe and to predict the future course of an epidemic of smallpox in 1840; another in mid-career did the same for the cattle plague in 1866 (Farr, 1840b; Farr, 1866). A third sort of statistical law described how mortality varied under the influence of changing environmental conditions. His elevation law for cholera described elsewhere in this volume is a good example (Eyler, Part II). Others are the two laws relating human mortality to population density that Farr announced, one early in his career and another shortly before he retired (Farr, 1843a, pp. 207–210 [419–26]; Anonymous, 1873; Farr, 1878–79; Farr 1878). The longevity of his interest in his density laws and the elaborate efforts he made to save the elevation law for cholera, even after his understanding of the transmission of cholera had changed, speak volumes for his belief in the importance of these statistical laws. For him, as for Edmonds, the laws were simple algebraic expressions that permitted him to generate a series of numbers that agreed with the observed series. As Edmonds had done, he presented them side by side to demonstrate the law. Mathematically simple though they might be, these laws confirmed for Victorian statisticians that vital phenomena were orderly and law abiding and that human health, no less than the subject matter of astronomy or physics was open to mathematical analysis. Such analysis, Farr believed, must precede any effective intervention.

Appendix

A note on sources

Farr's annual letter in the *"Annual Report of the Registrar-General of Births, Deaths, and Marriages in England and Wales"* is cited as Farr, *"Letter, nth A.R.R.G"*. This important source was reprinted in the British Parliamentary Papers, here abbreviated as *"B.P.P."* In some years the pagination differed between the separately published version and the version in the Parliamentary Papers. The version in *"B.P.P."* is cited, but when the pagination differs, the page number in the separately published version is given in brackets.

"On Prognosis"
(British Medical Almanack 1838; Supplement 199–216)

William Farr

Typed and edited by Gerry Bernard Hill

263, Chelsea Road, Kingston, Ontario K7M 3Z3, Canada

"On Prognosis" by William Farr

Prognosis, from πρω, before, and γνωσις, (γνοω know), knowledge, is literally translated by foreknowledge. Foretelling presupposes fore-knowledge; and prognosis is employed, in medicine, to designate the art of fore-seeing and foretelling the course and issue of diseases. It implies that vital phenomena succeed each other in a determined order; and that when one of a series is observed the existence of others may be inferred. The fundamental problem in medical prognosis is, from a given group of morbid phenomena, to determine the phenomena that will follow or that have preceded, and their mutual relations. The etymology restricts the application of prognosis to the future, but the idea of futurity is accessory. Hippocrates, in the second sentence of Prognostics, speaks of *predicting* "things present, things *past*, and things to come;" so that prognosis, in the etymological sense, is but a part of the subject. So important, however, is a knowledge of the future; so much more precious the power of foreseeing the events unaccomplished and controllable, than of telling things past and irremediable, that the emphatic term prognosis may still be employed, with the qualification that it shall include the science of the laws of succession of all morbid phenomena, whether regarded as past, present, or future.

Every medical man should be well versed in prognosis. It will enable him to take into consideration the subsequent phases of the malady, and rescue him from the system of expediency, where every symptom is treated as an isolated fact, and, according to the urgency of immediate circumstances, without regard to the subsequent states through which the patient must inevitably pass; while diseases often require to be treated, in the early stages, for phenomena not developed, and only acquiring intensity at a future period. This is the case with phthisis, the exanthemata, and fevers. An accurate prognosis in such cases gives the physician the advantages a general possesses, well informed beforehand of the enemy's forces, plans of battle, and order of attack. Hippocrates does not forget to enumerate one advantage of prognosis, which savours of the Greek cunning, the father of medicine sometimes discloses in turning the prejudices of his patients to account:

> *"By telling," he remarks, "the past, present, future, and recalling things the patient forgets, you gain his confidence, he places full reliance on your skill, and dares commit himself into your hands unreservedly. To cure all the sick is impossible; to predict which patients will die, which will recover, will screen the practitioner from blame."*

This is founded on a well-ascertained prejudice. Great credit is often gained by predicting the death of a patient where the bystanders perceive no danger. Nothing more forcibly impresses the minds of the common people; who have always treated their historians with calm indifference, their prophets with admiration and worship. It is, nevertheless, rare that the physician has to perform this mournful function, and to prophesy death. There is almost always a chance, and generally a strong probability of recovery. Nine times in ten he is the messenger of glad tidings; and it is seldom that he cannot point out some dawn of hope – some streak of light – when the horizon is darkest.

The reduction of the phenomena of disease to simple laws, susceptible of calculation, offers the same attraction as other fields of investigation; but its intimate connexion with human interests and sufferings gives it stronger claims on attention. To lessen the danger and duration of disease is the main object of medical science; this is the public function intrusted to the medical profession; but the laws of disease, the degree of danger, the extent and duration of morbid processes, must be determined before the relative value of remedial agents can be ascertained. Prognosis, then, naturally precedes Therapeutics in the order of study, and is preceded by Diagnosis. Many pretend to treat disease successfully with a very imperfect knowledge of prognosis; and to predict the death of patients without an accurate knowledge of the seat or nature of maladies. Nurses and empirics, with and without licences, are examples of these short-hand intellects.

In prognosis patients may be considered in two lights: in collective masses, when general results can be predicted with certainty; or separately, when the question becomes one of probability. If 7000 of 10000 cases of fever terminate fatally, it may be predicted that the same proportion will die in another series of cases; and experience has proved that the prediction will be verified, or so nearly verified as to leave no room for cavil or scepticism. The recovery or death of one of the cases is a mere matter of probability. Here, as Celsus has said, *medicina ars conjecturalis est*; but not in the shallow sense some persons imagine, that everything is at random in individual cases; for if medicine be guessing, it is at least the *Art of guessing*. The rate of mortality determined for 10000 cases applies, as a general standard, to each patient ; and the probability of death is 0.07, of recovery 0.93; the probability that the fever patient will recover is 93 to 7, raised or lowered by particular circumstances. This distinction applies to the prediction of all organic changes: collectively they can be predicted, where data exist, with certainty; individually their probability can be determined.

Prognosis may be extended to every kind of morbid phenomena; but, practically, it can only be applied, at present, to events of decided importance. The following are examples of several kinds of prognosis. Recovery may be predicted in cholera, fever, confluent smallpox, pneumonia, all acute diseases; for the general chances of recovery (at least under the age of 40) are equal to the chances of dying in these diseases; and generally as 2, 3, 4, and even 14 to 1. Death may be predicted in rupture of the intestine, phthisis, lumbar abscess. The probability of other diseases being developed in the course of the first may be determined: thus, local inflammations supervene in chronic diseases and fevers; perforation of the ileum occurs a certain number of times in the latter stages of typhus, of the pleura in pulmonary phthisis, and nearly always proves fatal. Haemoptysis is generally followed by phthisis; the pulmonary symptoms of phthisis by ulceration of Peyer's glands. Tubercular cachexia is the forerunner of phthisis (Clark). Dyspnoea from infancy, and clear sounding projections upon the chest, and over the clavicle, imply the existence of emphysema; whence may be predicted paroxysms of asthma, dilatation of the heart, oedema. Sometimes the recurrence of the same disease may be prognosticated; of epilepsy, insanity, apoplexy, catarrh, rheumatism, intermittent fever. The same method is applicable to these and other cases of the same kind; and to the whole facts included in the prognosis.

In prognosis (1) the patient may be considered, (2) the circumstances in which he is placed, and (3) the disease. The age, sex, temperament, habits, strength, intellect, passions, fall under the first head.

a. The patient

Age. It had long been observed that the rate of mortality is high in infancy, that it declines to the age of puberty, then increases, and in old age proceeds with increasing rapidity. Mr. Edmonds discovered the law regulating the mortality of the general population at all ages; he found that the mortality increased from puberty 3 per cent every year[1] up to 50–60; and 8 per cent afterwards annually up to the end of life. Dr. Southwood Smith gave in his excellent book the *Philosophy of Health*, a column of the mortality at different ages in cases of fever treated in the *London Fever Hospital*; but Mr. Finlainson by whom the calculation was made, withheld the data on which it was founded, merely stating that the observation comprehended 6000 cases. Mr. Edmonds proved that the rate of mortality in Dr. Smith's observation increased 34 per cent every ten years, (3 per cent annually) and also that the same law applied to sickness, and cases observed in the London Hospital.[2] From facts published by the

---

[1] Life Tables 1832. Supplement to British Medical Almanack 1837, page 130.
[2] Lancet, Feb. 27th and Sept. 3rd. 1836. British Medical Almanack 1837, page 138.

Factory Commissioners, I showed that among 2934 labourers in the East India Company's service, and persons employed in Factories, the attacks were nearly the same at all ages; and that the fatality of cases and the quantity of sickness, increased with age nearly at the same rate.[3] But as all the data were not given, or given in an unsatisfactory form, the value of these observations was much diminished.

In the spring of 1836, I collected, by the kind permission of Dr. Gregory, Physician to the London *Small Pox Hospital*, a series of 7851 cases, 2176 deaths of Small Pox, at every consecutive five years of age; a greater number of deaths than had entered into the previous observations. The facts are here given in detail; they have been carefully recorded by the officers of the institution; and though I went over the books but once, and the columns of deaths is far removed from the ages, there is probably no error of any consequence to the results. Two periods were taken: the first (20 years 1780–99) before vaccination had had any influence, the second embracing the 10 years ending in 1835.

The mortality of cases, at the age 0–5 years, was 41.97 per cent; it declined 19.12, and rose till at 50 and upwards it was 79.41. The minimum was attained at 10–15, at 12^1/$_2$ years of age – when the probability of recovery was 4 to 1; the probability of recovery was reduced to 2 to 1 at the age 20–30; to 1 to 4 after the age of 50. The fa-

Of 7850 cases of Small Pox, and 2475 Deaths at every five years of Age

Age	Cases				Deaths			
	1780–89	1790–99	1826–35	Total	1780–89	1790–99	1826–35	Total
0–5	0	16	240	256	0	1	104	105
5–10	43	37	184	264	9	10	45	64
10–15	258	169	190	617	40	41	37	118
15–20	871	766	666	2303	223	210	129	562
20–25	1083	870	812	2765	419	295	207	921
25–30	363	276	332	971	159	98	95	352
30–35	156	90	92	338	72	44	41	157
35–40	55	29	40	124	28	11	19	58
40–45	47	29	15	91	|	|	|	|
45–50	28	18	7	53	46	24	14	84
					|	|	|	|
50–	35	26	4	68	29	21	4	54
All Ages	2939	2329	2582	7850	1025	755	695	2475

---

[3] Macculloch's Statistics of the British Empire, Art. Vital Statistics, vol. ii, page 576.

Deaths in 100 cases of Small Pox at eight different ages

Age	Deaths per cent	Age	Deaths per cent
0–5	41.97[4]	30–40	46.54
5–10	24.24	40–50	58.33
10–15	19.12	50–	79.41
15–20	24.40	All Ages	31.53
20–30	34.07		

tality of the cases, beginning at puberty, (10–20), increased at rates very nearly represented by 34 per cent; as will be apparent on comparing the mortality observed every 10 consecutive years, with the mortality calculated from one basis. Some of the calculated numbers, that advance regularly, are above, others below the numbers directly observed.[5]

[Small Pox Hospital Data]*

	Age 10–20	20–30	30–40	40–50	50–
Deaths per cent (observed)	23.29	34.07	46.54	58.33	79.41
Deaths per cent (calculated)	24.66	33.12	44.46	59.70	80.11

The application of this principle to practice is very obvious: small pox is dangerous in infancy; safest at puberty; and from that age the danger increases *one-third every ten years*. Sydenham says, "that persons in the prime of life are in greater danger in smallpox, than women or children under fourteen."[6] This is all an observer so accurate could detect by the old methods of investigation.

The influence of age upon the mortality in *Cholera*, is exhibited in the following extensive series of observations, published from official Reports in the Austrian Medical Journal. The Reports were by Dr. J. Knoltz.[7]

---

* Titles in brackets have been added.
[4] (ed.) Should be 105: 256 = 41.02.
[5] To obtain the 5 calculated numbers, multiply 24.66 (λ1.3920) and every successive number produced by 1.343 (λ0.128). (ed.) λ denotes logarithm to base 10.
[6] Works, vol. 2, page 53. Edition, Wallis, 1788.
[7] Einige Notizen über die Brechdurchfall's Epidemie in Wien und auf dem platten Lande von Nieder Oesterreich in dem Jahre, 1831/2 betreffend. Aus dem Sanitäts Berichte des H. Dr. J. J. Knoltz. The mortality of Cholera was lower at all ages in the country (platten Lande) than in the city of Vienna: at the age 20–30 the mortality from Cholera (city and country 34.62) was scarcely greater than the mortality of smallpox in London (34.07 per cent).

Table showing the Deaths per cent and the Cases and Deaths of Cholera at eight different ages in Vienna and the country round in Lower Austria

Age	in Vienna			in the country		
	Cases	Deaths	Deaths per cent	Deaths per cent	Deaths	Cases
0–10	327	174	53.21	41.87	206	492
10–20	478	188	39.33	38.66	196	507
20–30	837	317	37.87	31.81	307	965
30–40	801	356	44.45	34.49	219	635
40–50	690	363	52.61	40.71	208	511
50–60	635	370	58.27	43.27	167	386
60–70	374	249	66.43	49.35	113	229
70–	220	171	77.73	52.00	65	125
All Ages	4360	2188	49.02	38.46	1481	3848

There are two anomalies in these observations; the mortality attains its minimum at the age 20–30; and it does not increase so fast as in other observations. The rate of increase every ten years is 16 per cent; and 1.1596 ($\lambda 0.06245$)[8] has been used to calculate the subjoined series of numbers running parallel with the facts observed.

Vienna

	Age 20–30	30–40	40–50	50–60	60–70	70–
Deaths per cent (observed)	37.87	44.45	52.61	58.27	66.43	77.73
Deaths per cent (calculated)	37.87	43.73	50.49	58.30	67.32	77.73

The rate of increase is nearly the square root of the rate regulating the mortality of small-pox and other diseases ($1.16 \times 1.16 = 1.3456$). But it would be unsafe to speculate on this isolated fact, unless the mode in which the observations were made had been detailed, in the Austrian report, with less official brevity. There has been everywhere a culpable disposition to deny the name of cholera to all cases not absolutely fatal; and so much dreaded the exaggerating the effects of treatment as to falsify science. This falsehood, like falsehood of every species, defeats its purpose. While

---

[8] (ed) λ denotes logarithm to base 10.

it diminished the number of cases of cholera, it augmented the mortality, the opprobrium of medical art, and the terror it was intended to allay. Is it not a fact that where the mortality was 49 per cent the severer cases only were reported, and that milder cases, a majority of which occur in early life, were excluded? This would diminish the number of favourable cases at 10–20, 20–30, and make the apparent rate of dying increase less rapidly with age.

Age appears to have the same influence on the duration of diseases as on the mortality ; cases become one third longer every ten years from puberty.[9] There is a certain class of diseases, of long duration, deemed incurable, where the morbid process only ends with life. The problem in prognosis is to determine the probability of cure; in a given time this diminishes 34 per cent every ten years, as I have ascertained from observations collected at Bethlem, by Dr. Haslam, in 1784–94[10]. Cases 1664, cured at all ages, 574.

Recoveries from Insanity

	Age	10–20	20–30	30–40	40–50	50–60	60–70
Recoveries per cent							
observed			29.0	41.0	34.2	24.0	17.5	12.9
calculated			56.9	42.3	31.5	23.4	17.5	13.0

The patients remained at Bethlem rather more than a year; this observation, therefore, shows the relative number of recoveries, at different ages, in a unit of time – in this instance, nearly a year. From the data preceding two principles may be established: (1) The rate of recovery in a unit of time diminishes 34 per cent every ten years; (2) The mean rate of dying per unit of sick time is the same at all ages. Future observation must show whether these are laws, or isolated facts.

There are few observations of sufficient extent and accuracy to show the influence of the patient's temperament, constitution, habits, &c, on the issue of diseases; and it would be useless to detail our empirical knowledge on these subjects. The mortality of cases in females is less than the mortality in males. This is established by many facts. The following is from an interesting pamphlet by Dr. R. Cowan:[11]

---

[9] See "British Medical Almanack" 1837, page 136. "Macculloch's Statistics of the British Empire." Article "Vital Statistics", page 284.
[10] See the facts in "Statistics of English Lunatic Asylums," by W. Farr.
[11] Statistics of Fever and Small Pox in Glasgow, April 28th, 1837.

Oct. 1835–6. – Fever Patients in the Glasgow Fever Hospital

	Cases	Deaths	Deaths per cent
Males	1116	180	16.1
Females	1141	110	9.6

b. External Circumstances

The influence of external circumstances and applications on the issue of diseases is unquestionable; on another occasion I will endeavour to ascertain how much residence in cities and crowded hospitals, exposure to cold and want increase the danger of disease; how much drugs and medicines diminish the mortality. The seasons do not appear to modify the mortality of small pox to any extent.

London Small Pox Hospital, 1780–9. Cases admitted, 2952, – Deaths, 1034

Months	Temperature	Dryness (Daniel)	Cases admitted	Deaths	Deaths per cent
Dec-Jan-Feb	38°	2°.2	760	266	35.0
Jun-Jul-Aug	60°	6°.9	814	271	33.3
Mar-Apr-May	49°	6°.4	634	227	35.8
Sep-Oct-Nov	50°	4°.0	744	270	36.3

c. Diseases

The *third head* of this inquiry is the most important: it does not refer to the previous state of the patient, or accessory circumstances, but to the type and course of diseases.

In fact, the first step in prognosis is generally to determine whether the individual is ill, and what is the nature of the malady; for the fate of the patient depends upon his actual state; and the probability of recovery is often regulated by the probability and accuracy of diagnosis. Thus, to distinguish some malignant tumours, tubercles in the lungs, ischuria renalis, from other types of disease, is the principal element, in such cases, of prognosis; for these diseases are fatal, while those with which they may be confounded are attended with little danger.

It is to be regretted that the relative mortality of different diseases is still unknown. To determine the mortality of diseases they should be followed from the beginning to the end; every death or recovery should be recorded; and this, though exceedingly simple, has been rarely done. The mortality of cases can only be accurately ascertained by practitioners, who see cases as they occur, slight or severe, and seldom lose sight of them to the end.

Diseases may be examined (1) in their tendency to destroy life, expressed by the deaths out of a given number of cases; and (2) in their mean relative force of mortality, expressed by the deaths out of a given number sick at a given time. The following observations illustrate the mortality of different diseases. They are from the Austrian official returns of epidemic diseases in Lower Austria, Austria on the Ems, Bohemia; and include 4–6 epidemics of each disease occurring between 1826 and 1832. The cholera in Galicia was the epidemic of 1831.[12]

	Cases	Deaths	Deaths per cent
Cholera (Galicia)	255774	96081	37.6
Fever (catarrhal, nervous, typhus)	1273	143	11.2
Dysentery	3961	418	10.8
Small-pox	14804	1588	10.7
Scarlet fever	2422	211	8.7
Hooping cough	8007	533	6.7
Measles	14051	327	2.3

Hence it appears that the probability of recovery from measles is as 97.7 to 2.3 (42 to 1); and that the chance of dying is three times greater in hooping cough, four times in scarlet fever, five times in fever.

The mortality in the *London Small Pox Hospital* in the fifty-six years from 1780 to 1835 has been deduced from a statement of the annual mortality published by Dr. Gregory:

Years	Cases	Deaths	Deaths per cent
1780–9	2954	1031	34.90
1790–9	2322	763	32.86
1800–9	1574	478	30.37
1810–9	1188	357	30.05
1820–9	2225	658	29.57
1830–4	1590	388	24.40
1780–834	11853	3675	30.99

---

[12] Medicinischer Jahrbucher, &c., vols. 3–10; observers Knoltz, Von Nadherzy Streintz, Slawikowski.

The decrease of mortality is due to the admission of a greater number of cases occurring after vaccination. In the ten years 1826–35, when 2593 cases were treated, 693 died = 26.73 per cent. 2264 of the cases distributed according to their character show that the mortality of cases where vaccination had not preceded still remained unabated.

[Small Pox Hospital Data]

	Cases	Deaths	Deaths per cent
Not vaccinated	1393	571	41.1
Vaccinated	789	46	5.8
Inoculated	9	2	
Other diseases	73	1	

This is the mortality of small-pox in cities; in the country it is lower, as will be perceived from the Austrian return. It is probable, also, that the proportion of persons vaccinated is greater in Austria, where the Vaccine Establishment is efficient. In the General Hospital of Vienna, 1834, 533 cases of varicella were treated, and 469 of variola. Of the latter, 82 of 160 not vaccinated died (0.51); 40 of 109 that had doubtful marks of vaccination (0.37); 25 of 200 vaccinated (0.125). Six of the 25 had putrid fever; 9 died of puerperal fever.

To determine the mortality of all attacks of sickness taken indiscriminately, army records furnish valuable data; for every case under the care of the Surgeon is entered, and followed to recovery, but not always to death, in chronic cases, as a certain number are invalided.

Cases treated in the whole of the Prussian standing-army, whether in or out of the Military Hospitals:[13]

Years	Total cases discharged	Cured	Died	Invalided	Missing
1821–30	1160719	1143081	12310	4571	157
Proportions	100	98.535	1.061	0.394	0.013
1831–2	550161	540611	7719	1725	76
Proportions	100	98.269	1.403	0.314	0.014

---

[13] Rust's *Magazin für die Heilkunde*, vols. 14–39.

The mortality computed on more than a *million* cases was 1.061 per cent, to which some of the invalided cases should be added. In the 2 years (1831–2) when cholera prevailed, the mortality of cases was raised 32 per cent. The Prussian soldiers are, on average, 20–25 years of age; they remain about 3 years in the service; their numbers in 1826 were estimated at 100000. If the mortality of patients at the age 20–25 is 1.061, the mortality at 50–55 should be 2.57 per cent. Attacks of diseases differ in intensity; some are so slight as to obtain no attention; for others, men consent to take physic; a third class incapacitates them for exertion. Itch, cutaneous and other slight diseases, run up the amount of cases in armies; syphilis constitutes perhaps 20 per cent of the attacks. This class of cases, and injuries got in quarrels, are not recognised by Friendly Societies; and medicine is taken in many cases that never fall "on the box," as the patients continue their employment. At the Liverpool Friendly Society this is clearly exemplified, where there were (1829–37) members equivalent to 23323 living 1 year; and 20251 entitled to relief.[14] The mortality of cases that fell on the box was 3.7 per cent; of the cases attended by surgeons 2.4 per cent; for only 40 applications for sick pay were made annually by 32 of 100 members, while 75 cases to every 100 members were attended by the surgeons, 28 at home, 47 at the surgeries.

The relative *force of mortality* is an unusual term; but it implies the rate of dying – the number deaths out of a given number, living a given time – and is required by the present state of science. The force of mortality in Sweden was 2282 this was the number of deaths out of 100 living a year – the assumed unity of time. Every population comprises two classes, the healthy and the sick; and it has been found that among adults there are two years of sick time to every death; in other words, that in a society where 1 dies annually 2 are constantly incapacitated by sickness. In Sweden, therefore, 4564 in 100 of the population constitute the sick, 95436 the healthy population. The deaths occur in the sick population; so the mean force of mortality may be taken at 0.50; of 100 living and sick 50 die annually. This is the average force of mortality in all kinds of sickness. Among the East India Company's labourers (= 20343 years of life) there were 328 years of sickness, and 973.5 years on the pension list; in the former 496, in the latter 161, deaths occurred.

Sick time 1391 years, deaths 657; annual deaths per cent 50.6.

The Liverpool Friendly Society [15]

Received sick pay 1 year 613; deaths 356; annual deaths per cent 58.1. On surgeons' books 1 yr. 912; deaths 408; annual deaths per cent 44.7.

---

[14] From a valuable return by J. Garthside, Esq. that shall be inserted entire in this or a future Almanack.

[15] The total deaths were 408, but 26 occurred in the half year after admission before the members could receive sick pay, which they were only entitled to in two months; as a correction, 52 deaths were deducted.

Prussian Army

	Years sickness	Ann. deaths per cent	Ann. invalids per cent
1821–30 (11 enumerations)	44810	27.47	10.2
1831–2 (3 enumerations)	18820	41.02	9.2

Assuming the mean strength of the Prussian army to be 100000, it follows that, in 1821–30, there were 0.015, in 1831–2 more than 0.18 constantly sick; that the absolute mortality was 1.23 in the first, 3.5 in the second period. The annual mortality among men, of every shade of sickness, was only 27.47 per cent.

In determining the relative force of mortality in different diseases, the same method is to be observed; the deaths must be divided by the sick time. As an illustration, it will be seen in the annexed table that 990 deaths occurred in a mean constant population of 41 individuals suffering from cholera. In a Cholera Hospital, containing 100 patients, on an average 2415 deaths would occur in the year. The second column, intended to represent the mean sickness from each particular disease, is the sum of the numbers *remaining* on December 31, 1826, 1827, 1828, 1829. To have made the numbers accurate, monthly enumerations should have been obtained of the numbers sick from each disease.

The table is deduced from a return given by Mr. H. Marshall, in the "Edinburgh Medical and Surgical Journal"[16], of the sickness among 69850 native troops in the Madras army. It must be considered rather an illustration than an accurate view of the facts. The relative force of mortality did not differ widely from that prevailing among the sick European troops, although the annual mortality was 0.048 of the strength among the latter, 0.014 among the former; and the constantly sick among the native troops was 0.0334; among the English troops, 0.0924. The last column but one shows the relative force of mortality in different diseases; cholera and apoplexy are at the top, syphilis is at the bottom of the scale. The *mortality* and the *force of mortality* will readily be distinguished, by comparing cholera with consumption; the *mortality* in the latter is 90–100 per cent, but its mean duration is two years, and the *force of mortality* is consequently nearly 0.50; the mortality in cholera is not 50 per cent, while the force of mortality is 2415, for cholera destroys in a week as many as phthisis consumes in a year. Phthisis is more dangerous than cholera; but cholera, probably, excites the greatest terror.

The form as well as the nature of diseases must be taken into account, in estimating the degree of danger. Thus, at the Small Pox Hospital, (1836) 81 of 205 conflu-

---

[16] Vol. XXXIX., pp. 124, 135.

Table of Sickness among the Native Troops of the Madras Army

	Cases	Sick a year	Die	Deaths in 100 cases	Deaths in 100 sick a year	Mean duration of cases in days
	[a]	[b]	[c]	[d]	[e]	[f]
Cholera	2142	41	990	46.2	2415	7
Apoplexy	76	3	51	67.0	1700	14
Dysentery	2285	136	198	8.7	146	22
Fever remittent	5067	185	244	4.8	132	13
continued	2627	71	73	2.8	101	10
intermittent	36436	1658	426	1.2	26	17
External inflammations	10803	381	52	0.5	17	13
Rheumatism	16387	1624	239	1.6	15	36
Ulcers	16482	1918	203	1.2	11	43
Syphilis	8668	970	55	0.6	6	41
All diseases						
Native troops	157796	9998	4041	2.6	40	23
English troops	84713	4371	2274	2.7	52	19

$d = c:a$; $e = (c:b) \times 100$.

ent cases terminated fatally; of the 116 remaining cases of modified confluent, and distinct variola, and varicella, two died of erysipelas and croup. Of 13 cases, confluent, malignant, and petechial, 12 were fatal.[17]

d. Periods of Disease

The laws of death and recovery, in different stages of disease, form the most interesting part of this inquiry. A very simple tabular construction enables us to determine the nature of these laws, and the probability of recovery at any period. Thus, I took 5268 cases of smallpox from the books of the Small Pox Hospital, and noted the deaths and recoveries (cols. D, E) taking place every five days from the date of admission. 3488 recovered, 1780 died. Of the 1780 fatal cases, 164 died in the first five days after admission, leaving 1616 cases to enter on the subsequent period; and thus, by subtracting the deaths every successive five days, (col. E) the number of fatal cases

---

[17] Dr. Gregory, "British Annals of Medicine".

Table of Sickness, showing, in Small Pox, the number of cases remaining at the end of every fifth day [C]: the numbers to recover [A] and to die [B]; also the numbers that recover [D], die [E], terminate in the next period

Days	To Recover	To Die	To Recover or To Die	Recover	Die	Terminate
0	A	B	C	D	E	F
5	3488	1780	5268	2	164	166
10	3486	1616	5102	5	737	742
15	3481	879	4360	37	552	589
20	3444	327	3771	176	153	329
25	3277	174	3451	321	70	391
30	2956	104	3060	487	39	526
35	2469	65	2534	535	23	558
40	1934	42	1976	466	14	480
45	1468	28	1496	384	9	393
50	1084	19	1103	246	3	249
55	838	16	854	367	4	371
60	641	14	655			
65	471	12	483	179	2	181
70	379[18]	11	390			
75	292	10	302	292	10	302
80	224	9	233			
85	173	8	181			
90	132	7	139			
95	100	6	106			
100	79	5	84			
105	60	4	64			
	200	20	220	added to the columns		

remaining at every stage was obtained (col. B) Column A was obtained in the same manner, by subtracting, successively, the number recovering every five days (col. D) The table is read thus: Of 5268 cases of small pox remaining at the end of the fifth day, 3486 will recover, 1780 will die; and two will recover, 164 will die, in the next five days, leaving 5102 on the list at the end of the tenth day.

The cases are from the London Small Pox Hospital (1780–99); the time at which they entered has been assumed to be the end of the fifth day, as this has latterly been

---

[18] Interpolated by successively multiplying by 0.76; which applies as high up the column as 1084. I have calculated a theoretical table that corresponds with the numbers observed.

the period of admission. The day of the disease, and the day of the eruption at the time of admission, have been entered in the books for several years, by Dr. Gregory, and this is the result:

Date	Cases [A]	Day of Disease [B]	Day of Eruption [C]	Interval in Days [D]
1827–31	1000	6333	3358	2975

[B] = 5333 + [A]; [D] = [B] − [C].

The *day of the disease* is one day more than the *duration of the disease*, which was, therefore, 5333 days at the time of admission. Omitting the fractions, patients enter the hospital at the end of the fifth day; at which period the table commences. The patients were not discharged till they had perfectly recovered, for fear of infection.

The probability of recovery is shown by the numbers of column A and column B, in juxtaposition. At the end of the fifteenth day there were 4360 cases – 3481 to recover and 879 to die. The chance of recovery is 3481 to 879 (4 to 1); at the 30th day the probability of recovery has risen; it is 2966[19] to 104 (29 to 1). The fraction expressing the probability of recovery is 2956/3060; the probability of dying is 104/3060; both probabilities added together make certainty.

The *probability of dying constantly decreases* in acute diseases; as the deaths take place at an earlier period than the recoveries. So the danger of being shot is greater at the beginning than in the middle of a battle; for a man alive in the middle of the day has escaped all the dangers of the morning.

This table possesses many other curious properties. I can here only call attention to two. It shows how long the disease will probably last from any given day; for 5268 cases are reduced to less than half the number (2534) by the 35th day. On the 6th day (end of the fifth) it is therefore *probable* the disease will have terminated by the 35th. On the 30th day it may be said that the disease will *probably* terminate in 15 days; for 3060 cases remaining at the end of the 30th, are reduced to 1496, or less than half, at the end of the 45th day. The probability that the patient will recover in the 15 days is (2956 − 1468)/3060 = 1488/3060; the probability that he will die in the time is 76/3060.

The *mean future duration* of the cases that attain the 5th, 10th, 15th, and every successive day is determined by adding the columns A, B, or C up to the number against

---

[19] (ed.) Apparently a misprint for 2956.

the day in question; dividing by that number, and subtracting 0.5 from the quotient. For example: the addition of col. C up to 3060 (this included) against the 30th day produces the sum 13880; which divided by 3060 is 4.433; reduced by subtracting 0.5 is 3.933 – or nearly 4 periods of 5 days. Multiply 3.933 by 5 and the product will be 19.7, the mean future duration of cases in days.

The mean future duration of (a) cases of recovery, (b) fatal cases, and (c) all cases of Small Pox; also (d) the probability of dying at the end of the 5th, 10th, 20th, 30th and 40th day is here given:

Day	Expected Duration of			Probability of Dying
	Recoveries	Fatal Cases	All Cases	
	a	b	c	d
5	41.5	12.0	31.5	0.3379
10	36.5	7.9	27.4	0.3168
20	26.9	11.0	25.5	0.0867
30	20.3	15.8	19.7	0.0340
40	18.4	22.6	18.5	0.0213

d = B:C in Table of Sickness, Small Pox (p.172).

The force of mortality in different diseases has been examined (page 208 [of the original publication]) it differs in intensity in the course of the same disease, according to a law which I have discovered in Small Pox. To determine the force of mortality at different periods, refer to the preceding table (page 210 of the original publication [see p. 172, Table of Sickness, Small Pox, this volume]): it will be perceived that 5268 cases remained at the end of the 5th day, 5102 at the end of the 10th day; and that 164 died in the 5 intervening days. The mean number constantly sick [see p. 175, Table of the deaths and recoveries out of 1000 patients], was the mean of the numbers at the beginning (5268) and the end (5102) of the period = 5315; so that 164 deaths took place in 5 days out of 5135[20] constantly sick, between the 5–10 days of Small Pox. This is equivalent to 6.39 daily deaths in 1000. The same method was pursued in calculating all the numbers in col. D; and the rate of recovery col. F.

The rate of mortality increased from the 5–10 days to days 10–15 when it attained a maximum (31.18); it decreased in a determined progression from the next period (15–20 days) to the end. The decrease begins to take place in geometrical progres-

---

[20] (ed.) Apparently a misprint, (5268 + 5102):2 = 5185.

"On Prognosis"

Table of the deaths and recoveries out of 1000 patients – this number being constantly kept up – in fourteen stages of Small Pox

Days	a Constantly Sick	b Die in 5 days	c Recover in 5 days	d Daily deaths in 1000 (observed)	e Daily deaths in 1000 (calculated)	f Daily Recoveries in 1000
5–10	5135 [5185]	164	2	6.39		0.08
10–15	4681 [4731]	737	5	31.18		0.21
15–20	4066	552	37	27.16	27.16	1.82
20–25	3611	153	167	8.48	8.48	9.25
25–30	3255	70	321	4.30	4.30	19.72
30–35	2797	39	487	2.79	2.78	34.82
35–40	2255	23	535	2.04	2.04	47.46
40–45	1736	14	466	1.61	1.58	53.68
45–50	1299	9	384	1.38	1.27	59.52
50–55	978	3	246	0.61	1.03	50.50
		10 days	10 days			
55–60 60–65	668	4	367	0.60	0.84 0.69	54.94
65–70 70–75	392	2	179	0.51	0.57 0.47	45.66

[Apparent misprints shown in brackets].

sion; but the tendency to decrease is met by another force that neutralises part of its effect. This is illustrated in the annexed diagram: where the lines against each day show the relative force of mortality – the quantity eliminated daily by death out of a given constant quantity (1000) sick on the 18th, 19th, &c. days of the disease. The curved line (a) describes the actual course of the rate of mortality, the dotted line (b) the course the rate of mortality would pursue if uninfluenced by a second force, tending to keep up the original intensity. This curve agreeing with the facts observed was calculated and any point being known the rest of the course can be deduced by a very simple process. (See diagram, p. 177).

The diagram was calculated from 4915 cases of Small Pox (age 10–35);[21] since then I have discovered a simpler formula applying from 10–15 to the end of the dis-

---

[21] British Annals of Medicine, page 74.

ease and its terminations. The results (col. E) all calculated from one basis, agree so exactly with the facts observed (col. D) as to leave little doubt that the force of mortality changes according to a fixed law (Table of the deaths and recoveries out of 1000 patients, page 212 of the original publication [p. 175 of this issue]). The nature of this law will be best understood by going over the calculation.[22]

The mean rate of mortality in the first period (days 15–20) is 27.16; and 27.16 multiplied by the rate of decrease, 0.312, is 8.48; the rate of decrease now changes to 0.508. To find the successive rates of decrease another rate must be employed; a rate regulating these rates. This second rate may be called the constant; it is here 1.626; the square root of 1.626 is 1.275, the next constant; and each successive one is the square root of the constant preceding. After deducing the roots of the constant, the successive rates are formed by them from the first; for 0.312 multiplied by the first constant 1.626, becomes 0.508; and 0.508 multiplied by 1.275, the square root of 1.626, becomes 0.647; so the successive rates of decrease are formed to the end of the series. The rates of mortality are determined by multiplying them by the rates of decrease; the rate of mortality at 20–25 days is 8.48; which multiplied by 0.508, produces the mortality of the next period, 4.30; and 4.30 multiplied by 0.647 = 2.78 the mortality of the next period. The constant – some power – or some root of it – regulates the whole series. The tendency to recover increases according to a determined law.

The Paris Board of Health gave the time at which 4907 fatal cases of cholera terminated as in col. B (see Table, p. 177); we have added col. A, the number remaining at

---

[22] The series of numbers in the Table of the death and recoveries out of 1000 patients, p. 212 [p. 175], may be calculated in many ways; the following is one by logarithms [λ].

Rate of Mortality λ		Rates of Decrease λ	Constant λ
27.16	1.43392		
	−1.49429	−1.49429	
8.48	0.92821	0.2112	0.2112
	−1.70549	−1.70549	
4.30	0.63370	0.1056	0.1056
	−1.81109	−1.81109	
2.78	0.44479	0.0528	0.0528
	−1.86389	−1.86389	
2.04	0.30868		

By dividing the constant by 2, this is continued. In ascending, the operation is reversed.

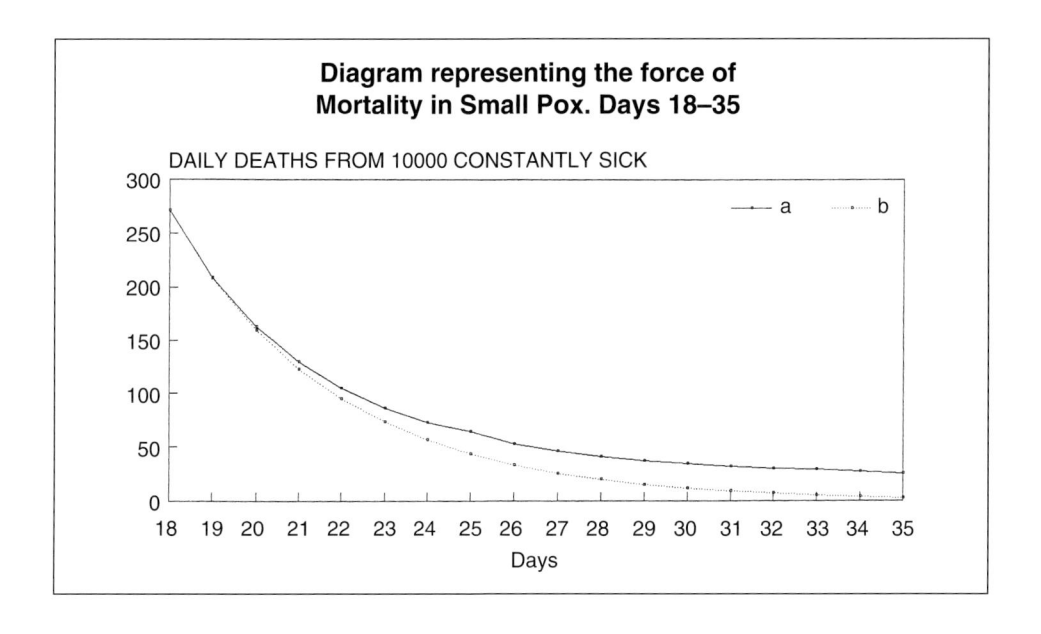

Diagram representing the force of Mortality in Small Pox. Days 18–35

DAILY DEATHS FROM 10000 CONSTANTLY SICK

Table of 4907 fatal cases of Cholera, showing the number remaining at each of 16 periods; and the number dying in the period following

Hour	A To die	B Dying[23]		Day	A To die	B Dying
0	4907	204	2384*	5	576	125
6	4703	615		6	451	79
12	4088	392		7	372	171
18	3696	1173		8	201	35
Day	A	B		9	166	36
1	2523	823		10	139	111
2	1700	502		15	19	19
3	1198	382		20	0	
4	816	240				

* (ed.) Number of deaths from hours 0–18.

---

[23] Rapport sur la Marche et les Effets de Cholera Morbus dans Paris, et le Département de la Seine.

Table of the Probability of Recovery from the severer Attacks of Cholera at the end of 12 hours, and 1, 2, and 3 days

	Cases	To Recover	To Die	Probability of Recovery
0 hours	10000	5093	4907	0.509 nearly 1 to 1
12 …	9181	5093	4088	0.555 … 1.3 to 1
1 day	7616	5093	2523	0.669 … 2 to 1
2 …	6793	5093	1700	0.750 … 3 to 1
3 …	6291	5093	1198	0.809 … 4 to 1

the end of every period, that it may be compared with the corresponding column in the Table of Small Pox.

The tendency to speak in weeks, and well known periods, produced the irregularity at the 7th day. Of the 171 thrown on that day, some died a day or two before, some a day or two afterwards. For the same reason it may be safely admitted that the deaths increased regularly on the first day. The daily rate of mortality in the first 12 hours was 16 per cent; in the next 12 hours (12–24) 37 per cent; in the second day 11 per cent; in the 3rd day 8 per cent, if the mortality of cases of cholera in Paris was 49 per cent – it could not have been higher – and none of the severe cases were cured in the first 3 days. The force of mortality attained its maximum in cholera by the 21st hour (18–24 hours); the maximum intensity in small pox is attained in days 10–15; in phthisis in 6–9 months. Taking a year as the unity of time, the relative maximum force of mortality – the deaths out of 100 constantly living – in the height of these three diseases is: cholera, 13614; smallpox, 1150; phthisis, 118. The danger of cholera decreases as the time advances; the longer a cholera patient lives, the more likely he is to live. The way in which the prognosis becomes favourable is shown in the table above.

These facts prove that in cholera the probability is generally not in favour of death; they also establish the importance of early treatment, for half the deaths happen in the first 24 hours. What the practitioner does he should do quickly.

The influence of age, sex, disease, different types of the same diseases, the period of disease in the prognosis have now been examined; the results are sufficiently decisive; they prove that these laws are active causes, to which the medical man should never forget to refer in practice.

Comments on the paper *"On Prognosis"* by William Farr: a forgotten masterpiece

Gerry Bernard Hill

263, Chelsea Road, Kingston, Ontario K7M 3Z3, Canada

The many contributions of William Farr, the "father of sanitary science" (Newsholme, 1899), to the development of classical epidemiology (the study of disease incidence) are widely acknowledged (Susser and Adelstein, 1975). Farr's role in the genesis of clinical epidemiology (the study of disease outcomes) is not so well known. It is hoped that by reprinting Farr's 1838 paper *"On prognosis"* this imbalance will be remedied. Farr published the paper in the British Medical Almanack, a journal which is not readily accessible to epidemiologists. Its existence was noted by medical historians such as Garrison (1929), Shryock (1979) and Eyler (1979), but it was not included in the collection of Farr's work edited by Humphreys (1885a).

"On prognosis" is an extension of the second of two papers published in the Lancet in 1835 (Farr, 1835), based on lectures on "hygiene" given by Farr at his home in Grafton Street, London. In this paper Farr quoted extensively from books I and III of *"Epidemics"* by Hippocrates. He tabulated, by day of disease, the crises of 41 cases of disease listed by Hippocrates. Farr complimented Hippocrates for including information on whether crises ended in death or recovery. Farr comments:

> "Whatever the Hippocratic doctrine (of critical days) may be, it is certain that in this country, in France, and in Germany, few diseases terminate of particular days, or at one period; *but I shall be able to show you that the termination or crisis of several, and probably every disease, takes place according to a determined law, which may at any time deduced, when observations are sufficiently exact and numerous* (emphasis added)." (Farr, 1835)

Farr's paper begins with quotations from another Hippocratic work, *"Prognostics"*, on the definition of prognosis and its importance to the work of the physician. However Farr does not follow his illustrious predecessor in describing the clinical signs of impending death. He emphasises the need for statistical estimates "in collective masses". This application of the law of large numbers, especially in the context of therapeutics, had been proposed earlier by Laplace (1814), and popularised by Louis

(1835). It was subsequently decried by Bernard (1865), and was not generally accepted until well into the 20th century.

In the main body of his paper Farr reviews the data then existing on the prognosis for various diseases, and the factors which influence disease outcome. The statistics cited by Farr are of considerable historical interest and are remarkable in the detail provided. Where, in this information age, can one find a table like that which Farr derived from the statistics on the prognosis of diseases in the Madras Army?

Farr was the first to distinguish between two measures of the tendency of a disease to destroy life: the ratio of the number of deaths to the number of cases in a given period; and the ratio of the number of deaths to the number of patient-years of sickness when patients are followed up to death or recovery. The first of these Farr calls simply "mortality", the second the "relative force of mortality". The current terms for these two measures are the case-fatality rate and the hazard rate. It is remarkable that the distinction between the two did not re-enter epidemiological parlance until the middle of the 20th century (Elandt-Johnson, 1975).

In his analysis of the effect of age on the case-fatality rate for smallpox Farr uses the approach developed by the actuary T. R. Edmonds, which assumes a log-linear relationship after the age of 10, i.e., the first difference of the logarithm of the rate is constant with age. Neither Edmonds nor Farr provide details on the method used to estimate this relationship. Today we would use least squares regression. The method of least squares to estimate the coefficients of a linear equation was introduced by Legendre in 1805, but Farr was not apparently aware of the technique. It is possible that Farr used the method outlined in Table 1 to analyse the small pox data.

As seen, Farr's estimates are very close to the least squares estimates. Thus Farr found a method of estimating a linear regression equation 50 years before Galton.

Table 1 – Log-linear regression of case-fatality of smallpox on age: comparison of Farr's estimate with least squares (Data from the London Small Pox Hospital, 1780–99 and 1826–35)

Age group	Log (fatality%)	Model	Farr's estimate	Least square estimate
10–20	$y_1 = 1.367$	a–2b	24.7	24.4
20–30	$y_2 = 1.532$	a–b	33.1	32.9
30–40	$y_3 = 1.668$	a	44.4	44.3
40–50	$y_4 = 1.766$	a+b	59.7	59.8
50–	$y_5 = 1.900$	a+2b	80.1	80.6

Farr's estimate of $b = (y_4 + y_5 - y_1 - y_2)/6 = 0.128$.
Farr's estimate of $a = (y_1 + y_2 + y_3 + y_4 + y_5)/5 = 1.647$.

However, later in the paper when analysing the cholera data from Vienna Farr uses the simpler method of interpolating logarithmically between the first and last age groups.

But without doubt the most innovative part of Farr's paper is his use of a double-decrement life table, with illness terminating by recovery or death, to estimate the recovery and death rates by period of disease in patients with smallpox. It was not until 1926 that Greenwood used single decrement life tables to estimate the natural duration of cancer. Even to this day no-one, to my knowledge, has used a double decrement table to estimate recovery rates and death rates in communicable disease. The idea of a competing risk between recovery and death, the former increasing and the latter decreasing with duration of disease, was a conceptual breakthrough. Of course Farr knew nothing about bacteria and immunity, but it is only recently that immunologists have used predator-prey models to simulate the competition between antigens and antibodies (Bell, 1973).

William Farr was the son of a farm labourer. He was largely self-taught. The little formal education he received was paid for by a retired cab-driver named Pryce, to whom epidemiologists should be eternally grateful.

Comments regarding *"On prognosis"* by William Farr (1838), with reconstruction of his longitudinal analysis of smallpox recovery and death rates

B. Burt Gerstman

Department of Health Science, San Jose State University, San Jose, California 95192-0052, USA

The editor has kindly asked me to comment from a statistical perspective on the historical article *"On prognosis"* by William Farr (1838). To place this article in context, I note that it was published about a year *after* the Registrar-General's office was established in 1837, and a year *before* Farr's appointment to his first official post as Compiler of Abstracts in this office, Farr later assumed the position of Superintendent of the Statistical Department in the Registrar-General's office, a position he held until his retirement in 1880 (Humphreys, 1885b).

The article *On prognosis* is notable in many ways. It reveals Farr's early insights into population-based epidemiologic principles, a fundamental understanding of longitudinal analysis, an interest in clinical research, and a commitment to explaining the course of health and disease in terms of "simple laws susceptible to calculation". It is no wonder that Susser and Adelstein (1975a) referred to Farr as "a founder, even the founder of epidemiology in its modern form".

Population-based epidemiologic principles

Farr's role in innovating population-based epidemiologic principles has been lauded by many prominent sources (Susser and Adelstein, 1975a; Langmuir, 1976; Lilienfeld and Lilienfeld, 1977). Examples of epidemiologic principles discussed in *"On prognosis"* include references to the spectrum of disease and "the epidemiologic iceberg" (Last, 1963), a clear distinction between risks and rates (Elandt-Johnson, 1975; Vandenbroucke, 1985), and exploration of rates by "person, place, and time" variables. In reference to the epidemiologic iceberg, Farr writes on page 169 (all page references will be to the re-publication as it appears in this book):

> *"Attacks of disease differ in intensity; some are so slight as to obtain no attention."*

In reference to the distinction between risk and rates, Farr writes (p. 167):

> "*Disease may be examined (1) in their tendency to destroy life, expressed by the deaths out of a given number of cases; and (2) in their mean relative force of mortality, expressed by the deaths out of a given number sick at a given time.*"

And later, on page 169, the mortality rate is described as the ratio of the number of deaths divided by the central (mean) number exposed to risk:

> "*The relative force of mortality is an unusual term; but it implies the rate of dying – the number of deaths out of a given number, living a given time – and is required by the present state of science.*"

In sections labeled "a. The patient, b. External Circumstances, c. Diseases, and d. Periods of Disease" (pp. 161–178), Farr explores morbidity and mortality rates by person, place, and time variables. For example, an interesting section on recovery from insanity is presented on page 165 in which Farr notes diminishing rates of recovery with age, but constant rates of mortality.

Longitudinal analysis

Farr's application of current ("cross-sectional") life table methods to vital statistics is well-known, but his analysis of clinical cohorts is less frequently cited (Hill, 1997). On pages 166–167, Farr writes:

> "*To determine the mortality of diseases they should be followed from the beginning to the end; every death or recovery should be recorded; and this though exceedingly simple, has been rarely done. The mortality of cases can only be accurately ascertained by practitioners, who see cases as they occur, slight or severe, and seldom lose sight of them to the end.*"

The importance of not losing sight of individual experiences "from the beginning to the end" underlies all longitudinal analyses and time-failure models, and forms the basis of cohort and case-control study methods (Miettinen, 1976a). That Farr was ahead of the time in applying time-failure principles in measuring human health and disease is illuminated in his *Table of Sickness* that appears on page 171. By working from first principles, and using methods most likely learned from the British actuary Thomas Rowe Edmonds (Eyler, 1980; 2002), Farr determines the extent to which two separate states (life and illness) persist in individuals. This allowed him to estimate probabilities of their complementary states (death and recovery) by describing the cohort's survival experience at its essence. In his *Table of Sickness*, Farr shows the number recovering (column A), the number dying (column B), and the number remaining sick (column C) in a cohort of 5268 smallpox patients. On page 173 Farr states

> "The probability of recovery is shown by the numbers of column A and column B, in juxtaposition."

By this, the autodidact Farr means the *odds* of recovery. Notwithstanding this semantical error, Farr properly calculates probabilities of survival and death, occasionally referring to them "fractions":

> "...at the 30th day the probability of recovery has risen; it is [2956] to 104 (29 to 1). The fraction expressing the probability of recovery is 2956/3060; the probability of dying is 104/3060; both probabilities added together make certainty" (p. 173).

Based on these calculations, Farr derives a remarkably modern inference:

> "The probability of dying constantly decreases in acute disease; as the deaths take place at an earlier period than the recoveries."

Today we would record this as evidence of *non-constant hazard*, a fact that would have been lost if data had been reduced to a too-simple comparison of proportions without accounting for time. Had graphical computing been available at the time, Farr might have expressed these results as an empirical survival curve (Figure 1) or, better yet, as incidence rates plotted over time (Figure 2).

Farr was also able to calculate the expected ("mean future") duration of disease for people who were to recover and for those who were to die, and for both groups combined (p. 173). His methods are akin to summing the number of person-days remaining in each subcohort ($_nT_x$ in current life table notation) and dividing this quantity by the number of people who began the interval. This allowed the calculation of the expected (mean future) duration of the state, or e_x in today's notation (Elandt-Johnson and Johnson, 1980). It should be pointed out that these expectations are superior to simple averages since they separate out survivors and decedents and deal with censored data in a relatively unbiased way (Morabia, 1996; Hill, 1997).

Scrutiny of Farr's Table of Sickness (p. 172) and Table of deaths and recoveries (p. 175)

Farr's *Table of Sickness* is a modified life table that follows outcomes in a cohort of 5268 smallpox cases. The table begins on day 5 following hospitalization, for the reason explained elegantly in the original article, with the cohort divided into those who

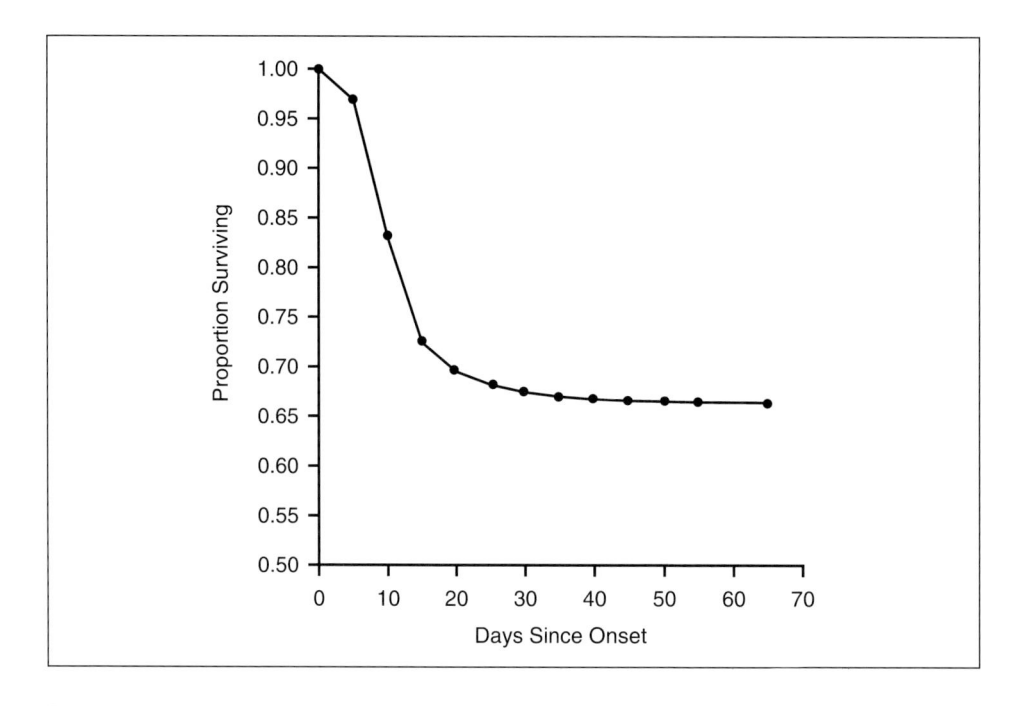

Figure 1
Survival following smallpox, based on Farr's Table of Sickness

ultimately recover (column A) and those who die (column B). Data are complete for 5-day follow-up intervals up to day 55. This is followed by two 10-day follow-up intervals (55–64 days; 64–74 days) before a final interval of indeterminate length is reported. There are no apparent losses before the final interval. Because data are incomplete for this last interval – the status of these individuals into the future is censored – Farr makes several assumptions so that he may complete his analysis. One of these assumptions is referenced in the form of a footnote to the table, where it is called an "interpolation". This interpolation assumes that, following the 55th day of illness, 0.76 of those bound to recover remain ill for at least an additional five days (i.e., 24% of those due to recover will do so within 5 days)* and that deaths (Column B) occur uniformly at 1 for every five days. Column C ("To Recover or Die")

---

* Although Farr does not fully explain the source of this interpolation, it can be noted that approximately three-quarters of those in Column A "survive" (that is, stay in their current state of illness) until the next interval starting at about day 40. For example, the survival proportion from day 40 to 45 is 1468/1934 = 75%; the survival proportion from day 45 to 50 is 1084/1468 = 74%; and so on.

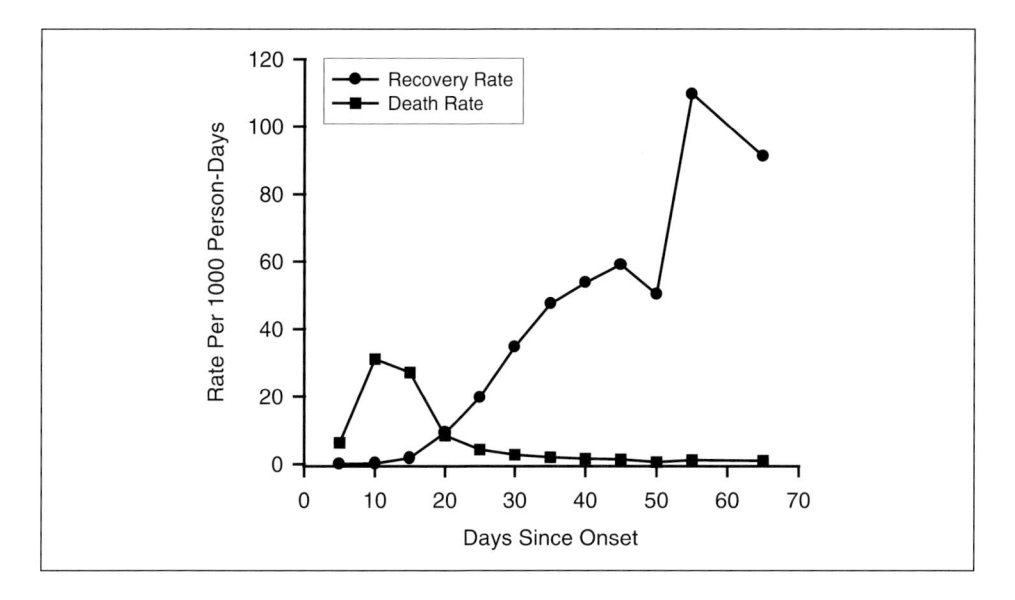

Figure 2
Rates of recovery and death in smallpox patients over time

contains those remaining alive but ill as of the beginning of the interval (simply the sum of column A and column B). Column D ("Recover") and column E ("Die") are the actual data from which all other columns are derived. Column F ("Terminate") is simply the sum of column D and column E.

The aforementioned *Table of Sickness* is used to build the *Table of the deaths and recoveries* on page 175. Column *a* in the *Table of the deaths and recoveries* contains the number of people *effectively* exposed to risk during the interval ("Constantly sick" in Farr's terminology). This is simply the average number of people who persisted in the state of illness until the next interval, assuming a uniform (or symmetrical) resolution of the current state. Farr makes an elegant description of how he calculated this number on page 173, but unfortunately makes an arithmetic error in two of his calculations. During the first interval, the average of 5268 and 5102 is 5185 (not 5135). During the second interval, the number of people effectively exposed to risk should read 4731 (not 4681). Otherwise, Column *a* in the *Table* is clean, apart from rounding errors.

Column *a* data in the *Table of the deaths and recoveries* serves as denominator data for the death rate (column *d*) and recovery rate (column *f*) in the table. For me, it is easier to see how these rates were calculated if we first determine the number of person-days in the interval as the product of the effective number exposed to risk (column *a*) and length of the interval (value in column *a* × 5 for 5-day intervals, value

Table 1 – Reconstruction of Farr's analysis of smallpox mortality and recovery

First day of interval		Cohort[a]	Recoveries[b]	Deaths[c]	Persistent illness[d]	Effective number[e]	Person-days[f]	Death rate[g] per 1000 p-days	Recovery rate[h] per 1000 p-days
	k		r	d	N	N'	T		
5-day risk periods	0	–	–	–	–	–	–	–	–
	1	5268	2	164	5268	5185.0	25925.0	6.33	0.08
	2	5104	5	737	5102	4731.0	23655.0	31.16	0.21
	3	4367	37	552	4360	4065.5	20327.5	27.16	1.82
	4	3815	167	153	3771	3611.0	18055.0	8.47	9.25
	5	3662	321	70	3451	3255.5	16277.5	4.30	19.72
	6	3592	487	39	3060	2797.0	13985.0	2.79	34.82
	7	3553	535	23	2534	2255.0	11275.0	2.04	47.45
	8	3530	466	14	1976	1736.0	8680.0	1.61	53.69
	9	3516	384	9	1496	1299.5	6497.5	1.39	59.10
	10	3507	246	3	1103	978.5	4892.5	0.61	50.28
10-day risk periods	11	3504	367	4	854	668.5	6685.0	0.60	54.90
	12	3500	179	2	483	392.5	3925.0	0.51	45.61
Remainder	13	3498	292	10	302				
TOTALS		3488	1780			160180.0			

a Initial cohort minus number of deaths from prior interval. Not reported by Farr, but needed to perform routine survival analysis and track the cohort.

b From Column D in Farr's *Table of Sickness*.

c From Column E in Farr's *Table of Sickness*.

d This is the number of people in which illness persisted. You can think of it as the number who remained hospitalized as of the first day of the interval.

$N_{k+1} = N_k - d_k - r_k$, where N_k = the number with persistent illness as of the first day of interval k, d_k = the number of deaths that occurred during this interval, and r_k = the number of recoveries that occurred during this interval. For example, $N_1 = 5268 - 64 - 2 = 5102$. This is reported as Column C in Farr's *Table of Sickness*.

e $N'_k = N_k - .5(r_k) - .5(d_k)$. Assumes mean time of recovery and death is mid-interval; Similar to column a in Farr's *Table of deaths and recoveries*.

f $T_k = N'_k \times 5$ for 5 day intervals; $T_k = N'_k \times 10$ for 10 day intervals

g Death rate per 1000 person-days = $d_k/T_k \times 1000$. This information is the same as column d of Farr's *Table of deaths and recoveries* (corrected).

h Recovery rate per 1000 person-days = $r_k/T_k \times 1000$. This information is the same as column f of Farr's *Table of deaths and recoveries* (corrected).

i "*On prognosis*" lists this value as 176 – a typesetting error.

in column *a* × 10 for 10-day intervals). In Table 1 of this commentary, I show how these death rates and recovery rates can be calculated.

"Simple laws susceptible to calculation"

Column *e* in Farr's *Table of deaths and recoveries* (labeled "calculated") contains hypothetical mortality rates based on an assumed geometric progression of occurrence. Three stages of mortality are posited: for days 5–10, for days 10–15, and from day 15 onward. Farr concentrates his effort on predicting the mortality progression from day 15 onward. When the observed rates flatten out, Farr superimposes an additional rate on the predicted rates ("a rate regulating these rates") to allow his model to better fit the data. This, too, Farr declares to act "according to a determined law" (see pp. 174–175). Farr then goes on to apply these law of progression to other populations (e.g., Paris) and other diseases (e.g., cholera, phthisis).

At this point it may be worth noting an important change in statistical reasoning since Farr's time. We no longer view statistical models as representing fixed *laws* of nature. Rather, statistical models are viewed as *tools* of science. Whether a particular model is true is irrelevant (Zeger, 1991). What counts is whether we obtain correct scientific conclusions if we believe in the fiction of the model. "The hallmark of good science is that it uses models and "theory" but never believes them" (Martin Wilk cited in Tukey (1962) on p. 7). We have no reason to believe that Farr's laws of morbidity may be applied uniformly across populations and diseases. We may even speculate that the cohort studied by Farr was a select one, not necessarily representing the experience of smallpox cases in the source population. Thus, the generalizability of results is tenuous. Health outcomes are influenced by multiple causal factors acting together, and the incidence of any outcome can be assumed to vary across populations, depending on the prevalence of its complementary factors (Rothman, 1976). Attempts to reduce rates of even a single disease to universal constants would today be considered short-sighted.

Acknowledgements

The authors expresses his appreciation to Dr. G. Hill and Dr. J. Eyler for their assistance with historical references and documents. He is also grateful to Dr. A. Morabia for suggesting the idea of a statistical review of Farr 1838 article and for publishing Farr's article in its original form, and to Dr. J. P. Vandenbroucke and Dr. J. Katz for their thoughtful and penetrating reviews of this manuscript.

Continuing controversies over "risks and rates" – more than a century after William Farr's *"On prognosis"*

Jan P. Vandenbroucke

Clinical Epidemiology, Leiden University Medical Center, PO Box 9600, NL-2300 RC Leiden, The Netherlands

More than a century after William Farr's 1838 publication "*On prognosis*", the difference between "risk" and "rate" was rediscovered by epidemiologists in the 1970s. The concept of the incidence rate over person-time continues to be misunderstood and has led to recent controversies.

In the second part of his 1838 publication "*On prognosis*", William Farr explained the "force of mortality", which nowadays we call an "incidence rate". He distinguished from "mortality", which we call "risk" or "cumulative incidence". The first is calculated over person-time and ranges from 0 to infinity; the second is a number between 0 and 1 without dimensions (Rothman and Greenland, 1998). In this commentary, I will trace the recent history of the distinction between "risk and rate", and recount how these concepts still lead to confusion and controversy.

A rediscovery

The distinction between "risk" and "rate" that was so well known to Farr was rediscovered in the 1970s in the USA (Vandenbroucke, 1985). In itself this is strange, since incidence rates had been used earlier in the 20th century in the UK and the USA. In the 1950s Richard Doll and Austin Bradford Hill used incidence per person-years in their studies of British doctors and smoking (Doll and Hill, 1956). However, they did not publish about the theory of this calculation. Hill did explain risks and life tables in his influential textbook on medical statistics (Hill, 1937), but only from the 7th edition onwards a few lines were devoted to incidence rates (Hill, 1984). In the USA the 1960 first edition of MacMahon's textbook on epidemiology used Doll and Hill's calculations on smoking and lung cancer to explain the person-years denominator (MacMahon et al., 1960). The example was retained in all later editions of that textbook. Nevertheless, the conceptual difference between "risk" and "rate" and their respective uses escaped attention.

Like Gerstman (Part II), I think that Elandt-Johnson (1975) should be credited for bringing the topic very clearly to the attention of "modern" epidemiologists in 1975. The distinction became the basis for Miettinen's (1976a) proposal that odds ratio calculations in case-control studies could be exactly the same as a ratio of incidence rates, without need for the "rare disease assumption". Thereafter, the distinction gained wide acceptance (Greenland, 1987a).

Continuing debates

Many persons remain confused about events per person-time. This was witnessed by a paper in the British Medical Journal in 1995, which called person-years "a dubious concept" (Windeler and Lange, 1995). The authors stated that incidence rates are meaningless because they are not probabilities. They described that person-years allow to use multiple events over time, which they thought was wrong. Actually, this is an advantage, and incidence rates are used for that purpose in infectious diseases. Also, they thought that the calculation is used to hide loss to follow-up – which in fact gives the same problem of bias, whatever incidence measure is used. Finally, they repeated the often-heard argument that incidence rates cannot distinguish between a few persons followed for a long time vs many persons followed for a short time. On the contrary, Farr demonstrated very beautifully in "*On prognosis*" how the time-dependency of incidence rates can be traced by dividing time into small periods (see the "*Table of the deaths and recoveries out of 1000 patients – this number being constantly kept up – in fourteen stages of Small Pox*"). Farr showed more than a century ago that it is perfectly possible to allow for the duration of follow-up and varying incidences over time with the person-years method.

Another strange episode on "risks and rates" was a critique on William Farr and Florence Nightingale in the Annals of Internal Medicine in 1996, entitled "100 apples divided by 15 red herrings" (Iezzoni, 1996). The author criticised publications on death rates in hospitals by Farr and Nightingale in the 1860s. The author rehashed the 130 year old accusation that Farr and Nightingale had used a "wrong" rate to overstate their political message about differences in death rates between hospitals. Farr and Nightingale had published death rates up to "90 per 100 per year" for particular hospitals for which they envisaged reforms. Interested parties at the time thought that these rates were impossible and thus wrong. Still, the explanation is straightforward: in hospitals several persons in succession occupy a single bed over a year, which yields 1 person-year of observation. Several persons might have died in that bed, which might even lead to death rates larger than unity. A simple solution to restore "intuitive credibility" is to calculate death rates per person-month or person-week: a death rate of 90 per 100 patient-years becomes 1.73 per 100 patient-weeks. The latter number would not as quickly have drawn accusations of "political spin", although it remains exactly the same in-cidence. Like the 19th century critics of Farr and Nightingale, the 1996 author concluded that these high mortality rates were used because of Nightingale's political agenda. Vandenbroucke and Vandenbroucke-Grauls (1996; 1997) took the defence of Farr and Nightingale.

Incidence calculations per person-week or per person-month are used nowadays for nosocomial infection rates in hospitals. This also took some time. Up to the early 1980s the Centers for Disease Control (CDC) in the USA propagated a so-called "rate" for the calculation of hospital infections: the number of infected divided by number of admissions (Haley et al., 1981). That calculation was already frowned upon in 1947 by Major Greenwood, at the London School of Epidemiology and Tropical Medicine (Vandenbroucke and Vandenbroucke-Grauls, 1988). Dividing the number of infected by number of admissions amounts to dividing the number of deaths in a population by the number of newborns over the same time period – which is neither an incidence rate, nor a risk. Even leading institutions seemed unaware that Farr and Nightingale had shown the right way of calculating incidence rates in hospitals in the middle of the 19th century (Vandenbroucke and Vandenbroucke-Grauls, 1988). This has changed (Freeman and McGowan, 1978), and in the early 1990s the CDC used nosocomial infection rates per person-time (Gaynes et al., 1991).

The difference between risk and rate gave raise to confusion and controversy, more than a century ago, and it still does. To those who have difficulty with the use of rates, the beautiful examples and explanations in "On prognosis" are still worthwhile reading.

Acknowledgement

I am indebted to Sir Iain Chalmers, Oxford, for the use of his collection of the several editions of Sir Austin Bradford Hill's "Textbook on medical statistics", and to Professor Christina Vandenbroucke-Grauls, Amsterdam, for guiding me through the nosocomial infection literature.

Understanding William Farr's 1838 article *"On prognosis"*: comment

John M. Eyler

University of Minnesota, Program in the History of Medicine, 511 Diehl Hall, Minneapolis, MN 55455, USA

In 1838, when William Farr published the accompanying article, he was a young general practitioner struggling to establish a practice near the bottom of London's highly stratified medical profession (Eyler, 1979, pp. 1–6; Peterson, 1978, pp. 5–39). To supplement his income Farr took in lodgers and gave lectures in his own home, and he turned to medical journalism. Beginning in 1835 he helped edit the British Medical Almanack, an annual review of the profession and its institutions and the journal that published his article *"On prognosis."* He also founded and edited his own journal the British Annals of Medicine, Pharmacy, Vital Statistics, and General Science, a weekly publication that ran from only January to August 1837. He wrote prolifically in these years in part to fill the pages of his journal. His vitriolic editorials in these years demonstrate his sympathy for radical reform of his profession. However, it was his articles on vital statistics had something novel to say, and in these early articles we can find the germ of ideas and methods he would develop during his long and productive career.

Before *"On prognosis"* appeared Farr had published five articles and a book chapter on vital statistics. Two were general overviews of the field (Farr, 1837d; 1837f, pp. 567–601). Two were direct progenitors of *"On prognosis"* and used a subset of the same data on smallpox (Farr, 1837a; Farr, 1837b, pp. 234–243). The final publications carried the methods he had demonstrated with clinical data for smallpox to clinical records from insane asylums (Farr, 1837c; Farr, 1837e). As a whole these early works by Farr demonstrate the lamentable state of vital data before the advent of civil registration. Civil registration of births, deaths and marriages began in England and Wales in 1837 as Farr was writing. Like the few other authors who dealt with health statistics before the results of civil registration became available, he was forced to rely of fragmentary, scattered, and often very incomplete published data: returns to Parliamentary investigative committees from friendly societies, a report by the Factory Commissioners, another by the East India Company, returns by the Army Medical Department on the health of troops, and statistical summaries published in British and foreign medical journals.

The longest of these early publications, his chapter on vital statistics for John Ramsey McCulloch's *"Statistical Account of the British Empire"*, provided a comprehensive review of this available data which Farr then synthesized for a general audience (Farr, 1837f). This was a prominent publication, and it probably helped secure for him a job at the General Register Office as Compiler of Abstracts in 1839. However, the most original and interesting of these early publications is *"On prognosis"* and his two predecessor articles in the British Annals of Medicine (Farr, 1837a, 1837b). He prepared these articles from the data he was permitted to abstract from the case records of the London Smallpox Hospital, and he used them to illustrate a method he called "nosography." By computing statistical laws for individual diseases, as he had done in these articles, Farr predicted boldly that physicians could both improve their ability make accurate prognoses and obtain a superior way of judging the efficacy of therapy.

These statistical articles can be understood in at least two ways. On the one hand, they reflect the broad general interest in statistics as tools of reform in the middle 1830s. These years were the zenith of the statistical movement in Britain, when statistical societies were formed in London and in several provincial towns by professional and other middle class men intent on finding objective, non-partisan means of promoting reform, mainly social but also professional reform (Cullen, 1975). On the other hand, these articles also are products of particular medical concerns. It is sometimes assumed that Farr developed his statistical approach under the influence of the Paris medical school, particularly Pierre Louis. This is not an implausible suggestion. After all Farr did spend some months at the Paris school, and in later life he recalled with pride his exposure to some of the famous Paris faculty. What he recalled most often, however, was the prominence the teaching of hygiene had in Paris in 1830 and how neglected it was in England (Farr, 1857–58, pp. 246; Farr, 1875, p. LXXIX). He did recall encountering Louis, but what he described was not Louis's numerical method but observing Louis lecture on typhoid fever (Farr, 1864, p. 179). We need to be careful in assuming what lessons Farr drew from his student experiences in Paris. An important recent historical study of the reaction of American students who studied medicine in Paris in these years emphasizes that what impressed them about Louis was his accessibility to them, his insistence on accurate observation, and his skepticism (Warner, 1998, pp. 8–9, 223–252). Like his American contemporaries Farr returned from Paris with an empirical and skeptical attitude. These qualities were certainly prerequisite for the development of modern biostatistics and epidemiology. Perhaps Louis's teaching suggested to some students, such as Farr, that medical problems could be objectified by using numbers. But can we go further and find the roots of Farr's statistical methods in Paris? I think not, and I believe that the case for Farr's statistical independence from Louis has been stated effectively and concisely (Hill, 1997). In fact, Farr's statistical methods bear little resemblance to those of Louis. In several ways they are superior. Among other things Farr recognized the hazards in small numbers, one of the features of Louis's study for which he was properly criticized (Matthews, 1995a, pp. 25–26, 30–34). On several occasions, most recently in this journal, I have argued that Farr developed his methods by following suggestions found in a series of publications by the English actuary Thomas Rowe Edmonds, most of which appeared in the Lancet between 1834 and 1837 (Eyler, Part IIb, 1980). Using the best available vital data Edmonds showed that human mortality varied each year through life in three geometric series. Using this so-called law of mortality and several preliminary assumptions, he could construct theoretical or model life tables that agreed quite well with the best tables drawn from experience. Following the 1831 English census, Edmonds was also able to demonstrate how his law of mortality could produce life tables for the general population and how, using age-specific mortality rates from these tables, the comparative health of portions the English population could be measured. More to the point of our discussion here, in 1835 Edmonds showed how he could use the same techniques to compute laws of sickness using records of the London Fever Hospital and of English and Scottish mutual benefit societies (Edmonds, 1835–36b; 1835–36e). Farr was well-acquainted with Edmonds. In 1835 both of them lived on Fitzroy Square in London, and Farr published two of Edmonds's articles in The British Medical Almanack (Edmonds, 1836; 1837). Farr also referred frequently to Edmonds's work in his own publications, including *"On Prognosis"* (Farr, Part II).

The following year Farr joined the permanent staff of the General Register Office to address the monumental task of turning the national death registers to good statistical and epidemiological use (Eyler, 1979). Farr did not forget his early interest in clinical statistics. In Lancet in 1862, he revisited the smallpox data he used for his article *"On prognosis"* and he argued again for the usefulness of computing statistical laws of recovery and death for groups of patients suffering from that same disease but undergoing different courses of treatment. He acknowledged that the age, sex, and condition of the patient all modified prospects of recovery and death and hence the statistical law of disease (Farr, 1837a, p. 79; Farr, 1862, p. 195). Further studies would be needed. He made only a very modest start in his article "On Prognosis" by computing a small set of case fatality rates by age group (Farr, Part II). In the articles we have been considering Farr was certainly most interested in presenting a method rather than final, definitive results. He evidently continued to hope into the 1860s that someone with hospital privileges would be as intrigues by the potential of "nosography" he was. Might the history of clinical trials have been different, if Farr had found a kindred spirit among the consultants at London's great teaching hospitals? We will obviously never know.

Methods of outbreak investigation in the "Era of Bacteriology" 1880–1920

Anne Hardy

Wellcome Trust Centre for the History of Medicine at UCL, Euston House, 24 Eversholt Street, London NW1 1AD, UK

Summary

The advent of bacteriological methods in the later 19th century has been seen, on the examples of America and Germany, to have been followed by a new laboratory-based, contact-tracing method of investigating outbreaks of epidemic disease. In Britain, however, this new approach never took firm root, and practising epidemiologists continued to follow an observational and deductive tradition in field investigations, rejecting any primary dependence on bacteriological methods. Alongside this persistent observational practice, there emerged a new statistical approach, based in Pearsonian biometrics, which allied itself with experimental laboratory techniques to develop a more systematic, theoretical trajectory for explaining disease outbreaks in the years after World War I.

At the International Health Exhibition of 1884, the President of the London Epidemiological Society outlined his society's objectives as follows (Epidemiological Society of London, 1884).

> "To watch pestilences; to study their mysterious ways, movements and changes, which are so often quite inscrutable even to the most experienced and learned; to become acquainted with their natural history; to track them step by step, as the hunter tracks the tiger and the wolf in all their concealments and devious lurkings, and thus to anticipate their attacks and discover means for their avoidance."

The very phrasing and terminology of this statement reflect much of the robustness and sense of purpose of High Victorian epidemiology. The period 1880 to 1920 is often regarded as one of abeyance and transition in the history of epidemiology, when the high Victorian discipline became submerged in the minute concerns of the new bacteriology, while the years after 1915 saw the emergence of new styles of epidemiology which foreshadowed its modern post World War II flowering, the transition from "a qualitative, descriptive procedure into a quantitative and analytical modern science"(Roth, 1976). This attitude is especially persistent among epidemiologists themselves.

For most practising epidemiologists, the Victorian contribution to their discipline is represented by John Snow and William Budd, who published their studies in the 1840s and 1850s, and history thereafter remains more or less of a vacuum until a more modern period. Yet a vigorous tradition of epidemiological study was established in the 1850s, in Britain at least, which produced a considerable body of literature in the years up to World War I. While there clearly were differences between England, Germany, and America in the pattern and timing of change in epidemiology after 1870, and it may well be that the English were notably slow in their responses to bacteriology, a closer examination of English epidemiology between 1880 and 1940 reveals not only a continuing emphasis on populations as opposed to individuals, but the development of new methods of outbreak investigation, a vigorous debate about the relationship between the different medical specialities of epidemiology, bacteriology and statistics, and a complex of professional, institutional and legislative developments which effected a substantial shift in the nature of the medical community involved with epidemiology. Moreover, it may be that different diseases provoked different epidemiological responses, taking the subject in new directions as it accommodated bacteriology and statistics in the first decades of the 20th century.

There are several factors external to the immediate history of the discipline which deserve consideration when we look at its neglected history between 1880 and 1914. First there is the continuing dominance in epidemiological mythology of Snow and Budd. Classic as their studies are, they have perhaps made it too easy to forget subsequent research which contributed to the shaping of epidemiology as a discipline, and to the establishing of its identity. Secondly, the impact of bacteriology on public health and epidemiology has rather been assumed than demonstrated – and recent research has indicated that it did not have a complete or immediate victory over older methods (Hardy, 1998). Finally, the period after 1880 saw a transformation in the kind of people who were interested and engaged in the practice of epidemiology. In the 19th century it was largely the concern of amateurs – of general practitioners like Snow and Budd, of medical officers of health responsible for controlling outbreaks of infectious disease, of military and naval physicians and surgeons interested in the wider context of their daily work. These men were not employed as epidemiologists; they practised it as part of their official duties. In England only a small and select group of men were professionally engaged in epidemiological investigation and research – the superintendents of statistics at the General Register Office, William Farr and his successors, and the staff of the central Medical Department (Eyler, 1979). Between its creation under John Simon in 1858 and its recreation as the Ministry of Health in 1919, the Medical Department investigated hundreds of disease outbreaks and occurrences in England and Wales, and sponsored a considerable programme of scientific research into the minute pathology of disease processes (Lambert, 1965). In this work, it was supported by the local medical officers of health, whose own concerns often provided the stimulus to investigation. From about 1900, however, the popular perception of England's most pressing public health concerns shifted from the infectious diseases to individual lives and their nature, nurture and management (Jones, 1994). This shift of focus entailed increasing administrative responsibilities, for maternal and child health, tuberculosis and veneral disease clinics, and eventually hospitals, and the medical officers' interest in epidemiology and medical research largely disappeared (Galbraith, 1966–67). At the same time, new medical specialities emerged whose representatives had claims on epidemiology and whose achievement of personal professional niches and creation of career pathways was eventually to establish a dramatically different occupational profile for practising epidemiologists.

These reflections can, perhaps, best be substantiated by examining the epidemiological investigations associated with one particular disease, or group of diseases. The salmonellas provide a useful window, partly because the causes of typhoid, the severest in man, were well enough understood by the 1890s for epidemiologists to be engaged in an extension of understanding rather than a basic search for clues; partly because the decline of typhoid as a public health problem was paralleled by the rise of its less virulent cousins as a cause of concern; and finally because by the first decade of the 20th century food-borne typhoid was replacing water-borne typhoid as a subject of epidemiological interest. On the one hand bacteriology modified and challenged the traditional techniques of epidemiology; on the other it extended its environmental concerns.

The integration of bacteriology, and a little later of modernising statistical methods into epidemiology was not accomplished without resistance on the part of epidemiology's practitioners. High Victorian epidemiology was, as William Coleman has noted, environmentalist in its concerns, and it was observational in its techniques (Coleman, 1987). The Victorians were above all field epidemiologists whose investigations of disease outbreaks and occurrences performed the dual function of resolving public health problems and extending their understanding of how diseases behaved. At its best, this epidemiology expressed itself in reports of a richly literary character, which incorporated a vast range of contextual detail of a human, social, topographical, geological, and even meteorological character. The investigators employed by the Medical Department in the 1880s and 1890s were past-masters of this type of epidemiology, and they were conscious and proud of their skills. Many of their investigations were, of course, of limited significance, but others were classics of their kind. In this genre, the report furnished by William Frederick Barry on epidemic typhoid in the valley of the Tees river in 1891is outstanding. At a time when there were still many who doubted the water transmission theory of typhoid, or who held that defective sanitary arrangements were more significant, Barry's Teesdale report reaffirmed and established the importance of unpolluted water supplies for public health (Hardy, 1998).

The report generated a renewed interest in typhoid incidence at the Medical Department, and right up until World War I its investigators reported on a long series of local typhoid outbreaks, which repeatedly emphasised the fragility of the new water distribution systems and their vulnerability to pollution, as well as drawing attention to the links between rural agricultural practices and urban disease, and the environmental hazards posed by dry conservancy systems. In these investigations the Victorian tradition was still very much to the fore, with the field investigations slowly building up a fuller long-term picture of the relationship between man, environment, and disease. In the earlier investigations of this series, bacteriology featured only occasionally as a handmaid to epidemiology.

Early in the 20th century, however, bacteriology began to assert itself, while the epidemiologists began to incorporate it into a developed picture of preventive action. Failing to unravel the mysterious distribution of typhoid in the city of Chichester in the late 1890s, Theodore Thomson noted the need for comparative local environmental studies of typhoid-prone places with others not so affected. "Such investigation", he observed, "would need to be supplemented by skilled research on the part of the statistician, the geologist, the chemist and the bacteriologist". In other words, epidemiology alone was not enough (Hardy, 1998).

In these years, as means of typhoid transmission other than through water became known, bacteriology began to assume a more significant role. In the early 1890s, it became apparent that certain foodstuffs played a regular part in causing sporadic cases and occasional outbreaks of typhoid. Shellfish, for example, became something of a cause celebre. In 1894 a sharp outbreak of typhoid in Connecticut was traced to oyster consumption, and the link was firmly established. In England, the association was confirmed by two major incidents in 1902, when participants in the annual mayoral banquets at Winchester and Southampton caught typhoid as a result of eating contaminated oysters. Here, the menu surveillance technique still used in food poisoning outbreaks today was first introduced (Hardy, 1998). These outbreaks provoked a spate of local epidemiological studies, which demonstrated, among other things, that the incidence of typhoid in the county of Essex was more than twice as great in the areas bordering the Thames, where polluted shellfish were freely gathered and consumed, as it was in the inland districts.

A very clear population concern was evident in these studies – medical officers were seeking to establish how far the continued prevalence of typhoid among populations in their districts was associated with the consumption of shellfish taken from polluted coastal waters. Bacteriology played little part in these assessments, since negative bacteriological evidence on the sewage pollution of waters carried a known possibility of being highly misleading, while there was no agreement among bacteriologists as to the precise significance of either the presence or numbers of *B. coli* and *B. enteritidis*; that is, no bacteriological standard existed or could in justice be applied (Houston, 1904). Such standards became available within a few years, and the epidemiological investigation of shell-fish related typhoid outbreaks, which continued enthusiastically up to 1914, gave way after the War to an increasingly specialised branch of bacteriology.

Meanwhile, bacteriology was opening up a new field of hazard in respect of foodstuffs, which was to increase in importance as the century advanced. This was the discovery of the vast spectrum of salmonella bacteria less virulent than typhoid, and their association with animal populations, especially of domestic animals. First indications of this huge reservoir of hazard came in 1880, when Edward Ballard investigated an outbreak of food-poisoning originating on the Duke of Portland's Welbeck Abbey estate (Hardy, 2000). Eight years later Gaertner demonstrated the pathogenicity of the bacillus which he named *B. enteritidis*, and the recorded history of the lesser salmonellas began.

For some years, however, there was confusion over whether these organisms were natural inhabitants of the animal gut, or whether they were introduced by accidental contamination during preparation, or whether they were present in animals as the result of animal diseases. Each of these possibilities indicated different methods of prevention but traditional epidemiology did not prove competent to settle these questions. However, in a series of experiments conducted for the Medical Department between 1908 and 1910, the microbiologist William Savage showed that salmonellas are not normal inhabitants of the animal gut, but that the micro-organisms are found in the muscle and internal organs of animals suffering from clinical or sub-clinical infections, and that such infections may also be introduced into foodstuffs externally, through unhygienic food-handling practices. This was epidemiology with a difference – but Savage's work both reflected and supported an interest in food-borne infections which had been building in the Medical Department since 1880. It was a public health interest that survived the War, and was continued by the Ministry of Health and the Medical Research Council in the inter-war period. Under the aegis of the latter, and with the assistance of another microbiologist, Bruce White, Savage was instrumental in the early 1920s in establishing the relationship between the various salmonella types and food poisoning, and in showing that domestic animals and vermin are important reservoirs of these organisms (Savage and Bruce White, 1925a; 1925b).

In the years immediately before the War, human reservoirs of typhoid, rather than animal reservoirs of salmonella, constituted the great public health issue; and provided the context for a series of English debates as to the relative merits and necessary relationships of epidemiology, bacteriology, statistics, and preventive medicine. The starting point for these debates was Robert Koch's theory that typhoid was due to an organism whose natural habitat was the human body, and the resulting campaign mounted in South-West Germany from 1903 to isolate typhoid sufferers, to search out all persons harbouring the bacillus, and to disinfect and destroy all infective material produced by these healthy carriers (Klinger, 1910). It was a policy which epitomised the bacteriological approach to epidemiology – the point of contact method (Leavitt, 1992). In England, however, such methods proved widely unacceptable when applied to typhoid at least until after the War. Indeed, several eminent British epidemiologists were sceptical about the significance of carriers in typhoid prevalence. William Hamer, in particular, set out to demonstrate that much of the German field evidence of the role of carriers in typhoid outbreaks was "unconvincing" when viewed from an epidemiological as opposed to a bacteriological standpoint. Five years later, when the final report on the South-West German anti-typhoid campaign was published, Hamer gave it a lengthy and destructive review, in which he argued from a traditional epidemiological and statistical standpoint the case against a significant role being played in typhoid endemicity by carriers (London County Council, 1912).

Hamer's reactions to the German carrier theory of typhoid were possibly extreme. Although an able mathematician, he was hostile both to bacteriology and to the new biometry and the biometrical approach to epidemiology which emerged in these years. His own epidemiology was traditional and humanistic: social change, population movements, and the peculiarities of different diseases were continuous themes in his work. His critical attitude towards the carrier theory was nonetheless consistent with a more general English preventive attitude: if such a carrier is found, what is to be done with him? (Clegg, 1913–14). Public health in Britain at this time still trod a fine line between the permissible and the impermissible in terms of the liberty of the subject, and even if treatment of the carrier himself fell to one side of that line, treatment of contacts most certainly would fall on the other. As Savage admitted, "the elaborate examination of excreta (on the German model)…certainly would not be tolerated" (Savage, 1907).

For a time, it seemed as if anti-typhoid inoculation, by a process developed by Sir Almwroth Wright, the "father of English bacteriology", might offer a solution. In practice, however, English mistrust of immunisation procedures combined with the consideration of personal liberty and very public disagreements among medical men as to the real value of the operation, ensured its virtual uselessness as a preventive measure. The debates over anti-typhoid inoculation illustrated, however, the encroaching into epidemiology of a new statistical methodology, that of biometry, which cast long shadows before it towards the later 20th century. On one trajectory, it was statistics rather than bacteriology that was to reshape the theory and practice of epidemiology in the long term. Several important figures in the bacteriology/epidemiology negotiation, like William Savage, were young bacteriologists carving out specialist careers; similarly, statistics were driven into English epidemiology by another striving young specialist, Major Greenwood. Greenwood has been a relatively neglected figure, but there is a case for arguing that he was one of its pivotal influences – less perhaps through his own original contributions than for the talents which he fostered as teacher and mentor.

It was Greenwood's own mentor, the biometrician Karl Pearson, who formalised the statistical attack on anti-typhoid inoculation. Almwroth Wright had sought to use statistical evidence in proof of the efficacy of the technique. Unfortunately, not only were his statistics very crude, but field experience seemed to demonstrate that the effectiveness of the technique was questionable (Matthews, 1995a). At this point Pearson provided a destructive statistical analysis of Wright's data. The technique then went back to the laboratory where another bacteriologist, William Leishman, sorted it out and finally produced both laboratory and statistical evidence, based on field results, of efficiency. With the outbreak of World War I in 1914, the whole debate resurged over the issue of whether British troops going abroad should be compulsorily inoculated against typhoid. In an argument considerably complicated by political, ethical, and military considerations, the statisticians once again set out to try to develop a method of analysis which would validate preventive and curative procedures to the satisfaction of both the statistician and the epidemiologist. In 1915, Greenwood, in association with the Cambridge mathematician G. Udney Yule, published an essay on the interpretation of inoculation statistics in which they demonstrated the fundamental tensions between statistical modelling and biological reality, concluding "that mathematical difficulties of method must not absorb the whole energies of the statistician" (Greenwood and Yule, 1914–15). If the new statistical methods were to be of value to epidemiology, biological reality must not be lost sight of.

Greenwood's campaign to bring new statistical methods into wider use and better repute in epidemiology and public health can be seen in part as an attempt to maintain and extend the population emphasis within epidemiology, and also as an active counterbalance to the ominous minutiae of the fashionable bacteriological model. Yet, as already indicated, point of contact epidemiology did not find extensive application in England; indeed, medical officers of health were reluctant even to use inoculation for fear that it would distract from the need to secure safe water supplies and proper sanitation. Between about 1900 and 1914. There was an ongoing debate within English epidemiology as to the uses and limitations of bacteriology and later of statistics, and these debates continued to some degree after the war.

After 1918, much of the dynamism of pre-war epidemiology in Britain disappeared. The Medical Department, for so long the central force of English epidemiology, was replaced by the Ministry of Health, and Arthur Newsholme, a dedicated epidemiologist, was replaced as Chief Medical Officer by George Newman for whom epidemiology had never been much of an interest. These changes, combined with the extending administrative responsibilities of the local medical officers of health, effectively put an end to the old epidemiological community as it had existed before the War. In the 1920s, a new, professional community of epidemiologists gradually emerged under the aegis of Major Greenwood, and achieved an institutional focus with the creation in 1927 of the Department of Epidemiology and Vital Statistics at the new London School of Hygiene and Tropical Medicine (LSHTM).

Continuity with the pre-war world was represented by Major Greenwood, and to a lesser degree by men like Hamer (Mendelsohn, 1998). Greenwood was perhaps the moving force in English epidemiology in these years, being appointed head of the Medical Research Council's Statistical Unit after the War, and first professor of the new department at the LSHTM in 1927. In particular, he joined William Whiteman Carlton Topley in the latter's attempt to develop the field of epidemiology along biological lines. Wartime experience of the great Serbian typhus epidemic focused Topley's attention on epidemiology. As a laboratory scientist, however, he found its lack of precision intellectually unsatisfying, and he began to explore it as a form of experimental biology (Greenwood, 1944).

Topley recognised two outstanding obstacles to the investigation of epidemic disease behaviour along bacteriological lines: that the diseases best suited to such inquiry were those in which the causal organisms were unknown (e.g., measles), and that it had proved impossible to reproduce in laboratory animals diseases as they occurred in man (Topley, 1919). Building on the work of earlier bacteriologists like Savage, Topley resolved the problem by using naturally occurring infections of animals to elucidate the mechanisms of infection and epidemicity. Thus a series of studies developed the concepts of herd immunity and of unstable equilibrium between host and parasite, and incidentally reinforced recognition of overcrowding as a potent force in the generation of epidemics. At an early stage in these researches, Topley realised the need for a statistician to analyse the data he was accumulating, and recruited Greenwood's assistance. In the early 1920s, therefore, bacteriology and statistics went forward together, as the latest research tools of a broader, more theoretical epidemiology than had been practised in England before the War. In this development, it seems likely that Topley's experience of epidemic typhus in Serbia – the experience of observing a major epidemic in a human population at first hand – was central in arousing his interest in general, as against local, epidemiological problems.

The immediate post-war years saw a change in English epidemiology for both intellectual and institutional reasons. The period between 1880 and 1920, however, was not as devoid of epidemiological enterprise as is often assumed. The impact of bacteriology on the English epidemiological tradition was rather less impressive than has been generally accepted, and the practitioners of epidemiology continued actively to evolve new methods for the investigation of disease and disease outbreaks, some of which involved bacteriology, but in a constructive and exploratory rather than a reductionist, contact-tracing, mode. Reductionist bacteriological methods encountered criticism and resistance from an already well established tradition, which accepted as sensible certain modifications to its practice indicated by bacteriology, but which drew back from embracing a wholesale bacteriological perspective on problems of disease. Less historically obtrusive, more insidious in its gradual inroads into epidemiological method, was the statistical methodology introduced by Major Greenwood and creatively developed by Austin Bradford Hill, which drew its inspiration from Pearsonian biometry. Under Greenwood's guidance, this achieved a subtle and influential accommodation with the statistical and observational traditions of high Victorian epidemiology in the inter-war years; under Hill it contributed to the methodological revolution which transformed epidemiology after the Second World War (Doll, 1994; Susser, 1985).

Statistical methods in epidemiology: Karl Pearson, Ronald Ross, Major Greenwood and Austin Bradford Hill, 1900–1945

Anne Hardy, M. Eileen Magnello

Wellcome Trust Centre for the History of Medicine at UCL, Euston House, 24 Eversholt Street, London NW1 1AD, UK

Summary

The tradition of epidemiological study through observation and the use of vital statistics dates back to the 18th century in Britain. At the close of the 19th century, however, a new and more sophisticated statistical approach emerged, from a base in the discipline of mathematics, which was eventually to transform the practice of epidemiology. This paper traces the evolution of that new analytical approach within English epidemiology through the work of four key contributors to its inception and establishment within the wider discipline.

"The object of the present *Grammar*", wrote Karl Pearson (1900, p. 515) towards the end of the second edition of *The grammar of science*, "has been chiefly to show how a want of clear definition has led to the metaphysical obscurities of modern science". Pearson did not explicitly delineate a statistical methodology in his text, but his call for clear definition provoked an enthusiastic response among many young, scientifically-minded men in the last decade of the 19th century, not least in a medical student named Major Greenwood (1880–1947), who had rather have studied either history or mathematics, but whose family tradition had compelled him into medicine (Hogben, 1950–51). It has long been recognised among historians of epidemiology that the quantitative methods and statistical philosophy of Karl Pearson (1857–1936) with W.F.R.Weldon (1860–1906), and Francis Galton (1822–1911) generated the processes by which the modern discipline emerged after World War II. The extent of the metaphysical confusion within which the process was generated has generally been underestimated: bacteriology, it is assumed, effectively displaced the existing tradition of epidemiological study, which was only gradually rediscovered in the years after 1910. This perspective overlooks the obduracy of epidemiology, however. Despite the challenge of bacteriology, despite the historicism and metaphysical obscurity re-introduced into the discipline by Charles Creighton, whose monumental "*History of epidemics*" appeared in the mid-1890s, despite the Pearsonian conviction that every biological event could be reduced to a mathematical formula, epidemiology retained a distinct identity, and consciously maintained and debated that entity, in the years between 1900 and 1940. In that debate, a crucial preparation for the development of the subject after 1945, Major Greenwood played a central part.

Before the 1890s, Victorian epidemiology had been a largely observational, environmentally-oriented science, which employed fairly simple statistical methods. The year 1894 proved something of a watershed, with the publication, on the one hand, of Creighton's History, which sought to illuminate disease causation and behaviour through the examination of past epidemics, and on the other of Emil Roux' successful anti-toxin therapy for diphtheria. The historical approach induced some epidemiological practitioners to go back to older sources, and to develop, from a reading of Hippocrates, Baillou, and especially Sydenham, a more metaphysical approach to problems of disease. The enticing technologies of bacteriology, by contrast, appeared likely to dispense with the need for epidemiology altogether; as one observer noted, once the germ had been found, "The next step is either to exterminate the germ or devise an antidote. This step having been taken, the epidemic disease ... is, or ought to be, of only historical interest" (Anonymous, 1921). The metaphysical approach developed, no doubt, in part as a reaction against epidemiology: those who espoused it tended to be sharp critics both of bacteriology and of the new statistical methods.

For statistics also played a part in this confusing equation. Between the devil of metaphysics and the deep blue sea of bacteriology lay a small band of practitioners who sought the general laws of disease through the application of mathematics, a discipline at once more rigorous and less reductionist than either. Victorian epidemiology had made judicious use of others' expert knowledge – of meteorology, of geology, chemistry, bacteriology, and statistics – but rather as consultant than as integral methodologies. It was, in the tradition of William Farr, a highly pragmatic epidemiology, dealing with the best available data and not straying far from them, using average death-rates, simple methods of statistical induction, and common sense, to draw conclusions – relationships – between illness and insanitary conditions (Greenwood, 1935). It was focused largely on local disease outbreaks, on patterns of disease on the ground, and entered into little speculation about issues such as epidemic waves, or the periodicity between outbreaks. Mathematics was not made use of in these investigations, nor were complex statistical analyses: there were few medical men – let alone epidemiologists – with the ability to deal in mathematical issues. Mathematics did not feature in the curriculum of the Victorian medical school, and the only "epidemiological" training then available was vital statistics taught on the Diploma in Public Health courses. Like the great majority of any given population, early twentieth-century medical men shied away from anything at all complex to do with figures.

There were, however, a handful of medical men who were attracted by mathematics as a means of epidemiological analysis, who were interested in trying to establish "natural laws" for the behaviour of disease. The near-universal movement towards new standards of scientific rigour, which had been gathering pace through the 19th century, invited criticism of epidemiology, which, bacteriology apart, contained little that could be described as scientific method. Statistical methods offered an alternative to bacteriology – and a methodology which could be integrated into the existing explanatory models without too evidently relegating the whole discipline to the mathematical practitioners. Indeed, the idea of supplying statistical methods to measure biological variation derived from Francis Galton, whose work influenced the Darwinan zoologist W.F.R. Weldon who, in turn, provided the impetus to Karl Pearson's development of the modern theory of mathematical statistics. Their work represented a new and challenging method of scientific verification and exploration (Magnello, 1996). For statistically-minded epidemiologists, the statistical tools which Pearson had created for curve-fitting and goodness of fit tests (for asymmetrical and symmetrical distributions), in addition to the series of correlation methods he devised, had a particular attraction. Having created the Biometric School at University College London (UCL) in 1893, by 1900 Pearson had devised the foundations to the mathematical theory of statistics and the journal Biometrika had also been founded by Weldon, Pearson, and Galton. Some three years later, Pearson established the Drapers' Biometric Laboratory at UCL.

It was in the first years of the new century that Greenwood approached Pearson for guidance on using statistics in medical research, so initiating one of two slender contemporary strands of interest in statistical epidemiology. At about this time also the second strand emerged, independently of the biometric stable, in the redoubtable person of Ronald Ross (1857–1932), discoverer of the mosquito transmission theory of malaria. Like Greenwood, Ross was a reluctant medical man, and also like Greenwood, pressurised by his father into the profession. Ross had wanted to be a painter, but he was also multi-talented: painter, musician, physician, and mathematician. Arriving in India in 1881, he spent most of his first six years in the Bengal Medical Service studying mathematics. Writing to G.H.F. Nuttall in 1899, just before he returned home, he asked, "Can you tell me whether immunity has been ever studied mathematically?" A few years later, as external examiner for the Diploma in Tropical Medicine and Hygiene at Cambridge University, he spent his spare time buying maths books in the town (Nuttall, 1932–35). Ross had no affiliation with the biometric school, although he appreciated its standing, and sought Pearson's assistance on quantitative matters regarding his work. In 1908, tackling the problem of the relationship between mosquito density and malarial infection in Mauritius, he used a simple difference equation in illustration, later developing applications of the technique in the second edition of his *"Prevention of malaria"*.

Ross's essay into quantitative epidemiology was closely associated with his interest in malaria. The discovery of the mosquito vector had, inevitably, resulted in unpopular attempts to reduce mosquito numbers as a preventive. It was, however, frequently observed that there was little apparent relationship between numbers of mosquitoes and numbers of malaria victims in a given locality; an observation which was used to argue that the amount of malaria did not depend on the number of mosquitoes, and that as an anti-malarial measure mosquito control was redundant. Experimental investigation being impractical, Ross set himself to examine the question by "a carefully reasoned analysis of the relations between the amount of disease and the various factors which influence it." His first attempt, using the inverse square law, was for Mauritian malaria; in the *"Prevention of malaria"* he extended his reasoning to the infectious diseases in general with a focus on time-to-time variations. He was subsequently asked to contribute a description of his methods to Nature (Ross, 1911).

Ross was no proselytiser of quantitative methods in the sense that Greenwood became; with his established reputation as an experimentalist, he did not need to be; he had no career to forge. He was, however, interested in general epidemiological phenomena, and in the business of scientific rigour; indeed David Bradley has noted as one of Ross's major intellectual legacies, "a rational and quantitative approach to communicable disease epidemiology" (Bradley, 1997). In his Nature article, Ross (1911) claimed to have established three laws of disease behaviour: that the disease (in this case malaria) cannot maintain itself unless the proportion of disease carriers is sufficiently large; that a small increase in carriers above this figure will cause a large increase in the disease; and that the disease will tend to reach a fixed value, depending on the proportion of carriers and the other constants. Ross expressed his doubt that such laws could be achieved except by "such mathematical attempts", and went on to extend their application: the equation showed that yellow fever could "scarcely be considered a disease of men at all", and explained both why certain diseases were absent in the presence of capable carriers, and the phenomenon of smouldering epidemics. He concluded with a generous swipe at existing epidemiological method:

"These studies require to be developed much further; but they will already be useful if they help to suggest a more precise and quantitative consideration of the numerous factors concerned in epidemics. At present medical ideas regarding these factors are generally so nebulous that almost any statements about them pass muster, and often retard or misdirect important preventive measures for years." (Ross, 1911).

Ross's mathematics were, however, too sophisticated for his wider audience, as Greenwood perhaps perceived, and his methods were only slowly, and at much later dates, taken up by other researchers (Hogben, 1950–51). His intervention in favour of quantitative methods in epidemiology was probably important in reinforcing a growing conviction among forward-looking medical institutions that mathematics was a potentially important epidemiological tool. The director of the Lister Institute of Preventive Medicine, Charles Martin, had in 1910 created a post for Major Greenwood as medical statistician; in 1914, the newly-established Medical Research Committee (MRC), funded under the National Insurance Act 1911 to investigate all conditions affecting the health of the people, created a similar post. The latter was filled by John Brownlee (1868–1927), also a Pearsonian disciple. Ross's reputation as a laboratory scientist of international standing lent authority to his endorsement of the mathematical approach: the British Medical Journal, for example, noted that his quantitative work was the more important because he was "neither an arm-chair worker nor a 'biometrician' – he was not "obsessed by a vision of the redoubtable Galton Professor of Eugenics", and his advocacy meant that statistical methods had now to be reckoned with seriously as a research technique for "the modern investigator". The journal concluded by quoting Ross directly (Anonymous, 1911):

"All epidemiology, concerned as it is with the variation of disease from time to time or from place to place, must be considered mathematically, however many variables are implicated, if it is to be considered scientifically at all."

Ross's views on epidemiology, despite his independent stance, strongly echo Francis Galton's dictum that "until the phenomena of any branch of knowledge have been submitted to measurement and number it cannot assume the dignity of a science" (Pearson, 1922). For epidemiology, the study on which preventive medicine was based, quantitative methods were essential if it was to have any claim to be a modern science.

The reception accorded to Ross's quantitative studies by the British Medical Journal make clear the extent to which the association with Karl Pearson was a double-edged sword for those wishing to apply biometric methods to medicine. On the one hand, the methods embodied the new science; on the other, they were irrevocably associated in many educated minds with scientific controversy over issues of heredity. For the preventive medical community in particular, hereditarian attitudes which condemned the past 60 years of public health effort as contributing to the deterioration of the British race, were highly sensitive (Porter, 1991). Pearson himself, by his remarks about the deterioration of British intelligence in his Huxley lecture for 1903, had raised hackles among the medical community. Moreover, in 1911–12, Pearson crossed swords with Arthur Newsholme, a leading medical officer and student of epidemiology, over the use of statistics in epidemiological studies. Biometricians with an interest in epidemiology, like Greenwood and John Brownlee needed to tread warily with the epidemiological and public health community, associated as they were with Pearson, regarded with suspicion by the non-mathematically minded, and medically speaking of parvenu status. As the British Medical Journal put it in 1911, the modern English school of quantitative methods had "suffered from not numbering among its members any experimental worker of world-wide reputation and perhaps also from the, largely accidental, associations in the public and professional mind between mathematical methods and the heated controversies respecting Mendelism and eugenics" (Anonymous, 1911). As Greenwood was repeatedly to record during the inter-war years, in the early 20th century biometrics and statistics were regarded as barely respectable by most medical men. Among the medical statisticians active before World War I, Greenwood, in particular, was consciously fighting a battle to establish medical statistics as a respectable discipline.

The dubious reputation of statistics in epidemiology in the first decade or so of the 20th century was not simply the consequence of widespread mathematical incompetence, or of its association with controversy. Since the 1870s, for example, the vigorous campaign against compulsory infant vaccination against smallpox had compounded suspicions about the use of statistics in medical argument, and these doubts had been reinforced by the fiasco of Almroth Wright's anti-typhoid vaccine in the Boer War. In a discussion of the anti-typhoid vaccine at the Royal Sanitary Institute in 1914, for example, Herbert Snow, an anti-vivisectionist London practitioner, used Wright's vaccine to illustrate his argument that,

> "*there was no note of scientific certainty from beginning to end... the case for inoculation was presented to them now on the strength of statistics. Disease-phenomena being extremely complex, medical statistics were apt to be most unreliable. Every doctor present knew that. At the hands of unscrupulous men they were apt to show all sorts of results. Most medical statistics were not worth the paper they were written on; one could cook them and fake them in any direction*" (Woodhead, 1915).

This general suspicion of statistics, which ran through the medical profession, existed in a more refined form among the established epidemiological community, who operated within the existing field-work tradition. The epidemiologists and public health workers already using statistics, even if in a fairly crude form, were not more receptive to biometric ideas: they feared that more sophisticated methods of analysis would result in a belief that, given sufficiently refined methods of investigation, "truth could be elicited from *any* data, however inaccurate or biased" (Greenwood, 1935). Coming from a highly environmentalist, observational, tradition, early twentieth-century epidemiologists were as wary of being over-ridden by statistical methods divorced from biological reality as they were of being subjugated to the minute concerns of the laboratory.

It was against this background of misunderstanding and suspicion that Major Greenwood began to carve out a career for himself as a medical statistician. Unlike John Brownlee, who pursued his interest in statistical epidemiology alongside a career in public health and clinical medicine until his appointment to the Medical Research Council, Greenwood early directed his efforts to a specific career in medical statistics. Even before his appointment to the Lister, one of his early publications carried the subscription, "From the London Hospital Statistical Laboratory". In his early 20s, working in Leonard Hill's laboratory at the London, reading the "*Grammar of science*", working under Karl Pearson in his Biometric Laboratory, Greenwood began to move towards medical statistics as a career, even though there were no easy openings for a young man with such an ambition. He quickly slanted himself towards epidemiology – the one branch of medicine where statistical methods were already in established use. Although his first publication, in which he acknowledged Pearson's assistance, dealt with the weights of human viscera detailed in the post-mortem records of the London, it already had an epidemiological aspect: it discussed the problems of working with hospital statistics, and concluded by stating that the intention had been to compare the experience of a normal or healthy group with a diseased "group of population" (Greenwood, 1904). Greenwood's second paper, with Theodore Thompson of the London Hospital, was on meteorological factors in acute rheumatism; his third on marital infection in respiratory tuberculosis. Although not recorded in the last (1905–06) membership roll of the old Epidemiological Society, he soon appeared as an active member of the Epidemiological Section of the new Royal Society of Medicine, publishing a first paper in the Proceedings for 1908. In 1907, he published his first paper in the new, dynamic, Cambridge-based Journal of Hygiene, a serial founded (in 1901) and edited by G.F.H. Nuttall, which reflected a distinct strand of epidemiological endeavour: rational, scientific and modern in tone, combining a markedly bacteriological approach with the epidemiological and statistical.

Before the First World War, Greenwood was a vigorous activist and propagandist in his own cause. Well aware of the pervasive medical mistrust of his personal intellectual and professional objectives, he sharpened his wits and his tongue, and acquired, as he later recalled, the "virtues and vices of a minority, a certain courage and a certain trick of over-emphasis [which] always characterise a fighting minority". At this time, he regarded himself primarily as a medical statistician. "I used to see in the statistician the critic of the laboratory worker", he later remarked revealingly, "It is a role which is gratifying to youthful vanity, for it is so easy to cheat oneself into a belief that the critic has some intellectual superiority over the criticised" (Greenwood, 1924). Greenwood's contest with Almroth Wright over the viability of the opsonic index in 1908–12 was characteristic of this phase, and was also nicely calculated to attract the attention of the wider medical community (Matthews, 1995b). It seems likely that Wright's outspoken disdain for traditional preventive medicine and epidemiology, typical of many bacteriologists at that time, added to Greenwood's determination to put the world to rights: the immediate future for any aspiring medical statistician lay – as Greenwood's appointment to the Lister in 1910 was to prove – in precisely those two sub-disciplines. Even at this stage in his career, Greenwood was adept at utilising the current preoccupations of epidemiology to assist his own arguments; with his latent historical sympathies, he quickly took on board the retrospective historical methodology re-introduced by Creighton in the 1890s, and integrated it into his own perspective. At the 17th International Congress on Hygiene, held in London in August 1913, he presented an "exhaustive" account of the history of scarlet fever and of epidemiology in the past 100 years. Discussing the problem of describing the evolution of an epidemic, he argued that in deciding such questions:

> *"a knowledge of epidemiological history, combined with a firm grasp of the statistical method were as essential parts of the outfit of the investigator in that field as was a grounding in bacteriology. It was ... along the lines of Dr Brownlee's work, in applying practically mathematical considerations to the question, that future progress must be looked for..."* (Anonymous, 1913).

In the discussion that followed, Greenwood claimed to be satisfied to find that all the speakers "more or less distinctly recognised" that careful descriptive analysis based on modern statistical methods was an essential part of epidemiology: "the popular impression that such studies have lost their value in the light of bacteriological science seems to be entirely erroneous".

By the eve of the First World War, Greenwood's position in the epidemiological community was established. He had his post at the Lister, he was an active member of the Epidemiological Section of the Royal Society of Medicine, and his list of publications was growing steadily. Political adroitness, and a willingness to take a stand against bacteriology gave him stature within his community, despite the misgivings of his epidemiological colleagues towards biometric methods. Sir William Hamer (1862–1933), a distinguished epidemiologist who worked for the London County Council, was for many years celebrated for having likened epidemiology to the Sleeping Beauty with bacteriologists as authors of the spell. In 1917, he portrayed Greenwood "glowing with epidemiological enthusiasm", in contrast to his own profound depression over the future of the discipline. Talking to Greenwood, he recorded:

> *"For a few brief moments there was revealed over the hills and far away a sunlit world of practical endeavour ... I was filled with hope, that, as the good sword of the new statistical methods was in his hand, he might hack a way through and awaken the Princess Epidemiology."* (Hamer, 1917).

Greenwood's success was in considerable part due to his ability to express himself clearly, and to communicate his statistically-based epidemiology in a variety of literary forms ranging from the immediately accessible to the highly mathematical. His historical sympathies and the fact that he was not a professional mathematician probably helped here: throughout his life he collaborated in his more mathematical-statistical projects with the Cambridge statistician G. Udny Yule (1871–1951). Yule first came into contact with Pearson as an engineering student attending Pearson's lectures on applied mathematics and mechanics in the late 1880s, and later became a

Demonstrator in Pearson's Biometric Laboratory. Yule's contributions to the modern theory of mathematical statistics include his introduction of least squares measures as a means of interpreting multiple regression (which has since remained an important tool for regression). His work on statistical measures of association in 1899 engendered further statistical developments for Pearson, who devised a series of methods to measure statistical associations and correlations for discrete variables between 1899 and 1909. Unlike John Brownlee, whose papers were so reliant on mathematical-statistics that only those trained in the Biometric School could read them, Greenwood took considerable pains to keep a significant proportion of his work in language comprehensible to ordinary educated people. He admired Yule for his ability to express difficult mathematical arguments in language accessible to attentive readers, and he acknowledged that Brownlee's "not very attractive" literary style might deter readers from his work. While Greenwood could, and did, produce rigorous mathematical-statistical papers on epidemiology, he was entirely capable, as his "*Epidemics and crowd diseases*" demonstrates, of writing with perfect clarity for the ordinary educated reader.

As for so many of his generation, Greenwood's perspective on his life's-work was altered by his experiences in the First World War. Although he did not see active service, having become a sanitary officer in the Royal Army Medical Corps before being seconded to the Ministry of Health and Welfare for statistical work, Greenwood came to see the war as a melting-pot for academic research and its personnel: "The events of the great war", he noted in 1919, "have led to the co-operation of isolated investigators now…". (Greenwood, 1919).

Of even greater significance for his personal perspective, experience of the terrible influenza epidemic of 1918–19 forced a re-evaluation of the value of statistical methods: from this time onwards, the identity of Greenwood the medical statistician blurred imperceptibly into that of Greenwood the epidemiologist, as he realised that neither statistical techniques nor laboratory investigation could satisfactorily describe disease behaviour, that what was needed was to "learn more of the grammar of the language of epidemiology" (Greenwood, 1932).

The years 1919–20 also brought fresh professional associations. He was appointed to the new Ministry of Health as medical officer in charge of statistical work, and acquired new involvements with the National Institute for Medical Research and the Medical Research Council, in whose Hampstead premises he had his office. In 1920, moreover, he began his association with W.W.C. Topley (1880–1942), whose own wartime experience of the Serbian typhus epidemic of 1914–15 had turned him from a straightforward minute pathologist into an experimental epidemiologist, pursuing the laws of epidemic behaviour among populations of laboratory animals. For both Greenwood and Topley, first hand experience of major epidemics resulting from mass population movements occasioned by war were critical in shaping their postwar research concerns. For nearly 20 years, from circa 1920 to the outbreak of World War II in 1939, the two collaborated in an extraordinary enterprise of experimental epidemiology, with Topley designing the laboratory experiments and Greenwood and his statistical protegés providing the analytical expertise.

A continuing theme of Greenwood's reflections on the relationship between epidemiology and statistics, and one reason why he found experimental epidemiology so attractive, was the difficulty of balancing mathematical-statistical constructions against biological events. This problem was also, of course, that at the crux of general medical scepticism of the value of statistics and was, in the 1930s, to preoccupy Greenwood's protegé and later successor, Austin Bradford Hill, as he began to drive statistical methods into clinical practice. Both Greenwood and Brownlee had, for example, been attracted by Pearson's family of frequency curves, which was capable of describing effectively both asymmetrical and symmetrical distributions (which included the normal curve), so enabling statisticians to deal with a wide range of frequency systems. According to Greenwood, Brownlee took this work further than any other contemporary epidemiologist, with the objects of first graduating the statistics, and then, if possible, of classifying epidemics on the basis of the type of curve found. The results were fairly satisfactory as far as graduation was concerned, but he found it impossible to obtain any useful classification. The only clear result was that Pearson's Type IV curve (the family of asymmetric curves) was found more commonly than any other. As Greenwood remarked, "The more fundamental problem of epidemiology, viz., that of discovering the laws of which the epidemic, whether viewed in its temporal or spatial relations, is an expression, could scarcely be solved in this way" (Greenwood, 1916). By using Pearson's method of curve-fitting, Brownlee eventually obtained a curve which effectively described certain symmetrical epidemics, but he could not obtain any function which accounted satisfactorily for the marked asymmetry characteristic of many epidemics. Ross's theory of happenings, which similarly attempted a mathematical law of epidemics with an *a priori* method, was not vastly more successful in Greenwood's view, even though he considered that Ross had achieved important results in the genesis of an asymmetrical curve with general application. "It is too early", he cautioned, "to speak with confidence". Once restrictions were relaxed, he warned, the analysis would inevitably become more intricate and, "having devised an *a priori* law, one must devise, usually by [Pearson's] method of moments, a way of applying the law to statistical data" (Greenwood, 1916). Thus, Greenwood also emphasised the utility of Pearson's family of curves for fitting empirical distributions to one of Pearson's theoretical distributions. Greenwood was one of the few epidemiologists capable of understanding Ross's calculations at this time; it has been suggested that he found Ross's methodology too theoretical to be practicable as a way forward for contemporary epidemiology (Hogben, 1950–51).

The use of mathematical-statistics for medical data concerned Greenwood in another, more practical, way at this time. In the early months of the war, Greenwood and Yule were engaged in a fairly comprehensive investigation of the inoculation statistics of cholera and typhoid, which led them into a consideration of the theoretical problems associated with their interpretation. As part of this inquiry, they used firstly Pearson's chi-square goodness of fit test (of 1900) to determine how well an observed distribution compared to the theoretical distribution. They chose this test because it provided a criterion to determine if the probability that any difference between the incidence- or fatality-rates of the inoculated and uninoculated were statistically significant. They found that those who were inoculated recovered from typhoid and thus there was a lower mortality rate in these patients. They argued that the "case in favour of anti-typhoid inoculation as a practical means is very strong" (Greenwood and Yule, 1914–15, p. 120). They wanted to determine next the ratio of "advantage of immunisation process as the difference between fatality rates" using data from cholera. They used the tetrachoric correlation coefficient and found mainly moderate correlations (ranging from 0.35 to 0.53) with one high correlation (0.83). In the final section of the paper, they wanted to know whether the cholera or the typhoid inoculations produced better immunisation results. To examine their data they used Pearson's product-moment correlation (which was very similar to Pearson's tetrachoric correlation coefficient) to determine if there was a statistically significant difference between the results from typhoid and cholera. The results in the final section were disappointing as they could not determine which set of inoculations was more efficacious. "The general lesson to be learned", they concluded, "is that mathematical difficulties of method must not absorb the whole energies of the statistician". Pearson and his pupils had provided a solution for many mathematical difficulties, but "Dr Brownlee and Dr Maynard alone, so far as we are aware, have assigned a due measure of importance to the biological difficulties of interpretation which present themselves in connection with such inquiries" (Greenwood and Yule, 1914–15, p. 189).

By 1916, therefore, Greenwood was already moving into a position from which he viewed the efficacy of mathematical statistics, as applied both to epidemiological theory and to laboratory medicine, with some reservations, as being too detached from the biological reality of disease behaviour. His experience of the terrible influenza epidemic of 1918–19 compounded these doubts, as he tried to make sense of the raw data of the outbreak. Looking back to that event in his Herter Lectures of 1931, Greenwood recalled,

> "I [had] thought that with the sharp tools of statistical research Pearson had forged and a certain emotional faith in eugenics, we should reach epidemiological truth. Confronted with a mass of data, good, indifferent, bad, which the great epidemic of 1918–19 provided, upon which it was my duty to report, I realised my ignorance and helplessness." (Greenwood, 1932, pp. 19–20).

That helplessness, in his first year as the first official Government statistical expert, must have been somewhat traumatic, forcing a re-evaluation of his professional stance. In a paper delivered in 1924 at the Institute of Pathology and Research at

St Mary's Hospital, on Almroth Wright's home ground, he noted, "In some ways I value [the statistical method] more, in others less, than I did as a youth" (Greenwood, 1924). Although, he continued, he had not yet reached the point where he thought statistical criticism of laboratory investigations useless (as did, for example, Almroth Wright), he now placed "enormously more" value on direct collaboration, on the making of statistical experiments, and on the "permeation of statistical research with the experimental spirit". His collaboration with Topley furnished one of the many examples of the virtue of using life tables for epidemiological problems: the life tables and "shop-arithmetic" of William Farr were all that had been applied to the data of Topley's controlled mouse populations. By these means, however, "it is almost certain, that we shall reach a clearer insight into the phenomena of epidemic disease than generations of unintegrated experimental and statistical work have achieved; armed with that knowledge, we may be able to interpret the record, both minute and defective, of human history" (Greenwood, 1924).

Although Greenwood emphasised the importance of statistics to his St Mary's audience, he also stressed that different diseases might call for different investigative methods. Treading carefully, in a political situation of some delicacy, he noted the potential value of the element of heredity as an explanatory factor in the causation of some diseases. "Even the most convinced adherents of the environmental as opposed to the genetic origin of ill health", he now wrote, would hardly deny that Pearson's investigations of the factors influencing the ill-being or well-being of children had given a clearer insight into the roles of different possible and probable causes of ill-health. "Nature *does* present us with skeins not to be unravelled by the most habile experimenter, cases where the A, the B, and C *cannot* be studied in isolation". In such cases, the calculus of correlations was an invaluable tool (Greenwood, 1924).

The inter-war years saw Greenwood persistently working over the problematic relationships of biology, statistical method and natural law. In a well-established, if perhaps increasingly old-fashioned, scientific tradition, he seems still to have been preoccupied with the possibility of establishing natural laws of disease behaviour if only a correctly balanced biological/statistical accommodation could be achieved. In this sense, he was neither an original nor a creative epidemiologist – as both he and others noted, his long-term contribution to the subject was rather in the careers he fostered, in the department he established at the London School of Hygiene and Tropical Medicine (LSHTM) after 1927, in the scientific profile he maintained for epidemiology. While he continued to enjoy his work with Topley, and counted it as his most important research achievement, he did not take his discipline forward methodologically in these years. He worked with existing statistical tools, he did not modify, refine or develop them significantly. Summing up the state of the discipline in 1935, he could only remark: "There is no real doubt that the present standard of descriptive accuracy is far higher, and the analysis to which the data are subjected are less superficial, then even twenty-five years ago" (Greenwood, 1935, p. 65). Despite the enormous quantities of data provided in the past century by death registration and disease notification, despite the "hecatombs of animals" offered on the altars of experimental science, the new discipline of mathematical statistics had not succeeded in resolving the questions which had exercised epidemiologists for generations: the problems of secular variation, of changes of type, of methods of spread. Epidemiologists in the 1930s could not even explain why death-rates from tuberculosis had fallen, or why the virulence of scarlet fever had diminished.

Greenwood's central preoccupation here was the problem of elucidating the fundamental laws of disease – the epidemiologists' holy grail. He thought that the available series of disease-data were not long enough by comparison with the infinitely longer history of human populations to be of use; but that there was already so much medico-statistical information that choices for analysis had to be made, and even a choice involved so many further variables that the available statistical tools were not sophisticated enough to achieve satisfactory analyses. The central problems of epidemiology in searching for fundamental laws were, he considered, imperfect statistical methods and the range of significant factors in disease causation:

"The statistician, however mathematical, has no magic spell which frees Dame Nature to treat him differently from other men. She always answers truthfully the question you ask her, not the question you meant to ask but the one you did ask." (Greenwood, 1935, pp. 66–67).

Although the lectures from which these ideas were drawn were for public health men, and designed to generate a general interest in epidemiology rather than to stimulate innovative epidemiological research, Greenwood's reflections do indicate the limitations of his own brand of epidemiology. To free up epidemiological inquiry, techniques to account much more precisely for unknown or obscure variables, and more sophisticated methods which would allow equations involving the further powers of variable, had to be evolved. *"Epidemics and crowd diseases"*, although not a specialist textbook, still reveals the limitations of English epidemiology as represented by Greenwood on the eve of World War II. Although in terms of statistics and experiment, epidemiology had extended its perspectives since the Victorian period, the book was in many respects recognisably in the same tradition, emphasising the observation of biological events, stressing the importance of collaboration between different specialist workers, insisting that statistical methods should not play a dominant role. "I am a statistician by training," Greenwood had observed in 1931, "I emphasise the statistical aspects ... I do not wish to suggest that they are therefore the most important" (Greenwood, 1932, p. 28).

Within Greenwood's department at the LSHTM, however, a revolution – it is fair to call it that, although it also had roots in the United States – was brewing. Austin Bradford Hill (1897–1991), son of the physiologist Leonard Hill, who had fostered Greenwood's own research career, had been one of Greenwood's earliest protegés.

Debarred from a career in medicine by tuberculosis and the loss of a lung, Hill had studied economics at Greenwood's suggestion in the aftermath of World War I. After qualifying in economics at the University of London in 1922, Hill found a place in the Medical Research Council's Statistical Unit managed by Greenwood. Under Greenwood, the Unit became closely associated with the new department of epidemiology and vital statistics at the LSHTM after 1927, and in 1933 Hill was promoted to a Readership at the School. He was to succeed Greenwood as Professor in 1945, and to assume the directorship of the Statistical Unit.

Hill's early research career was unremarkable. He had begun by intending to pursue a career in epidemiology with a special interest in occupational medicine. Greenwood, too, had developed an interest in this subject during the first war, and before the second war Hill was largely occupied in collecting and analysing data relating to occupational illness – of London bus drivers, printers, cotton weavers and spinners, and asbestos workers; he was also involved in the Topley and Greenwood experimental epidemiology project. These surveys, as Richard Doll later observed, were characteristic of their period, using routinely collected morbidity and mortality data, and attempting to elucidate them by means of population surveys. The originality of Hill's approach to epidemiology, and his stature as a creative epidemiologist, only began to become apparent after the second war, when he had succeeded Greenwood as professor. His development of the traditional survey methods, of the methods of case-control and cohort studies, and his guidelines for drawing conclusions about causal relationships, were all part of a wider upsurge of creative energy in the discipline of epidemiology which distinguished the post-World War II period (Susser, 1985). None the less, much of the creative thought and planning behind some of the later innovations took place before the War.

Bradford Hill's introduction of randomisation into the clinical arena, his development of the modern randomised clinical trial, the prospective and case-control studies on smoking and lung cancer completed with Richard Doll, have tended to overshadow his other contributions. However, the "trial run" of randomisation took place in the epidemiological field, before the advent of streptomycin provided the opportunity of extending the technique into clinical medicine. Mervyn Susser (1985) has designated the prophylactic trials of vaccines as epidemiologists' "own firm round". It is a designation which Bradford Hill did much to make possible. In Britain in particular, a century-long tradition of opposition to immunisations laid every vaccine introduced up to 1940 and beyond open to both lay and medical suspicion and condemnation, and in the course of this long-standing argument statistical assessments of efficacy had come to be viewed with particular mistrust. This was not a uniquely British phenomenon, but the British were perhaps the most extreme among the European peoples in their cautious reaction to vaccines. The inter-war years had, however, seen an acceleration of research in immunology, with vaccines for tuberculosis, diphtheria and whooping cough being actively developed and tried. While both the tuberculosis and diphtheria vaccines had their problematic aspects, whooping cough vaccines proved significantly more difficult to manage in the developmental stages. The impetus for developing a satisfactory vaccine was strong, for the disease was still a notable killer of infants and young children, besides being a most distressing illness for both victim and attendants. Hill's interest in whooping cough dated from at least the early 1930s, when his first disease-specific publication dealt with the disease (Hill, 1933). When in 1942 the Medical Research Council broached their intention of trying out whooping cough vaccines with a view to extended preventive action against the disease, Hill took the opportunity of introducing the randomisation feature into these large-scale trials.

Hill's originality lay, of course, in his application of statistical randomisation to preventive medicine, and in his successful promulgation of Pearsonian statistics for medical research and specifically for clinical trials. Hill was, however, somewhat in contrast to Greenwood, basically interested in medicine rather than in history or statistics; he intended from the start of his career to be an epidemiologist, and he would have preferred to be remembered as an epidemiologist rather than as a statistician. Before 1940, it is possible to examine developments in British epidemiology to a great extent in isolation from developments in European and American epidemiology, as has been done in this essay. Greenwood, of course, had his contacts with American epidemiologists and biometricians – and in particular was a close friend of Raymond Pearl (who had his training in Pearson's Biometric Laboratory) – but as an academic discipline, epidemiology was a newly emerging one, and did not solidify its institutional structures and objectives in research and training until the 1940s in either England or America. When he succeeded Greenwood at the London School in 1945, Hill rapidly created a department of young research workers whose statistical and epidemiological expertise far outstripped anything in Greenwood's pre-war department. The Second World War marks a "convenient watershed" in the history of epidemiology (Susser, 1985), on which can be hung the transition from pre-occupation with infectious diseases to a recognition that chronic diseases and a range of other biomedical problems are important in the compass of the discipline. It also marks the definitive transition from an empirical to a statistical methodology. Significantly, Hill renamed his LSHTM department "Medical Statistics and Epidemiology". This change of emphasis may not have been fully approved by Major Greenwood. As early as 1924 he had envisaged the possibility that at some future date, "a brilliant young mathematician, building on higher foundations laid by Karl Pearson, will assert that in medical, or in any other biological research, the judgement of the biometrician must be final; he must be the ultimate court of appeal". It was not a prospect which appealed to Greenwood. Summoning, with some irony, the shade of the old adversary who so vehemently objected to the imposing of statistical discipline on medical judgement, he noted that when that time came, "I shall be found enlisted under the banner of Sir Almroth Wright ... the statistician must be the equal not the predominant partner" (Greenwood, 1924, p. 156).

Chohort analysis: W.H. Frost's contributions to the epidemiology of tuberculosis and chronic disease

George W. Comstock

The Johns Hopkins University, School of Hygiene and Public Health, Washington County Health Department, Box 2967, Hagerstown, MD 21742-2067, USA

Summary

Although Wade Hampton Frost was not the first to develop cohort analysis, it was the posthumous publication of his study of age and time trends of tuberculosis mortality that directed attention to this method of analysis. Frost's developing interest in and contributions to the epidemiology of chronic disease are reviewed in connection with a summary of his professional career.

Although Wade Hampton Frost's bibliography contains 57 scientific publications, only four of them deal with tuberculosis (Maxcy, 1941). This small proportion hardly suggests a major interest in or influence on the field of tuberculosis. However, a review of his biography shows that these four papers represent the culmination of a teaching career aimed at developing theoretical bases for epidemiology and expanding its limits.

Frost was born on the third of March, 1880, in rural Virginia, the son of a country doctor (Maxcy, 1941). His pre-college education was obtained at home under the tutelage of his mother except for a final two years in boarding schools. He entered the University of Virginia, and was granted his medical degree in 1903. Following the lead of many graduates of that institution, he sought a post in one of the Uniformed Services. In 1905, he was appointed Assistant Surgeon in the Public Health and Marine Hospital Service (now the Public Health Service). He was first assigned to one of the medical care facilities of the Service, as was customary for newly commissioned officers. With the exception of a temporary assignment to help investigate a yellow fever epidemic in New Orleans, and another to examine immigrants at Ellis Island, he spent several years in Baltimore, first at the U.S. Marine Hospital and then at the Training School for the U.S. Revenue Cutter Service (now the U.S.

Coast Guard). Two summers were spent on extensive cruises with the cadets, first to the New England area and then to Europe and North Africa.

In 1908, the arcane workings of the Service fortuitously resulted in an assignment that proved to be extremely fortunate for Frost, for the Service, and for public health. His new post was the Hygienic Laboratory (the forerunner of the National Institutes of Health) where he associated with some of the best investigators of the time. Maxcy, Frost's successor at Johns Hopkins, says Frost emerged from four years' service in this environment "a trained and highly competent investigator in epidemiology" (Maxcy, 1941). He was then assigned to posts that gave him opportunities to apply his new skills to studies of the health problems related to stream pollution, to poliomyelitis, and to influenza. This last assignment brought him into a life-long collaboration with Edgar Sydenstricker, the first national public health statistician (Kasius, 1974). Together they struggled with the problems of analysing morbidity surveys and family studies. Their solutions laid the groundwork for Frost's later work with tuberculosis.

In 1919, there came another major turning point in Frost's career. William H. Welch, the first director of the newly established School of Hygiene and Public Health of the Johns Hopkins University was able to obtain Frost's assignment to the School as Resident Lecturer in the Department of Epidemiology and Public Health Administration. In 1922, he was appointed Professor and Chairman of the Department. Three years later, in 1925, Epidemiology and Public Health Administration became separate departments, Frost remaining with Epidemiology as Professor and Chairman. During his first decade at the School, Frost was largely occupied in defining the field of epidemiology (Frost, 1923; 1927), developing appropriate courses of instruction, and working with his students on problems related to diphtheria, the common cold, and other acute infectious diseases.

During the 10 years from 1928 to 1938, the last decade of his life, he began to turn his attention to diseases of longer duration. What led him to expand his interests cannot be ascertained, but it seems reasonable to assume that Frost's inquisitive and logical mind would eventually lead to speculation about applying epidemiologic methods to chronic diseases. That such a transition did occur can be documented from his published and unpublished writings (Fee, 1987). Elizabeth Fee, in her history of The Johns Hopkins University School of Hygiene and Public Health, has three illustrative citations (Fee, 1987). In 1919, Frost's definition of epidemiology was "the natural history of the infectious diseases, with special reference to the circumstances and conditions which determine their occurrence in nature" (Fee, 1987). This was broadened but still restrictive in 1927: "It is (…) good usage to speak of the epidemiology of tuberculosis; (…) and also to apply the term to the mass-phenomena of such noninfectious diseases such as scurvy, but not to those of the so-called constitutiona diseases, such as arteriosclerosis and nephritis" (Fee, 1987). By 1937, he referred to "epidemiology as comprising the whole of the unremitting effort being made to clarify the relation between the disease and disabilities which men suffer and their way of life" (Fee, 1987).

Frost also left no indication of why he selected tuberculosis as the principal springboard for his venture into the field of chronic diseases. Maxcy surmises that there were several reasons (Maxcy, 1941). First, tuberculosis was then a major cause of death and disability. It was the sixth leading cause of death in 1930 (Linder and Grove, 1947), accounting for 6.3 percent of all deaths in the United States (U.S. Public Health Service, 1944). Frost also had a personal reason for appreciating its importance. In 1917, he had been diagnosed as having incipient pulmonary tuberculosis and had spent several months in a sanatorium (Maxcy, 1941). Furthermore, in making a break with traditional epidemiology, it is not unreasonable to concentrate on a single disease, especially one like tuberculosis that was both infectious and chronic. Ruth Puffer, one of Frost's major collaborators in his tuberculosis studies, suggests that he initially selected tuberculosis and rheumatic fever in order to compare the familial characteristics of these two chronic and infectious diseases (Puffer, 1946). Her suggestion is supported by the doctoral theses and publications of his students and colleagues (Maxcy, 1941). Two dealt with families of rheumatic fever patients and far more, 18 in number, had tuberculosis as their subject (Maxcy, 1941, and theses on file in Department of Epidemiology, Johns Hopkins School of Hygiene and Public Health).

It is likely that the emphasis on tuberculosis was influenced by the accessibility of new and challenging data for analysis. Dr. E.L. Bishop, Commissioner of Health for the State of Tennessee, was concerned about the high tuberculosis mortality rates in his state, and puzzled by the unusual concentration of tuberculosis deaths among elderly persons and rural residents (Zeidberg et al., 1963). With the help of the Rosenwald Fund, he began to study tuberculosis in the little town of Trenton. When the type of analyses employed in investigations of acute infectious diseases did not seem to make sense, Bishop sought the help of his former teacher, Frost. After reviewing Bishop's findings, Frost identified some deficiencies and set down a detailed plan for a subsequent investigation (Zeidberg et al., 1963). Requisites of the new study included its being based on an unselected series of tuberculosis cases reported to the state from a single rural county of about 25000 persons. Detailed histories were to be taken of the cases and their families, and the subsequent incidence of tuberculosis. Comparisons were to be made with families without tuberculosis. In addition, Frost recommended tuberculin skin tests of the families, and for comparison, similar testing of children in the community schools.

Before embarking on such an ambitious investigation, Frost recommended a pilot survey in Kingsport. This was supported by the Rockefeller Foundation, and included virtually all the black families in the town (Frost, 1933). Rather than setting out to follow these families for the many years required by the long incubation periods commonly seen in tuberculosis, Frost suggested a retrospective approach by obtaining "simple facts (i.e. deaths and tuberculosis cases) as lie within the knowledge and memory of the average householder" (Frost, 1933). To analyze the data, Frost made adaptations to the life table methods used by Elderton and Perry in their prospective studies of the fate of persons discharged from tuberculosis sanatoria (Elderton and Perry, 1910) and by Weinberg in his study of the fate of children with tuberculous parents (Weinberg, 1913). Surprisingly, Frost does not cite the earlier work by Lawrason Brown, a clinician at the Adirondack Cottage Sanitarium in Saranac Lake, New York, and E.G. Pope, an actuary and patient at the Sanitarium (Brown and Pope, 1904). Frost's addition to these early applications of survival analysis was to recognise that the techniques could be applied to historical data and to show how to do this (Frost, 1933). His approach was subsequently used in studies of the risk of tuberculosis among families of tuberculosis patients in Philadelphia by Persis Putnam, a biostatistics graduate of the Johns Hopkins School of Hygiene and Public Health (Putnam, 1936); in Cattaraugus County, New York by Jean Downes, a colleague of Edgar Sydenstricker (Downes, 1935); and in Williamson County, Tennessee by Ruth Puffer, one of Frost's students (Puffer, 1946; Zeidberg et al., 1963).

The Williamson County Study was the major field study of tuberculosis in the United States during the 1930s and 1940s (Zeidberg et al., 1963). Its design was based on the prior experience in Trenton and Kingsport, and was laid out in considerable detail in a 1931 memorandum from Frost (Zeidberg et al., 1963). In addition to the use of historical survival analysis, a major feature was an adaptation of Chapin's secondary attack rate (Cassedy, 1962). In a chronic infectious disease like tuberculosis, there could be multiple cases within a single family. In such instances, it was often impossible to differentiate "primary" and "secondary" cases. To avoid this uncertainty, Frost suggested that the first case to be identified be called the "index case". Like primary cases in acute infections, index cases were to be excluded from calculations of risk associated with living in a tuberculosis family. Although not a perfect substitute for the primary case, the index cases could be clearly defined, and the attack rate among the other members of the household could be treated like a secondary attack rate.

Frost's first paper dealing with tuberculosis was basically an exposition of how to apply survival analysis to historical data, using the findings from the Kingsport survey mainly for illustrative purposes (Frost, 1933). The risk of dying from tuberculosis was found to be twice as high among families exposed to a tuberculous member than among families not so exposed, a finding very similar to those of Weinberg in an earlier prospective study in Germany (Weinberg, 1913). The Kingsport data also showed that the highest case rates occurred among young children, adolescents and young adults, and the elderly. This pilot study served its purpose. It allowed Frost and his students to develop methods for handling historical data and suggested some interesting findings to be investigated further in the Williamson County Study. Unfortunately, definitive results from the Williamson County Study would not be available until after Frost's death in 1938.

Perhaps the most widely cited of Frost's four papers on tuberculosis was the one on cohort analysis (Frost, 1939). This was found in his desk drawer and published after his death. The material had been presented to the Southern Branch of the

American Public Health Association and apparently laid aside to await additional data and analyses (Maxcy, 1941). To illustrate cohort analysis, Frost first arranged tuberculosis mortality rates from Massachusetts, supplied by his friend Sydenstricker, in a table with age on one axis and year of death on the other (Table 1). Arranged in this way, one could quickly see the age-specific mortality for each of the available years on one axis, and the time trend for each age group on the other. What proved to be most interesting in this instance were the rates in the cells of the table that lay on the diagonals, starting with the youngest ages and earliest years. These "diagonal rates" were analogous to tuberculosis mortality rates experienced by a group of persons born in a specified time period, the "cohort". They represented the tuberculosis death rates that were those experienced by each cohort of persons as they simultaneously aged and passed through time. One had to assume, of course, that immigrants and emigrants were generally similar in their risks of dying from tuberculosis.

As he studied the diagonal "cohort" curves, Frost first noted that in every cohort, the highest rates occurred among infants and very young children, and also among young adults. After this second peak, the tuberculosis death rates tended to decrease with age. The latter finding was in marked contrast to the death rates in any specified year in which the highest rates occurred among older persons.

Frost also noted that the pattern of high rates in infancy, lower rates among children, high rates again in young adult life, and then falling with increasing age was similar for each cohort, although rates at every age became consistently lower in more recently born cohorts. Frost concluded that the present high rates in old age must be "residuals of higher rates in earlier life". If the cause of the decreasing rates was that the frequency of exposure to tuberculosis had become progressively less, the similar age patterns for each cohort gave no indication that postponement of infection to later years caused more serious disease as Frost had once feared, based on his experience with acute infectious diseases (Frost, 1937). Thus, a theoretical objection to postponing infections with *Mycobacterium tuberculosis* was rebutted by this finding.

The findings in Frost's cohort analysis of tuberculosis death rates now appear to be the resultant of two different trends: a decreasing risk of becoming infected with time and a consistent pattern of change with age. His findings were in marked contrast to those of Andvord who had published cohort analyses of tuberculosis death rates in Norway six years prior to Frost (Andvord, 1930). Andvord's cohort curves were virtually identical with the age specific curves for each year during his observation period (Comstock, 1985), presumably because tuberculosis infection rates were not changing appreciably during the early years of this century in Norway. In retrospect, it is difficult to see why Andvord felt that rates for cohorts offered any advantage over age-specific death rates.

Although Frost referred to Andvord's paper, one wonders if Frost did not develop the idea on his own, only later finding Andvord's work. This speculation is supported by the similarity of Andvord's age-specific and cohort curves. If Frost's introduction

Table 1 – Deaths rates* per 100,000 from tuberculosis, all forms, for Massachusetts, 1880 to 1930, by age and sex, with rates for cohort of 1880 indicated

Age	1880	1890	1900	1910	1920	1930
Males						
0–4	|760		578	309	209	108	41
5–9	|43 \	49	31	21	24	11
10–19	126 \	115 \	90	63	49	21
20–29	444	361 \	288 \	207	149	81
30–39	378	368	296 \	253 \	164	115
40–49	364	336	253	253 \	175 \	118
50–59	366	325	267	252	171 \	127
60–69	475	340	304	246	172	95
70+	672	396	343	163	127	95
Females						
0–4	|658		595	354	162	101	27
5–9	|71 \	82	49	45	24	13
10–19	265 \	213 \	145	92	78	37
20–29	537	393 \	290 \	207	167	92
30–39	422	372	260 \	189 \	135	73
40–49	307	307	211	153 \	108 \	53
50–59	334	234	173	130	83 \	47
60–69	434	295	172	118	83	56
70+	584	375	296	126	68	40

* They were obtained as follows: For the years 1910, 1920 and 1930 – based on US. Mortality Statistics – deaths from tuberculosis, all forms. For the years 1880, 1890 and 1900, the rates used are calculated from data compiled by the late Dr. Edgar Sydenstricker from the state records. Because of differences of classification in deaths, it has been necessary to base the rates on the deaths recorded as "tuberculosis of the lungs" to get comparable data for these years. The rate calculated from the state records for "tuberculosis of the lungs" has been multiplied by a factor based on the proportion such deaths bore to those from tuberculosis, all forms. This factor varied with the year and age considered.

(Permission has been granted to reproduce Table 1. The original appeared in (Frost, 1939).

to cohort analysis had come from Andvord's work, it is hard to see why he would consider cohort data an improvement over the more readily available age-specific curve for a recent year. His correspondence with Sydenstricker further strengthens the assumption that he arrived at cohort analysis independently (Maxcy, 1941). In it, he gives no hint of the idea having been suggested to him by anyone else. That Andvord's report might have served to raise doubts about the generalisability of cohort analysis is indicated by a comment to Sydenstricker that in spite of having obtained similar results with data from England and Wales and also the United States, Frost still wanted to "get together material for a somewhat more orderly study later" (Maxcy, 1941).

Frost's other two papers on tuberculosis had essentially the same theme, namely what would be needed to control the disease and the probability of eventual eradication (Frost, 1937; Frost, 1935). He emphasised that the principal goal was the avoidance of infection. His contemporaries must have considered it nearly impossible to avoid tuberculous infection at a time when almost all adults in much of the country reacted to the strong dose of tuberculin, a reaction then considered indicative of tuberculosis infection (National Tuberculosis Association, 1940). Now, reactions to a strong dose of tuberculin are considered to be almost entirely the result of non-tuberculous mycobacterial infections (American Thoracic Society, 1969). But even though Frost could not have known this, he did know that close and prolonged contacts with infectious cases were more likely to result in tuberculous disease than casual contacts. He therefore emphasised the desirability of reducing the dose of infection by isolating as many infectious cases as possible in sanatoria. Another feature of tuberculosis that he felt favored its human hosts was the fact that most infections with tubercle bacilli were rather quickly walled off. These organisms could only become infectious if they were located in the lung where some, as a result of some uncommon circumstance, were able to erode through the encapsulating tissue and escape into an airway. Finally, he noted that the steady fall in tuberculosis death rates in Western countries was evidence that each case of tuberculosis was, on average, giving rise to less than one new case. Thus, "the biological balance is against the survival of the tubercle bacillus", and "the eventual eradication of tuberculosis requires only that the present balance against it be maintained" (Frost, 1937). Looking forward to a future when tuberculosis might become uncommon, Frost anticipated the modern disease control technique of concentrating more and more on infectious cases, advising "that the protection thrown around these infectious cases and their immediate contacts be not relaxed, but steadily and progressively increased" (Frost, 1937).

To Frost's credit, it should be pointed out that he realised that isolation of cases and surveillance of contacts could impose major hardships on patients and their families.

"If we are to require the isolation of open tuberculosis as a matter of public protection, it becomes a public responsibility to bear not only the cost of medical

care, but the whole cost to the patient's family, or as large a share as may be required. Moreover, it should be recognised that what is needed is not bare maintenance on a minimum or average 'relief' standard, that it is not sufficient merely to prevent their dropping lower in the economic scale; it may often be necessary to raise them to a higher level." (Frost, 1937).

Even with less frequent and shorter durations of hospital care at the present time, Frost's words still need to be heard and heeded.

It is hard to assess Frost's influence on the field of tuberculosis. A search through a nonrandom selection of books on tuberculosis reveals only scattered brief references to the age selection of tuberculosis and to his statement about the biologic balance being against the tubercle bacillus. Many epidemiologic textbooks, if they mention Frost at all, do so only in relation to cohort analysis. In my opinion, Frost's published work has had very little effect on phthisiologists and only a slight effect on epidemiologists. His influence appears to have been on his students, a high proportion of whom rose to high positions in public health. Through them, he had some influence on tuberculosis but very much more on epidemiologic thinking in all fields of public health. Frost was interested in tuberculosis as a means to an end, an area in which to develop methods for understanding and eventually controlling all the ills of mankind. He and his students gave us all a good start.

A short history of pathology registries, with emphasis on cancer registries

Benedetto Terracini[1], Roberto Zanetti[2]

[1] University of Torino and Regional Centre for Cancer Prevention of Piedmont, Via Santena 7, 10126 Torino, Italy
[2] Cancer Registry of Torino and Regional Centre for Cancer Prevention of Piedmont, Via Santena 7, 10126 Torino, Italy

Summary

In the 1950s, major technical problems for ensuring quality and effectiveness of population based registration of cancer and other conditions had been faced and solved. Nevertheless, the classical epidemiological texts published in the 1960s and the 1970s gave little attention to and showed limited enthusiasm for population-based registries of pathology. The latter, in fact, have been marginal to the dramatic evolution of basic conceptual issues such as study design and causal inference. Consideration might increase with the use of registries in order to assess quality of care in a public health perspective.

In looking retrospectively, marked changes occurred since the 1960s in distribution between countries and continents of cancer registries to the dataset known as "Cancer Incidence in Five Continents" (where worldwide data from cancer registries of quality converge). The number of countries with cancer registries approximately doubled vs. a fivefold increase in both the number of active cancer registries and the total population served by registration. Nevertheless the increases were concentrated in developed countries whereas in developing countries there was a substantial decrease in registration, attributable to the political and economical situation.

Background

The terms used in the present article are those indicated by Last (1988). A *registry* is a file of data concerning all cases of a particular disease or other relevant condition in a defined population, so that the cases can be related to a population base. The register is the actual document and the *registry* is the system of ongoing registration. A survey is an investigation in which information is systematically collected: it must not necessarily be population based and is not a continuous ongoing exercise. In fact, the borderline between the mechanisms and purposes of surveys and registries is not always sharp. For instance, in the US, in the past, cancer and stroke surveys fulfilled functions which nowadays would be attributed to permanent registries.

A number of roles have been traditionally recognised to population-based disease pathology registries (Tuyns, 1978). The primary function was (and is) the description of the frequency of disease in a population or in a set of sub-populations. Comparisons of rates with those produced by other similarly designed registries or within sub-populations served by the same registry provide clues for or evidence in favour of etiologic hypotheses. In fact, registries are also a database for investigating the natural history of disease. In public health, they have unique role for measuring the efficacy of screening programmes and for evaluating the effectiveness, coverage and overall quality of care.

The spectrum of health-related circumstances other than the occurrence of death or overt disease whose registration may be useful is wide and heterogeneous. Etiological studies may benefit from registries of persons having experienced exposure to alleged or proven risk factors, either endogenous (e.g., twins) or exogenous (e.g., occupational exposures, environmental accidents). Similarly, identifying and counting – within a population – persons suffering from restricted individual performance, bed disability, inability to work etc. may be the purpose of a registry and contribute to health planning. It has been pointed out that for a registry the important point is to find a gauge whose definition is consistent (Riley, 1993). This can be easy for standard gauges relying on diagnostic evidence, whereas in some circumstances individuals and societies make different decisions about the threshold between occurrence and non occurrence of health-related events – e.g., inability to work (Riley, 1993).

In the present context, attention will be addressed to measurements of the number of persons with overt disease. It is nowadays commonly accepted that a pathology-specific registry is justified in a given historical and societal framework when two conditions are met. Firstly, its *product* is of use in public health and/or for clinical and epidemiological research. Secondly, it can function effectively, i. e. the logistics for describing what it is expected to describe is adequate. Underlying *sine qua non* conditions include: (1) the specification of operational standards in order to characterise the individuals liable to registration; (2) the exhaustiveness of their identification (including estimates of cases lost to registration, if any), (3) the availability of adequate denominators in order to estimate rates; and (4) a favourable cost-benefit balance.

In fact, the term "registry" has been used to indicate the collection of individual nominal data within different contexts. Many initiatives were designed with the aim of assembling and managing data for the purpose of etiological or clinical studies, the estimate of occurrence on a population basis being a by product of the exercise. This has been the case of the registry of neurological diseases at the Mayo Clinic in Rochester, Minnesota (Kurland et al., 1982), which has been retrospectively extended back to 1907. Procedures of record linkage (of increasing sophistication throughout the decades) with the files of other institutions have been applied to such an extent that measures of disease occurrence in the area of Rochester and related trends have been available for almost half a century (Kurland et al., 1982).

Conversely, projects originally addressed to disease specific measurements evolved in other directions. In 1971, WHO launched a project for registering the occurrence of stroke over a 4-year period in 17 areas in Europe, Asia and Africa (Thorvaldren et al., 1995). This initiative led to what nowadays is known as MONICA. In fact, the representativeness of the population and the comparability of findings between areas has been problematic. In some countries MONICA evolved to more elaborated experiences: this occurred in Finland, where linkages between a variety of databases have been undertaken in the last decade, with the perspective of a reciprocal validation with mortality data (Tuormilehto et al., 1996).

The role of disease registers in the transition to modern epidemiology

Admittedly, the expansion of population-based registries and surveys has been relatively marginal to the dramatic evolution of epidemiological thought during the last decades. Basic conceptual issues such as study design and causal inference seem to have been in the forefront of modern epidemiologists to a much greater extent that the refinement of registration techniques (among which the current possibility of storing and processing a huge number of files is a major but not the exclusive one) and the updating of nosological classifications. As recently as 1985, in his seminal review, Mervin Susser, while focusing on the theories and techniques used to cope with the changed spectrum of diseases and on the relevance of population research, barely mentioned disease registries (Susser, 1985).

During decades, disease registries were felt to be less promising tools for epidemiological research than long-term community studies (the origins of which can be traced to Sydenstricker's study in Hagerstown, Maryland, in the 1920s (Sydenstricker, 1926)) or prospective studies on cohorts of persons exposed to exogenous agents. This lack of enthusiasm transpires from the major epidemiological texts published up to the 1970s, with the exceptions of books addressed to the epidemiology of conditions particularly liable to registration (Lilienfeld and Lilienfeld, 1980). The alphabetical index of the first edition of the "Epidemiological methods" of the Harvard School of Public Health (MacMahon et al. 1960) does not include the term "register" or "registry". The text mentions and acknowledges the role of two disease registries, i.e., cancer registration in Connecticut and the pulmonary tuberculosis register in Copenhagen (no mention of the Danish Cancer Registry!), but does not address the methodological problems inherent to the collection, processing and interpretation of data.

The introductory chapter of the second edition of "Principles of Epidemiology", (Taylor and Knowleden, 1964) addressed in general terms the issue of mechanisms (and shortcomings) of notification of infectious and industrial diseases and cancer registration. Clinical follow-up and measure of the results of therapy is specifically mentioned as a purpose of cancer registration (started in the UK in 1947 by the General Register Office) whereas it is acknowledged that registration "may ... provide information of epidemiological interest (but) at present it has not been used for this purpose". Approximately in the same period, another "classical", Morris (1970) commented that morbidity studies were becoming a main interest of public health since mortality seemed to be progressively less useful in the diagnosis of community health. Nevertheless "the cancer register and some hospital figures for psychosis apart, there are little data even on a national scale of the incidence and prevalence of the chronic diseases that now dominate the practice of medicine". Morris acknowledged the potentialities of the National Cancer Registration Scheme in England and Wales, but he pointed out the shortcomings – for aetiological research – created by the limited number of individual data which were recorded. While emphasising the need for a community (as opposed to hospital) approach, the scenario depicted by Morris, was that of a chronic disease register (as opposed to a registry addressed to a specific condition) in order to study the transition of subclinical to clinical conditions.

Probably, there were two reasons for this limited interest in population-based pathology-specific registries. One was scepticism on the ability of registries to produce reliable and exhaustive data. The other was mistrust for a practice which had proved to be able to work but which was still looking for a function. This was well expressed by Harold Dorn (who was a pioneer of the national cancer survey of cancer in the US, and later of international comparisons of incidence rates), in 1950, at the 77th meeting of the American Public Health Association:

"Universal reporting, wherever it has been partially successful, has been required for administrative or legal purposes. This is true for ... infectious diseases and occupational diseases. The statistical data resulting from the registration arise as by-products of the system and are not the primary reason for its existence. As yet, the principal reason for the reporting of chronic diseases has been the statistical data which would be obtained. Until registration of cases of disease can be justified for reasons other than the statistics which will result, the universal reporting of chronic disease is not likely to be a useful source of morbidity data." (Dorn, 1951).

In fact, Dorn (1951) intended to be more benevolent than critic: he was searching for justifications for registries (or large surveys) of chronic diseases to exist and went as far as to hypothesise "direct services" to be given to suspected cases in such an exhaustive form that record keeping would be tantamount to the creation of a registry producing morbidity data. Dorn was also concerned by the logistic and financial problems created by the huge volume of records, the possible heterogeneity in quality of data, if registration was exhaustive or – alternatively – the bias the likely selective identification of cases.

Rather than reviewing systematically the conditions for which population-based registration has been suggested, attempted or implemented, in the next paragraph, we concentrate on the history of cancer registration. This choice does not merely reflect our field of investigation. Indeed, cancer has probably been the condition for which the cultural gap nicely described by Harold Dorn half a century ago has been abridged to a greater extent. Perhaps more than for other conditions, it has become clear that the "descriptive" function of cancer registries is only a part of the game: their product has been the object of the application of sophisticated techniques based on elaborated conceptual thought, such as analysis of time trends and survival data, as well as international coordination, thanks to the International Association of Cancer Registries (IACR) and to the International Agency for Cancer Research (IARC) (Wagner, 1991).

It is acknowledged on the other hand that comparable efforts regarding a number of conditions such as congenital malformations, diabetes, neurological disease and others have been effective in producing epidemiological and clinical knowledge in those areas.

Cancer registration

The beginning

In the first decade of the twentieth century, surveys measuring the point prevalence of cancer were reported from a number of European countries (Wagner, 1991), including one in Baden in 1906, in which physicians were required to report all cases observed within a period of one year. These "censuses" failed to reach their purpose, because of the high number of missing reports and the inability to match those obtained from different sources regarding the same individual. It was also soon realised that compulsory notification would be unfeasible.

In Europe, permanent registration systems were implemented in Hamburg in 1926 and in Mecklenburg in 1937, both being discontinued during the second World War (Lilienfeld and Lilienfeld, 1980), in North America, permanent registries were started in 1927 and 1935, respectively in Massachusetts and in Connecticut, whereas the first national survey on a significant sample of the US population (10 metropolitan areas) was carried out by Dorn in 1937–38 (and repeated in 1947–48) (Dorn and Culter, 1959). It has been suggested by Dorn (1951) that the implementation of health surveys was influenced by the achievements of the application of statistical methods in social research.

By the end of the forties, the four population based registries (those serving the populations of Hamburg, Connecticut, New York and Denmark, the latter having been created by J. Clemmesen in 1943) and the survey system (10 metropolitan areas in the US) had faced and solved most technical problems (exhaustiveness/representativeness, merging of data from different sources, nosological classifications, use of appropriate statistical indicators etc.). The concepts underlying these achievements have been valid for the subsequent half century. The first experiences of using nominal rosters of cancer patients for analytical studies or for linkage with other registries are dated in the late 1940s (Busk et al., 1948).

One of the many merits of the late J. Clemmesen was that of convening on September 1946 a meeting of experts (in those days, they would not qualify themselves as epidemiologists but rather as "experts on cancer statistics"), who debated about the usefulness of population-based cancer data and compared the respective advantages and disadvantages of registries and surveys (Clemmesen, 1974). The group acknowledged the potential for descriptive epidemiological information of mortality statistics and clinical findings: rates for a number of cancer sites varied according to occupation and social status, the number of deaths classified as carcinoma of the lung was increasing in several countries, geographical differences regarding carcinoma of the stomach had become obvious and a number of studies had associated cancer of the cervix and cancer of the corpus to ethnicity and parity. Thus, incidence and mortality statistics should not be considered as alternatives: the latter are largely credible but the former can provide information on treatment and follow up. In conclusion:

"the collection of accurate statistics of cancer incidence and mortality among different ... people and ... countries may lead to important indications for experimental (sic! – ndr) studies ... (whereas) the information (provided by mortality statistics) ... is becoming increasingly inadequate, owing to growing numbers of patients successfully treated and thus not registered in the statistics of death. (Thus), we ... make the following suggestions:

1. *Great benefit would follow the collection of data about cancer patients from as many different countries as possible.*
2. *Such data should be recorded on an agreed plan so as to be comparable.*
3. *Each nation should have a central registry to arrange for recording and collection of such data.*
4. *There should be an international body whose duty should be to correlate the data and statistics obtained in each country."* (Clemmesen, 1974).

These recommendations had a great impact. The World Health Organisation, in 1950, created a Subcommittee on the Registration of Cases of Cancer (World Health Organization, 1950). Within a few years, European Nordic countries, Great Britain and Canada launched programs which led to national coverage of registration (Wagner, 1991). The model followed in the US was different: no national coverage was attempted, whereas a number of county- or statebased registries were created and the surveys on samples of the population were converted – in the early 1960s – in the Surveillance, Epidemiology and End Results (SEER) program which has regularly produced incidence and survival rates broken down by ethnic groups.

Modern times

Whereas the public health impact of cancer registration was immediately perceived in North America, UK and European Nordic Countries, in other industrialised nations, such as Southern European countries, expansion of cancer registration occurred later and was slower. A major reason for this was the limited availability of epidemiologically-oriented skills within programmes for cancer control. In addition, in those countries, the medical milieu was reluctant to accept the role of exogenous agents in cancer aetiology and the need for investigations in this area. This attitude also reflected a paralysing interpretation of medical secrecy and some reluctance in adopting internationally validated classifications of disease. These problems were shared by most Southern European countries, where, in the early 70s, a handful of pioneers (including some clinicians) realised that an exchange of experiences would have been profitable. Their effort led to the creation of the Group for Cancer Registration and Epidemiological Studies in Latin Language speaking Countries, which has successfully accomplished its mission during the last 28 years (it has also been engaged in the identification of exogenous cancer risk factors typical of these countries).

The need for international comparisons was implicit in the cultural pressure for the creation of cancer registries. The first world-wide analysis appeared in the 1960s, with the stimulating and ambitious (for those days) title of "*Cancer incidence in five continents*" (Doll et al., 1966). This marked the beginning of a series of publications appearing at 5-years intervals, taken care of by UICC, IARC and IACR (International Association of Cancer Registries, which was created after the International Cancer Congress in Japan in 1966). In 2002, the series has reached its 8th update (Parkin et al., 1997). Contrary the publication of mortality data by WHO, this editorial programme does not simply and passively accept data, but revises them and controls their quality. Two by-products of this strategy have been a world-wide standardisation of the activity of registration and the provision (in recent times through IARC) of technical advice to developing cancer registries.

In the early 1960s, 32 registries in 29 countries served 3% of the world population: at the end of the century, 186 registries in 57 countries served 9% of the world population (Figs. 1–3). Within this conspicuous increase, the relative contribution of cancer registries operating in developing continents has decreased in time, leading to the inequalities reported in Table 1. This dynamics has been driven by at least two components. One is the political and economical situation (which explains the appearance and disappearance of registries of small and medium size in Africa and South America). The other component is structural: the current overall picture has

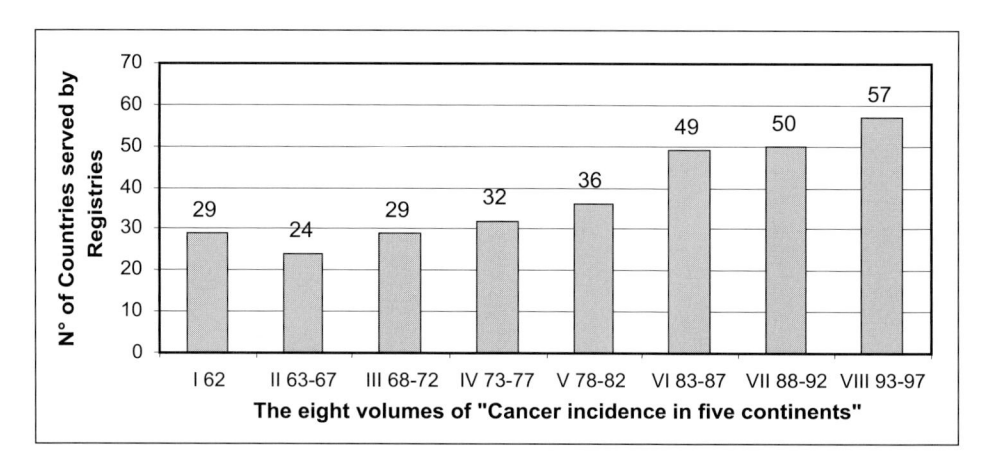

Figure 1
Number of countries served by population-based cancer registries reported in the volumes of "Cancer incidence in five continents" 1960–1992 (Doll et al., 1966; Doll et al., 1970; Waterhouse et al., 1976; Waterhouse et al., 1982; Muir et al., 1987; Parkin et al., 1992; Parkin et al., 1997; Parkin et al., 2003).

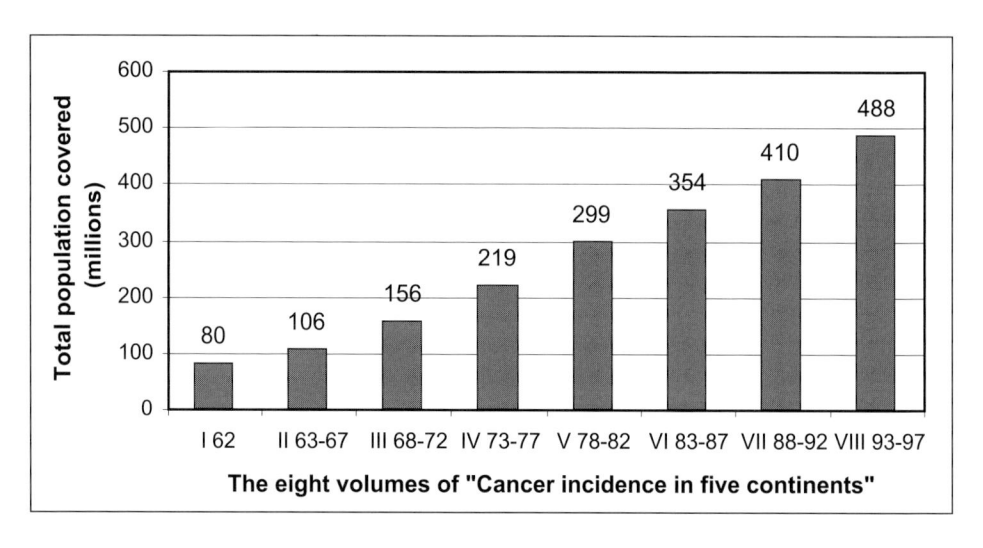

Figure 2
Total population served by population-based cancer registries reported in the volumes of "Cancer incidence in five continents" 1960–1992 (Doll et al., 1966; Doll et al., 1970; Waterhouse et al., 1976; Waterhouse et al., 1982; Muir et al., 1987; Parkin et al., 1992; Parkin et al., 1997; Parkin et al., 2003).

Figure 3
Number of population-based cancer registries reported in the volumes of "Cancer incidence in five continents" 1960–1992 (Doll et al., 1966; Doll et al., 1970; Waterhouse et al., 1976; Waterhouse et al., 1982; Muir et al., 1987; Parkin et al., 1992; Parkin et al., 1997; Parkin et al., 2003).

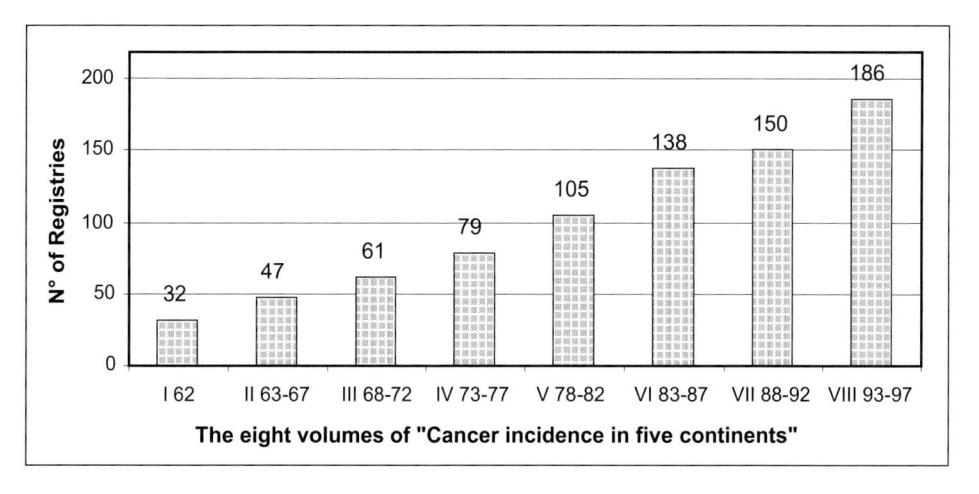

Table 1 – Geographical coverage by cancer registries around 1997 (from Parkin et al., 2003)

Area	Number of registries	Population served by registration (millions)	Total population around 1997 (millions)	% served population
Africa	6	7.2	743	1.0
Central and Latin America	11	15.4	489	3.1
Canada and US	26[a]	93.6	298	31.4
European Union	66	125.1	374	33.5
Other Western European Countries[b]	11	8.9	12	74.6
Other Europe	15	53.4	343	15.6
Asia	43	161.3	3552	4.5
Oceania	11	23.1	29	79.7

[a] Including SEER (Surveillance Epidemiology End Results) covering approximately 10% of the U.S. population.
[b] Norway, Switzerland, Iceland.

derived, in temporal order, by the national registries in Northern Europe in the 1950s, registries in North America and Japan in the 1960s, some large registries in Asia and national networks of registries in southern Europe starting in the 1970s. The current tendency to growth zero is partly attributable to the reduction in resources but also by the awareness that in a number of circumstances, incidence and prevalence estimates can be obtained indirectly from mortality and survival data, through validated methods (Parkin et al., 1993; International Agency for Research on Cancer, 1995).

Comparing the geographical distribution of cancer registries in 1960 and in 1990 shows a strong polarisation in areas of major economical development. Elsewhere, registry implementation has been discontinuous and unstable, in both time and space. Whereas decades ago developing areas were supported (also in terms of public health programs) by the industrialised countries from which they traditionally depended, more recently registration seems to depend from local initiatives, which find support in a complex programme launched by IARC some 10 years ago (International Agency for Research on Cancer, 1995).

Throughout half a century, there has been an increasing production of conspicuous descriptive data by cancer registries. The fact that the use of nominal files for analytical studies (either etiological or clinical) has been more limited derives from several reasons. On one hand the design of most analytical studies does not require the files of a central registry, even if this implies duplication of data collection. In addition, the circumstances for the implementation of analytical studies (formulation of a hypothesis and availability of the epidemiological skill required to carry out the study) do not necessarily coincide with the presence of a registry or with an adequate update of the data which it contains.

Investigations on temporal trends have been a natural consequence of "ageing" of registries (those of Connecticut and Denmark have reached their 50th anniversary!). Adequate statistical tools have been available since the 1970s. Limited international comparisons produced in 1980 (Magnus, 1981) led to a more recent and methodologically rich comprehensive world-wide analysis of temporal variations of cancer incidence and mortality (Coleman et al., 1993).

At first sight, studies on geographical heterogeneity within the areas served by cancer registries would seem to be the natural evolution of their activity. Whereas "maps" and descriptive studies have been reported by many registries, it must be acknowledge that they did not add much to findings from corresponding analyses on mortality. In fact, with a few exceptions, confirming the existence of alleged clusters of incident (or lethal) cancers proved to be much more difficult than originally hoped as well as their interpretation in terms of association with environmental exposures (Elliott et al., 1992).

In the early 1980s, it became apparent that cancer registries provided the basis for a number of "clinical" uses, i.e., other than the production of incidence data and clues for etiologic studies. Originally, the major effort was directed towards the evaluation of programs for the early diagnosis of cervical cancer with Pap-test, whereas more recently the attention was addressed to the evaluation of the efficacy of diagnosis of asymptomatic breast cancer through mammography (Tomatis, 1990).

A natural expansion of this approach was the idea that population-based survival rates of cancer patients could be used as an indicator (not the only one, obviously) of the quality of cancer care in a given area and that cancer registries could have a major role in this direction. In fact, during the 1970s and early 1980s this potential was perceived in the US by SEER and by some registries in Northern Europe but not elsewhere. The limited interest for this approach may have reflected the lack of resources for a systematic follow-up of the living status of the registered individuals. It can be traced back, however, also to an inadequate cultural co-operation between epidemiologists and clinicians, particularly in continental Europe. A major step to overcome the latter has been the Eurocare project, which published its first results in 1995 (Berrino et al., 1995). Undoubtedly, variations in survival after a diagnosis of cancer between populations served by registries must be interpreted with much caution. Nevertheless, the underlying comparisons may provide leads to the evaluation of cancer care (the same may well apply to other lethal conditions).

The contemporary era

Comparing the geographical distribution of cancer registries in 1960 and at the end of the century indicates a strong polarization in the areas of major economical development. The expansion has been greatest in Asia: no registry from China was included in the first three editions of "*Cancer Incidence in Five Continents*": subsequently, they increased from 2 to 10. Similarly, only one registry from India was included up to the 4th edition, whereas there were 9 in the latest edition. Data from 5 registries in Thailand appeared in in the 8th edition, vs. none until 1982. On the contrary, coverage in areas where the economical conditions have worsened (Sub-Saharan Africa and Latin America) has barely remained at the same levels in 30 years. Whereas decades ago developing areas were supported (also in terms of public health programs) by the industrialised countries from which they traditionally depended, more recently registration depends from local initiatives. Naturally, initiatives have been weaker in countries whose economy has been stagnant, although they find support in a complex programme launched by IARC some 10 years ago (International Agency for Research on Cancer, 1995). Although registration in developing countries does not always reach the standards required for inclusion in "*Cancer Incidence in Five Continents*", much information has been collected thanks to encouragement from IARC. Another achievement of IARC has been the production of estimates of incidence rates (through models based on the application of algorithms to mortality and incidence rates) in areas which are not covered by formal registration.

The paucity of epidemiological contributions from Arab countries in North Africa and Middle East does not reflect the economical level of those countries, some of which afford a sizable level of public expenditure. The few available estimates (Algeria, Kuwait) suggest that the Islamic lifestyle could reveal highly protective against many types of cancer; information from a wider set of regions should provide much information on this hypothesis.

In Europe, a major achievement in the uses of cancer registries has been the "Eurocare" programme which has provided unique survival data on cancer patients on a population basis (Berrino et al., 2003). However, the duality of programmes between the two "milieu" (incidence and survival publications) has not been very efficient, and prospects are grim, given the decision of the European Union in 2003 to stop the financial support to both, "Eurocare" and "ENCR" (European Network of Cancer Registries).

Programmes for the early diagnosis of cancer in asymptomatic persons is reflected in incidence rates and cancer registration has become an important public health tool for the evaluation of screening programmes . The implementation of such programmes has been heterogenous across countries, and again they have developed to a greater extent in industrialised areas. This has to be taken into account in geographical and historical comparisons of incidence rates, due to the fact that screening programmes can "inflate" incidence figures, through increasing diagnoses and anticipating them.

In conclusion, through the decades, cancer registries have found a number of functions, thus reversing the state of affairs which was feared by Harold Dorn half a century ago.

Cohort studies: history of the method

Sir Richard Doll

CTSU, Harkness Building, Radcliffe Infirmary, Oxford OX2 6HE; UK

Summary

The term "cohort study" was introduced by Frost in 1935 to describe a study that compared the disease experience of people born at different periods, in particular the sex and age-specific incidence of tuberculosis and the method was extended to the study of non-communicable disease by Korteweg who used it 20 years later to analyse the epidemic of lung cancer in the Netherlands. Such studies are now best described as generation studies or generation cohort studies to distinguish them from the common type of study that is now carried out that consists in defining groups of individuals distinguished by some variable (such as place of residence, occupation, behaviour, or environmental exposure) and following them up to see if the incidence or mortality rates vary with the selected variable. This type of study is now one of the most important tools for epidemiological investigation. Initially called prospective studies, because the information characterising the individuals in the cohorts was recorded before the onset of disease, they are now preferably called cohort studies and distinguished as prospective cohort studies, if the information obtained relates to the subjects at the time the study is started and they are then followed, or retrospective cohort studies, if the information characterising the individuals was recorded sometime in the past (for example, the receipt of radiotherapy, or entry to a specific occupation).

Studies of either type have the great advantage that they avoid all the most important sources of bias that may affect case-control studies, but the disadvantage that because incidence rates and more specifically mortality rates are commonly low, large numbers of subjects have to be followed for several (if not many) years to obtain statistically significant results.

Several early prospective studies are described: Namely, those of 34000 male British doctors, 190000 male and female American citizens with different smoking habits, some 5000 middle aged residents of Framingham with different blood pressures, blood cholesterol levels, etc, and 13000 children born in the UK in one week in 1946 with different family backgrounds.

Nothing biological is constant, certainly not language, and the meaning of cohort studies has evolved over time. In this chapter, I examine first the type of study that was originally called a cohort study and then, with the development of epidemiology, the evolution of the term to include a large and important section of all epidemiological work. In doing so, I describe in some detail a selection of the early studies of each of the main types that we now recognise and I conclude by giving examples of the modifications that have been introduced to make cohort studies more flexible and more fruitful. I do not, however, include any discussion of refinements in purely statistical techniques as applied to cohort studies; these are described in detail by Breslow and Day (Breslow and Day, 1987) in their monograph on statistical methods in cancer research.

Generation cohort studies

Tuberculosis

The first type of investigation to be called a cohort study was one in which the trends with age in the sex-specific incidence of tuberculosis were compared in groups of men and women born at different dates. Such groups were called cohorts by Frost, the leading American epidemiologist of the day, who used this term in a personal letter to Dr Sydenstricker in 1935. The letter was published in 1939 after Frost's death as a footnote to a paper entitled "*The age selection of mortality from tuberculosis in successive decades*" in which he had used the technique. In this paper, Frost (Frost, 1939) discussed the meaning to be attached to the fact that the age distribution of the mortality rate attributed to tuberculosis varied between 1880 and 1930, as is shown for males in Figure 1, reproduced from Frost's article. He noted that after the childhood peak at 0–4 years of age the mortality declined to a minimum at 5–9 years and then rose to a second peak that occurred progressively later with the passage of time, at 20–29 years in the data for 1880, at 30–39 years in the data for 1910, and at 50–59 years in the data for 1930. These changes, Frost thought, did not correspond to reasonably probable changes of like extent in the rate of exposure to infection and he preferred to think that the predominant factor in the movement along the age scale was a change in human resistance. He pointed out, however, that, if looked at from a different point of view, the change in the pattern of the age distribution might be more apparent than real. For, if the pattern is examined for men and women who were born at different dates, it is seen to be the same throughout. This is shown in Figure 2, again reproduced from Frost's (Frost, 1939) article, which shows that the second peak occurs at the same age (20–29 years) for each cohort irrespective of date of birth. The progressive increase with the passage of time in the age at which the second peak occurs in cross-sectional data from different years can be interpreted as the result of the fact that the high rates in old age at the later dates are just the residuals of higher rates in earlier life.

This technique, described as a cohort analysis by Frost (Frost, 1939) and associated with his name, had, however, been used by Andvord (Andvord, 1930) in Nor-

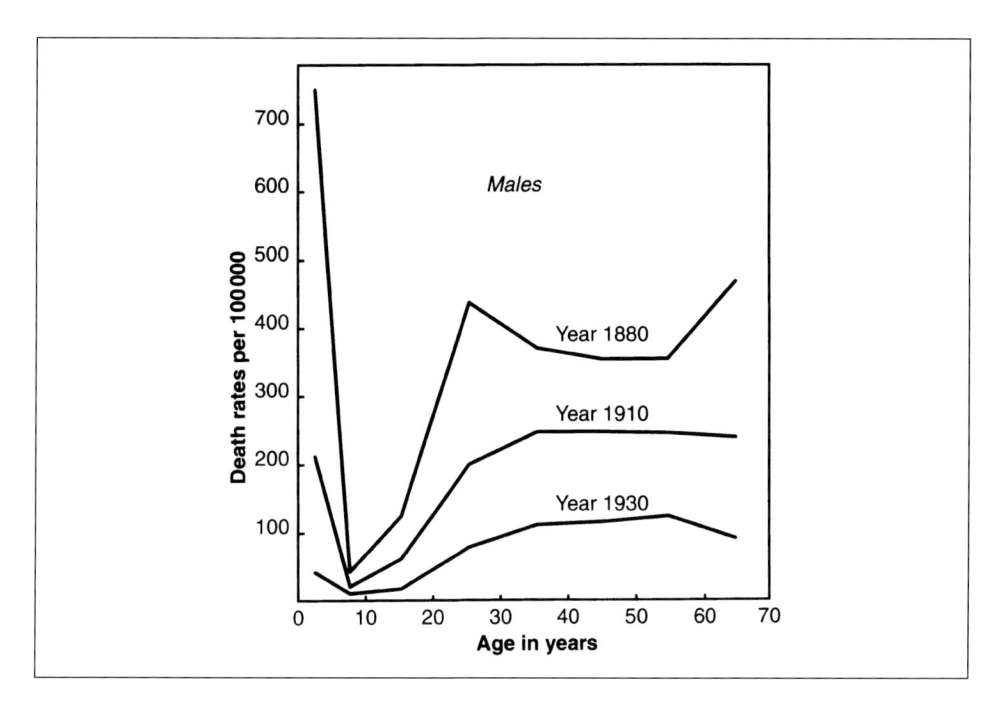

Figure 1
Age-specific mortality from tuberculosis among men in Massachusetts in 1880, 1910, and 1930 (Frost, 1939).

way, nine years earlier and described as a study by "generations". Andvord had, in fact, analysed the mortality rates from tuberculosis in England and Wales, Denmark, Norway, and Sweden in exactly the same way as Frost had done with the rates for England and Wales and Massachusetts. His data for Norway from 1886–1900 to 1926–27 are shown in Figure 3. His conclusions, as expressed in the English summary to his article, bear repeating in full.

"*By studying these tables and diagrams, we shall find it most conspicuous, that mortality of tuberculosis, shown within generations, has the distinct resemblance of undulatory motion, a wave, which during several decades of years has been upon its sinking phase nearly all over the civilized world. In England this fall in the tuberculosis death-rate in infancy commenced about the middle of the last century, while in Norway such a fall in the infancy death-rate is scarcely traceable till the eighties.*

If we compare the diagrams of the countries in question, it is very conspicuous that they show a most prominent accordance in their main features. The fall is gradual and regular from one generation to the other, each new generation hav-

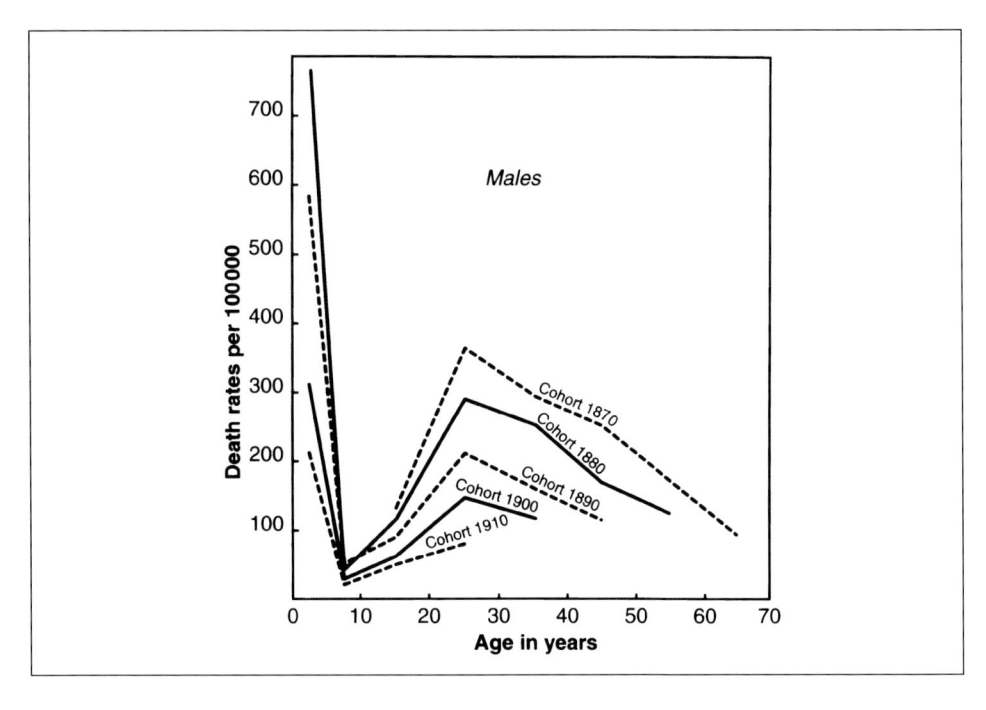

Figure 2
Age-specific mortality from tuberculosis among men in Massachusetts, plotted by year of birth (Frost 1939).

ing evidently received greater powers of resistance than the preceding one to the tuberculosis virus. Each generation shows its own characteristic diagram, because the frequency of infection in infancy seems to indicate the mortality death-rate in later years of life, a fall in mortality in infancy being invariably followed by a similar fall 20–25 years later among adults." (Andvord, 1930).

Consequently, as Frost (Frost, 1939) noted, Andvord was able to suggest that the analysis by generations formed a rational basis for extending estimates of future mortality at higher ages in the most recent cohorts.

Lung cancer

This technique of analysis by generation was not extended to the age specific incidence or mortality rates of non-infectious disease for some 20 years, until Korteweg (Korteweg, 1952) used it to examine the temporal changes in the mortality from lung cancer, without, however, realising that the method had been used previously in the

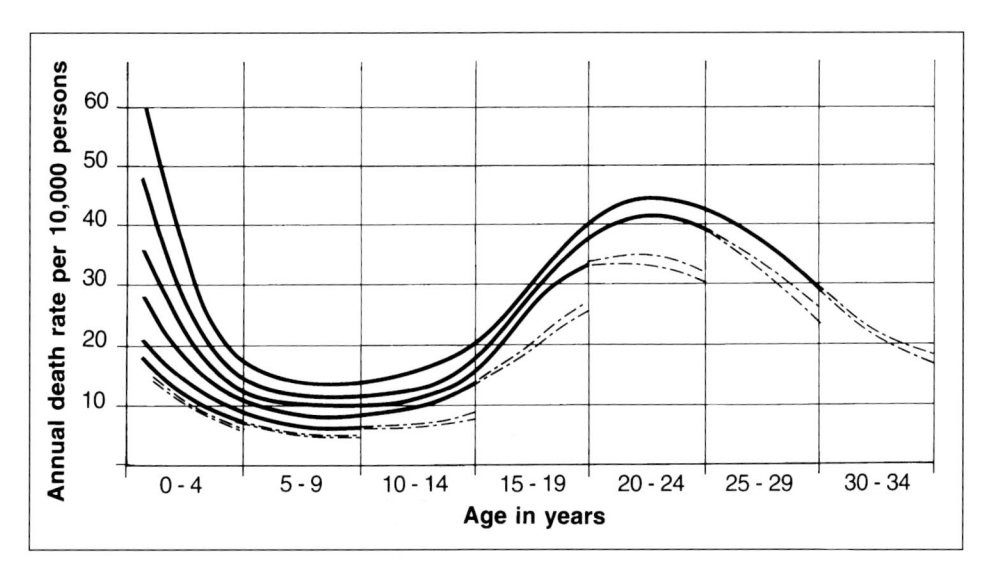

Figure 3
Age-specific mortality from tuberculosis among men in Norway between 1896–90 and 1926–27, plotted by year of birth (Andvord,1930).

study of tuberculosis. Korteweg had been struck by the difference between the pattern of the age-specific mortality rates for lung cancer in males and that for all other cancers in males considered as a group. The former had a maximum, in the data for England and Wales in 1945, at ages 55–64 years, while the latter showed a progressive increase up to 75 years and over. Was this decrease in the cancer death rate at a relatively early age something that was a characteristic of lung cancer, he asked, or was there some other explanation? Dormanns (Dormanns, 1936) he noted, had already suggested that the pattern might be an effect of the increase in lung cancer that had occurred over the previous 30 years, and Korteweg tested this hypothesis by comparing the mortality at each age with that at other ages in the group of persons born at about the same time; in other words he examined the mortality in cohorts defined by date of birth. When he did this he found that the peculiar pattern of the age-specific mortality rates for lung cancer, shown for four different dates in Figure 4, disappeared and the pattern came to resemble that for the combined group of all other cancers. This is shown in Figure 5, in which, to facilitate comparison, he gave the age-specific rates as proportions of their sum. From this he concluded that the decline in the mortality from lung cancer in old age was a consequence of the extraordinary increase in the environmental factors that caused lung cancer, which showed their full effect first at young ages, and that the mortality in old age would go on increasing, even when it had stopped increasing in youth, until the pattern in any given year came

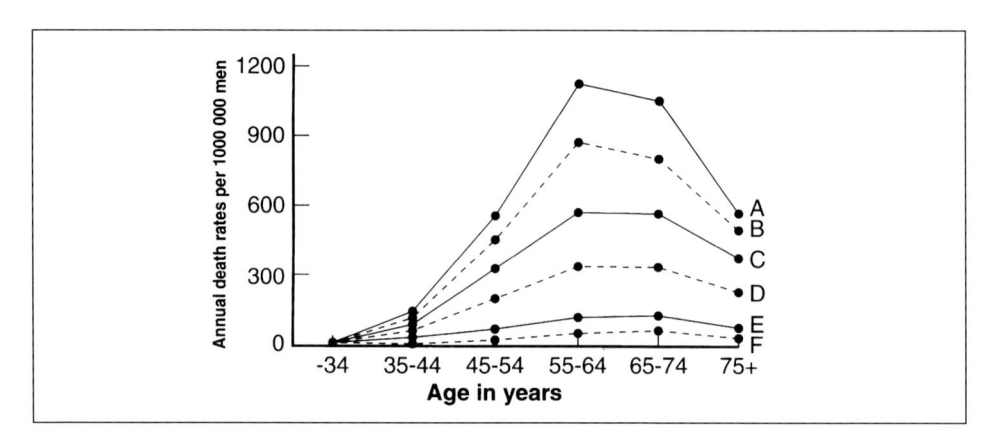

Figure 4
Age-specific mortality from lung cancer among men in England and Wales: A in 1945, B 1940–44, C 1936–39, D 1931–35, E 1921–30, F 1911–20 (Korteweg, 1952).

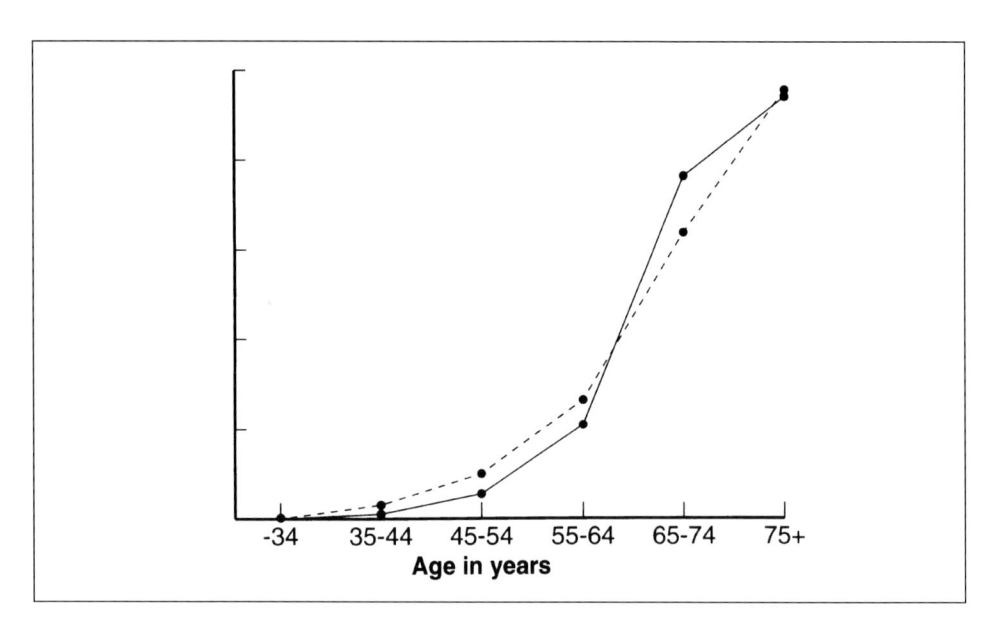

Figure 5
Age-specific mortality from lung cancer and from all other cancers among men in England and Wales in 1945, expressed as proportions of their sum: lung cancer —, all other cancers - - - (Korteweg, 1952).

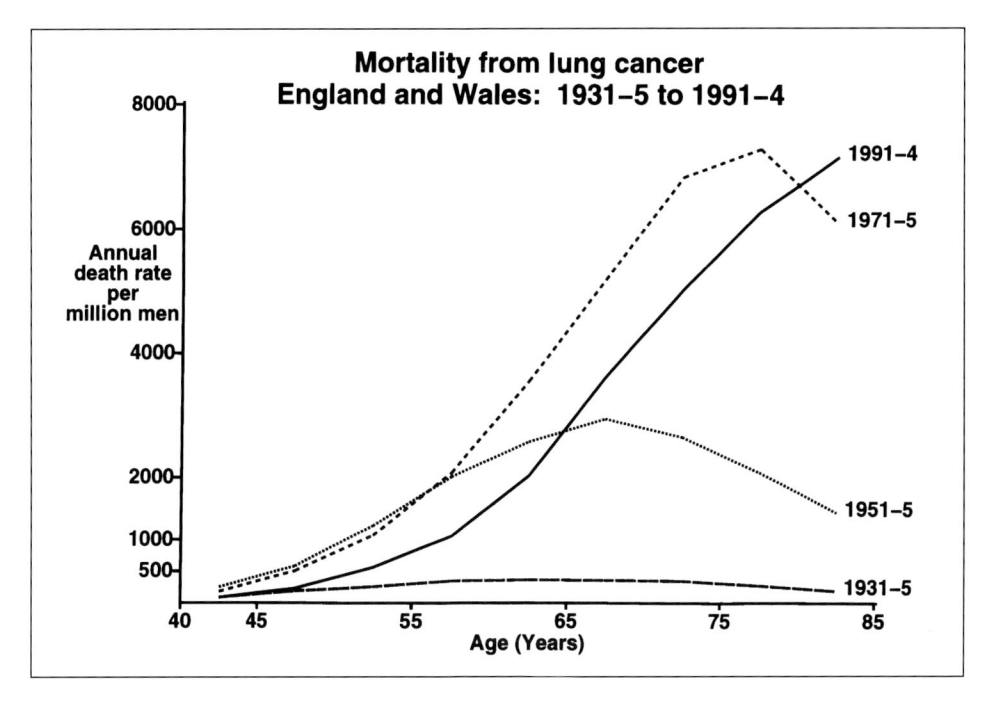

Figure 6
Age-specific mortality from lung cancer among men in England and Wales in 1931–5, 1951–5, 1971–5, and 1991–4.

to resemble that seen in Figure 5. This prediction was born out in the British data in the course of the next 30 years (Fig. 6) but Korteweg sadly did not live to see it.

In presenting this analysis, Korteweg attributed the increase in lung cancer to "irritating factors", and made no reference to cigarette smoke, which I know, from discussion with him, he believed to be the principal cause of the disease. The expression of his belief in the harmful effects of tobacco had, however, aroused so much antagonism in the Netherlands that he preferred not to mention tobacco in his article in the hope that his explanation of the pattern of the age-specific rates and its implication for the importance of an external "irritating factor" would be more readily accepted.

Cohort studies: modern definition

Some 10 years after Korteweg's paper, the term cohort study began to be given the much wider meaning that it now has: namely, any study in which groups of people with defined characteristics are followed up to determine the incidence of, or mortality from, some specific disease, all causes of death, or some other outcome. The risk of these outcomes can then be compared either with some outside standard, such as the incidence or mortality recorded for all people of the same sex and same age distribution over the same period nationally or locally, or it can be compared internally between different sections of the cohort defined as having different characteristics. According to the Dictionary of Epidemiology, sponsored by the International Epidemiological Association and edited by Last (Last, 2001) alternative terms for cohort study are follow-up, longitudinal, and prospective studies[1]. These according to Liddell (Liddell, 1988) in his review of the development of cohort studies, embrace at least four classes, depending *inter alia*, on whether the members of the cohort are presumed healthy or diseased at the onset of the study, whether the difference between different sections of the cohort is determined by past events or by the investigator, the nature of the characteristic that determines membership of the cohort or of its sections, and the type of outcome in the follow-up period that is of interest. While this is logically defensible, it makes the definition of a cohort study undesirably wide and I shall exclude from consideration controlled trials and clinical studies of the progress of disease, both of which are included in Liddell's definition.

Cohort studies, even of the limited type that I shall consider, constitute one of the most important elements of modern epidemiology. The annual risk of death and the annual incidence of the most important diseases are both fortunately low and cohort studies consequently commonly require large numbers of people to be observed over long periods, so that they may be complex to organise and expensive to carry out. They have, however, one enormous advantage over case-control studies, in that they avoid several important sources of bias which may be introduced by the subjects when they know that a specific disease has occurred, by the investigator in questioning when he or she knows whether a subject is a case or a control, and unintentionally in the selection of the controls, because the subject's exposure to whatever is the factor of interest is recorded *before* the outcome is known and the controls are whole defined populations or contained within the cohort. There remains, of course, the possibility of diagnostic bias, if those responsible for diagnosing the outcome know the groups in which the affected individuals are placed; but this is seldom important, for diagnoses in cohort studies tend to the made in the ordinary course of medical practice independently of the investigators.

---

[1] The Dictionary says the term is synonymous with concurrent, incidence, follow-up, longitudinal, and prospective studies, but as I am not familiar with the term "concurrent study" and as the Dictionary goes on to say that alternative terms are the three cited, I have preferred to omit concurrent and incidence.

Prospective cohort studies

Studies which, in retrospect, may be called prospective cohort studies have probably been carried out since the beginning of the century, if not before. Liddell (1988) cited as examples the studies of Farr (1885) and Snow (1854) that led to the discovery of the cause of cholera and those of Goldberger in the second and third decades of this century that led to the discovery of the cause of pellagra, but these seem to me to be more accurately described as case-control studies or surveys and included, in Goldberger's case, in preventative trials (Terris, 1964). This in no way detracts from their importance or the validity of the evidence that they obtained. Whatever they are called they remain outstanding examples of epidemiological research and have an established place in the history of preventive medicine. Weinberg's (1913) study of the mortality of children born to tuberculous parents, which was cited by Frost (1933) but which I have not been able to trace, may have been a prospective cohort study by the strictest modern definition. It was, however, almost certainly small and the large studies that we now usually envisage under this head were not developed until after the Second World War, when they were initiated independently and more or less contemporaneously in the UK and the USA.

British doctors study

By a stroke of good fortune, I was associated with their development in the UK, through my association with Professor Bradford Hill, who had asked me, at the end of 1947, to assist in a case-control study aimed at finding out the cause of the great increase in the mortality attributed to lung cancer in England and Wales over the previous 30 years. This had led to the conduct of a case-control study which was published in 1950 in which we concluded that (*I quote*) "cigarette smoking is an important cause of carcinoma of the lung" (Doll and Hill, 1950). This conclusion was accepted by Sir Harold Himsworth, Secretary of the Medical Research Council, but by very few other scientists at the time, who were unaccustomed to the idea that firm conclusions about causation could be drawn from case-control studies, and it was clear that if the conclusion was to be widely accepted the conclusions would have to be checked by some other method of enquiry. The obvious way, Bradford Hill suggested, was to obtain the smoking habits of a large number of individuals and to follow them forward to see if the prediction could be confirmed that the cigarette smokers among them would have a higher mortality from lung cancer than the non-smokers and that the heavy cigarette smokers would have a higher mortality than the light smokers. Bradford Hill suggested that doctors would make a suitable population to study as they might be more interested in responding to a questionnaire about smoking habits than most other people, that having had a scientific training they might be more accurate in the description of their smoking habits, and, most importantly, that they would be relatively easy to follow up, because of the need to keep their names on the Medical Register for legal reasons.

With the help of the British Medical Association we wrote to all the 60 000 doctors on the Medical Register at the end of October 1951 and resident in the UK and obtained replies to a single enquiry from 40 000. We should certainly had have a higher response rate if we had written again to the non-responders (as we did to a sample 10 years later) but it took a year, with the little help that we had, to open all the letters and to get the responses coded on Hollerith punch cards. The questionnaire used was extremely simple and covered only one side of a piece of quarto paper. No more than seven questions were asked, the number depending on the subject's classification as a current smoker, ex-smoker, or lifelong non-smoker, something that has sometimes been attributed to Bradford Hill's teaching that questionnaires should not ask more than five questions. This was not, in fact, what Bradford Hill taught. What he did teach was that before including any question in a questionnaire the investigator should ask himself five questions about the necessity for including it.

Initially we relied for follow-up on the staff of the Office of the Registrar General of births and deaths (the national bureau of vital statistics) to provide copies of the death certificates of men and women whose occupations recorded on the certificate were given as medical practitioner or some equivalent term. For causes of death we accepted the underlying cause as described on the death certificate except when lung cancer was given as the underlying or contributory cause, when we sought detailed information about the basis on which the diagnosis was made from the doctor who signed the death certificate. We counted as lung cancer only those cases in which the diagnostic criteria were adequate and grouped all lung cancers together, irrespective of whether they were given as underlying or contributory causes. In the event, the great majority of cases were amply confirmed and we seldom found any reason to change the diagnosis[2].

The data obtained in this way enabled us to publish a preliminary report of the results of the follow-up with less than three years' observations. In this paper (Doll and Hill, 1954) the numbers of deaths in the 34 000 men with different smoking habits were simply related to the original numbers in each smoking category, standardised only for age. The rates so obtained for men aged 45–74 years were expressed as percentages of the rates for all men and compared with the comparable percentages estimated from the previous case-control study of patients with and without lung cancer in London. The results, which are summarised in Table 1 with

---

[2] Of 222 cases described as lung cancer on death certificates in our 10 year follow-up data (Doll and Hill, 1964) the diagnosis of only 10 (4.5%) proved unacceptable, the change of diagnosis being made by a chest physician who served as a consultant and was kept in ignorance of the individual's smoking habits.

Table 1 – Standardised death rates from lung cancer of men aged 45–74 years in relation to the most recent amount of tobacco smoked (Doll and Hill, 1950; Doll and Hill, 1954)

Study	Rate as per cent of that in all men			
	Nonsmokers	Smokers of:		
		1–14 g/day	15–24 g/day	25+ g/day
"Backward" study of patients' histories	6%	79%	112%	203%
"Forward" study of mortality of doctors	0%	68%	133%	199%

the same terminology that we used in the 1954 paper, amply confirmed our prediction.

The study was described as "prospective" on the grounds that when the smoking habits were obtained we were looking forward for the occurrence of disease in the future (Doll and Hill, 1954), while the case-control study that we had previously carried out was called retrospective because the occurrence of disease was known and we sought information about smoking habits that had occurred in the past. Such studies continued to be called respectively prospective and retrospective until Brian MacMahon in the USA suggested characterising them as cohort and case-control studies (McMahon et al., 1960), on the grounds that studies very similar to our prospective study could be carried out by determining the cohort from records of past exposure and following the subjects to the present day, thus allowing cohort studies to be either prospective (like the doctors smoking study) or retrospective like the occupational studies to be described shortly. Lilienfeld proposed the alternative of prospective and historical cohort studies, but this lost the simple contrast and did not catch on and MacMahon's terminology has come to be most used.

Two years after publishing the preliminary results of our prospective cohort study of British doctors, Bradford Hill and I published the results of following them for five years (Doll and Hill, 1956) by which time the prediction regarding the risks of lung cancer was confirmed beyond reasonable doubt and four other causes of death were also seen to be related to smoking: namely, coronary thrombosis (or as I should now prefer to say, myocardial infarction), chronic bronchitis (or chronic obstructive lung disease), peptic ulcer, and pulmonary tuberculosis. For this report we calculated what would now be called the man-years at risks in each smoking group by the relatively simple method of counting the numbers of men living in each five year age group at the beginning of each year of the study, taking the average for each year, and summing over the whole period for all ages. Standardised mortality rates were then calculated by the direct method for each category of smokers, using the total number of man-years at risk in each age group as the standard population. The discovery that, with increasing numbers, some other causes of death were also found to be related to smoking, suggested that it would be worth continuing the study for longer, until many more deaths had been observed and more causes could be studied separately. It has, consequently, been continued, by now for over 40 years, with information about changes in smoking habits being obtained on five intermediate occasions.

By 1956, however, it had become clear that reliance on reports of death from the Registrar General was inadequate, as not all doctors were so described on their death certificates and we had sought additional information about deaths from the General Medical Council, which kept a register of qualified doctors for legal purposes, and from the British Medical Association. We did not, however, at that time seek to check that all those not known to be dead were still alive and it was only later that we took to writing to individuals, partly to obtain information about changes in smoking habits and partly to discover unreported deaths.

Doctors, as Bradford Hill thought would be the case, have been easy to trace and after 20 years only 101 out of the original 34440 men (0.3%) were unaccounted for. At that time 2459 were known to be living abroad, 102 asked not to be followed further – one saying he was fed up with being our guinea pig – and 15 had been struck off the medical register for unprofessional conduct. Continued follow-up for a further 20 years of the other 21688 known to be alive and resident in the UK resulted in a loss of only another 118 (0.5%). The results after 40 years were reported in 1994 (Doll et al., 1994). Thirty causes of death were by then found to be positively related to smoking, but the most interesting finding was perhaps the difference in survival of different categories of smokers, which could now be analysed from 35 years of age to over 100. 50% of heavy cigarette smokers (of 25 or more cigarettes a day) had died in middle age – which we may now optimistically define as from 35 to 70 years of age – against 20% of non-smokers and only 8% survived to 85 years of age against 33% of non-smokers (Fig. 7). Men who gave up under 35 years of age, who, in this population, had smoked for an average of only 10 years had an expectation of life that was indistinguishable from that of non-smokers (Fig. 8) but even those who stopped at 65–74 years of age (mean 71 years) had age-specific mortality rates beyond 75 years that were appreciably lower than those who continued (Fig. 9) and the rates would certainly have been lower still if it had been possible to exclude those who stopped specifically because of smoking-induced ill-health.

American Cancer Society study

In the USA a very similar study was begun independently a few months after the British doctors' study by Hammond and Horn (1954) on behalf of the American Cancer Society. It was initiated, so Hammond told me, with the express purpose of disproving a causal relationship between cigarette smoking and lung cancer, which

Doctors' life-table

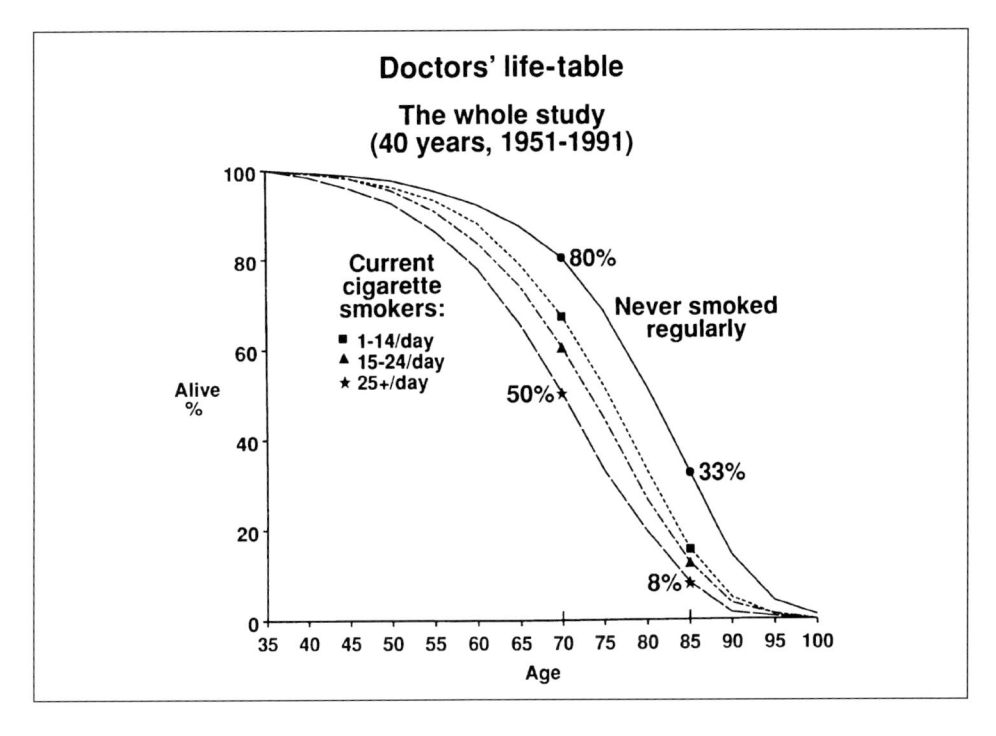

The whole study (40 years, 1951-1991)

Figure 7
Survival of British doctors from age 35 years by smoking habits: lifelong nonsmokers —, cigarette smokers, smoking 1–14 cigarettes a day ·····, smoking 15–24 cigarettes a day –··–, 25 or more cigarettes a day ---- (Doll et al., 1994) (Reproduced with permission of the BMJ Publishing Group).

had been suggested not only by the case-control study in Britain to which I have referred, but also by the association recorded in several case-control studies in Germany and the USA, most notably in that reported by Wynder and Graham (1950).

With the help of volunteer supporters of the American Cancer Society, Hammond and Horn obtained smoking habits for nearly 190000 men aged between 50 and 69 years who were friends of the volunteers and follow-up data were obtained approximately biennially by the same volunteers. Causes of death were obtained from death certificates and the diagnosis of cancer was checked by information obtained from personal doctors, hospitals, and tumor registries. A preliminary report in 1954 *confirmed* the predicted association with lung cancer and showed an association between smoking and coronary thrombosis, which was less close but potentially more important because of the large numbers of cases (Hammond and Horn, 1954). Four years later, after a mean follow-up period of 44 months, a major report was published which gave death rates for each of the four five year age groups studied and the ratio between the number of

Doctors' life-table
Age stopped: <35

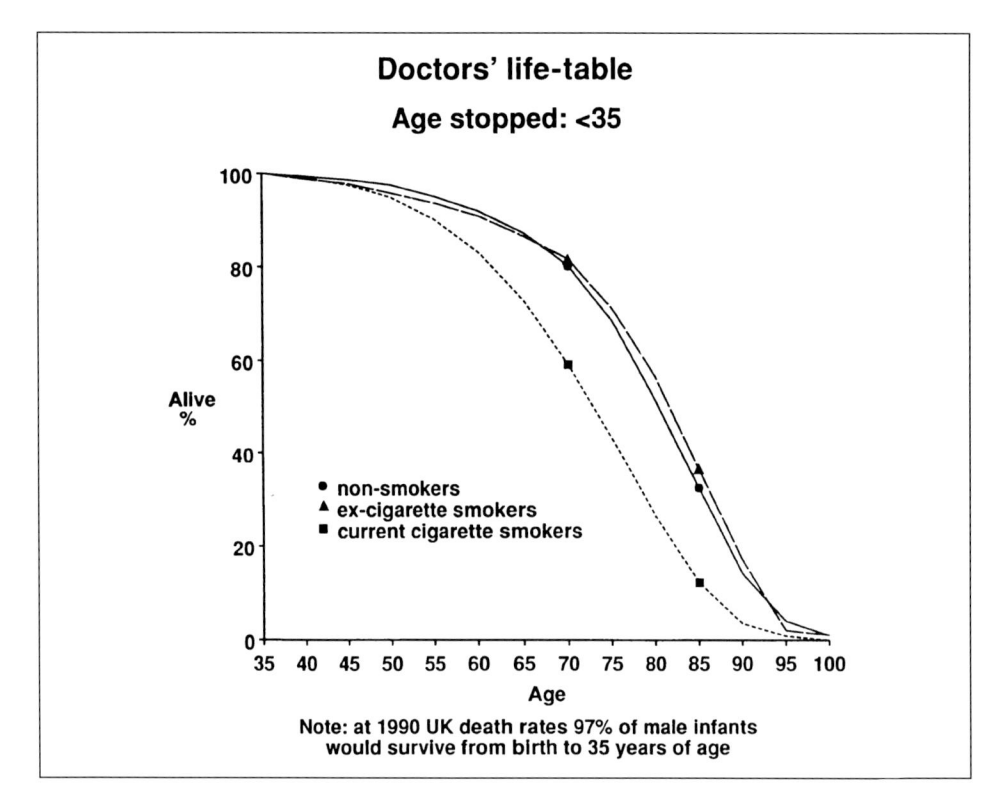

Figure 8
Suvival of British doctors from age 35 yrs by smoking habits: lifelong nonsmokers —, cigarette smokers stopped under 35 yrs of age –▲–, continuing cigarette smokers ··■·· (Doll et al., 1994) (Reproduced with permission of the BMJ Publishing Group).

deaths observed and the number expected from the rate in non-smokers for 32 diseases or groups of diseases (Hammond and Horn, 1958). Altogether nearly 12000 deaths were observed and it was possible to compare the ratios of the numbers of deaths observed from many different causes and the numbers expected from the experience of the non-smokers, for cigarette smokers smoking different amounts, for pipe smokers and cigar smokers, and for men who had stopped smoking for different periods. Excess mortality ratios for cigarette smokers were observed for 14 causes of death or groups of causes, with particularly high ratios for lung cancer (10.4 to one) and cancers of the upper respiratory and digestive tracts (5.1 to one). In total, the mortality among cigarette smokers was increased by 57% and over half of this was attributable to the excess of deaths from coronary heart disease, despite the mortality ratio being only 1.7, because the disease was relatively so much more common as a cause of death than any other.

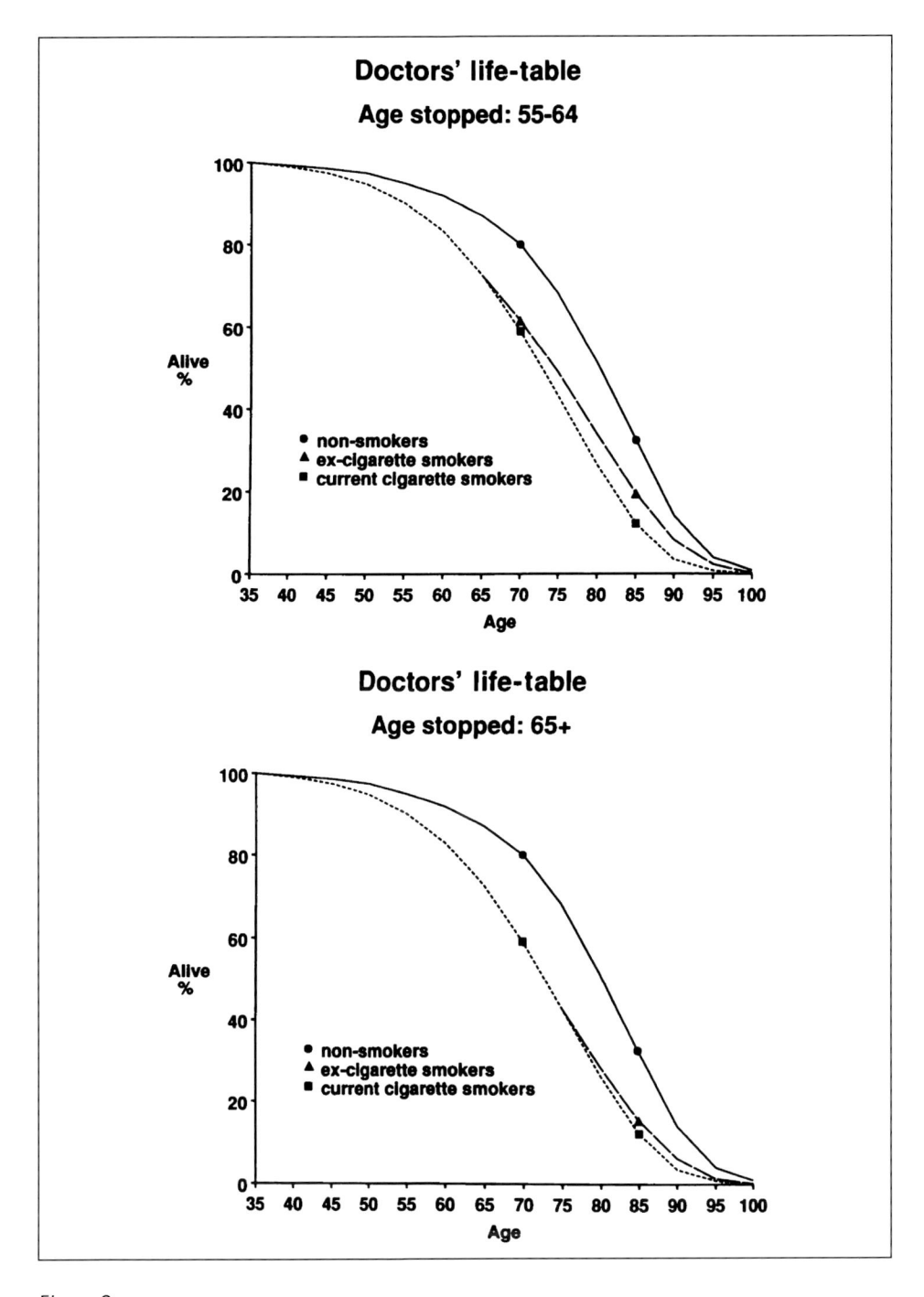

Figure 9
Survival of British doctors from age 35 yrs by smoking habit: lifelong cigarette smokers —, cigarette smokers stopped 65–74 yrs of age –▲–, continuing cigarette smokers ··■·· (Doll et al., 1994) (Reproduced with permission of the BMJ Publishing Group).

This study was remarkable for two reasons. First, because it was so large; the cohort of nearly 190000 being by far the largest of its type until it was overshadowed by the American Cancer Society's study of a million men and women in the 1960s. Secondly, because of the care that was taken to check the diagnoses of the 2350 neoplasms referred to on death certificates, information being obtained about 95% (2242). Only six of the diagnoses of a neoplasm were found to be incorrect and 79% of the cancers said to have caused death were microscopically proven.

Framingham study

Two studies had, however, antedated both these in their inception, although the results of one were not published until later and the other was envisaged only with immediate short-term aims. The cardiovascular risk disease study that was begun by Dawber and his colleagues in 1949 (Dawber et al., 1951) was different in character from the two smoking studies, as the cohort was much smaller, but instead of the individual members being asked just to complete a questionnaire they were also subjected to a detailed clinical examination, gave blood samples, and had an electrocardiogram. Moreover, it was planned that surviving members would be re-examined every two years. Originally the cohort was intended to be a random sample of all residents of the town aged 30–59 years, but the response rate of 69% was thought to be too low to provide a big enough cohort and 740 volunteers were added to it. On first examination, 81 subjects were found to have evidence of coronary heart disease and the cohort eventually consisted of 5128 subjects without evidence of coronary heart disease, of whom a little over half (55%) were women. Apart from the standard demographic details the information obtained from each respondent included serum cholesterol and several other blood lipid indices, blood pressure, weight expressed as a percentage of the norm for sex and height, electrocardiographic findings, respiratory efficiency, and smoking habits.

After eight years, 85% attended for the fifth round of examinations, 11% failed to attend but were known to be alive, 4% had died and only 19 (0.4%) were lost to follow-up (Kagan et al., 1962). During the previous eight years, 245 were found to have developed indications of coronary heart disease. The risk had been greater in men than in women, had increased in each sex with age, blood cholesterol, systolic (and diastolic) pressure, the presence of left ventricular hypertrophy, cigarette smoking, and decreasing respiratory capacity. Several of these factors, moreover, acted synergistically and the risk among men aged 30–59 years at entry was found to have increased progressively with the number of the leading predictive factors (namely, serum cholesterol 245 mg per 100 ml or more, blood pressure more than 165/95, and smoking 20 or more cigarettes a day). When all three were present the risk became 12 times greater than when none was present (Fig. 10). Adiposity, however, had lit-

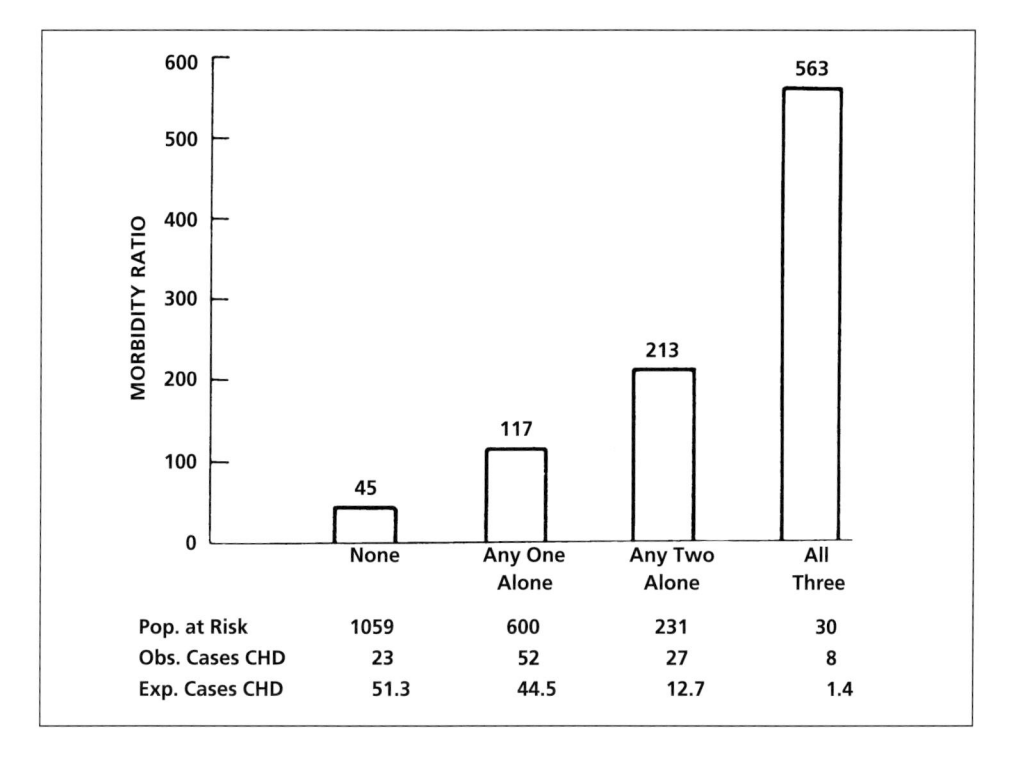

	None	Any One Alone	Any Two Alone	All Three
Pop. at Risk	1059	600	231	30
Obs. Cases CHD	23	52	27	8
Exp. Cases CHD	51.3	44.5	12.7	1.4

Morbidity ratios: None 45, Any One Alone 117, Any Two Alone 213, All Three 563.

Figure 10
Incidence of coronary heart disease in men aged 35–59 yrs followed for eight years, standardized for age, by number of risk factors present (serum cholesterol 245 mg per 100 ml or more, blood pressure higher than 165 mm Hg systolic and/or 95 diastolic, smoking 20 or more cigarettes a day) (Kagan et al., 1962).

tle or no effect when the leading factors were taken into account, unless it was gross (that is, 30% or more above the median).

This study, like the study of British doctors, was continued for many years and reached much the same conclusions about the effects of smoking. After 34 years' follow-up, the investigators emphasised, in particular, the great effect of smoking on the risk of cardiovascular disease. Major innovations, they wrote, have occurred over the past decade in the treatment and prevention of cardiovascular disease. They added:

> "However, none of these advances offer as much benefit as avoiding or quitting smoking. Because of its powerful independent effect, its continued prevalence in over one fourth of the [US adult] population, and the ability to eliminate it as a risk factor, cigarette smoking deserves the highest priority among preventive campaigns against cardiovascular disease." (Freud et al., 1993).

The continuation of the study for so long and the repeated clinical examinations enabled it also to make some unique contributions to medical knowledge. Thirty years of follow-up enabled it to differentiate the association between cholesterol levels at different ages. Under 50 years of age on first examination, increasing levels were associated with increasing mortality without any evidence of a threshold. At older ages, however, the relationship was confounded by an association of decreasing levels with increased mortality due, at least in part, to an effect of the presence of disease predisposing to death (Anderson et al., 1987). More important, perhaps, are the observations on the extent to which physiological features of the individual, such as blood cholesterol and blood pressure, persist over time. These have recently been examined by Clarke et al. (Clarke et al., 1999) and show much less stability than, I suspect, has previously been assumed.

The 1946 birth cohort

The other early post-war study was begun in 1946 as a simple cross-sectional survey to provide answers to questions about the availability, use, and effectiveness of the maternity services in Great Britain, specifically to find possible reasons for the apparent decline in fertility rates (Population Investigation Committee, 1948). It was conceived by James Douglas, a physician with a special interest in social medicine and public health, who sought to find out what might be discouraging families from having children. It aimed to involve all the women who gave birth in one week in March 1946 and actually recruited 13687, 91% of the total. The post-war baby boom quickly made questions about fertility less urgent, but the information resulting from the maternity survey was of acute interest to the National Health Service, which was to begin in July 1948, and it was realised that the families could provide the basis for a cohort study to assess the impact of family and social conditions on subsequent personal development, and behaviour on children's health. A random sample of over 5000 children was consequently drawn, stratified so as to increase the proportions born to agricultural and non-manual workers, and the members have been followed ever since, with periodic personal visits, interviews, questionnaires, medical examinations, school reports, and psychological tests. From 1969, special enquiries have also been made about the cohort members' own children at four years of age and reading tests have been applied to them at eight years of age.

The early results mostly concerned the impact of family relationships and educational facilities on personal development and behaviour (Atkins et al., 1981). Parental level of interest, for example, was found to be even more important in determining children's reading ability than social background. Subsequently, interest began to focus on factors related to social background and to disease incidence, such as the relationship between early chest illnesses, local smoke pollution, and overcrowding in the home and the occurrence of chronic cough in young adult life (Kiernan et al., 1976). Now, a fifty-one year follow-up is planned for 1997 when special attention will be paid to the links between low birth weight, poor early social environment, and the development of hypertension and other diseases of middle-age to test Barker's hypothesis that fetal nutrition affects the risk of cardiovascular and some other diseases in adult life (Barker et al., 1993; Barker and Osmond, 1986).

The numbers of children in the study were too small to answer many questions that such a study could potentially answer. It demonstrated, however, that collaboration could be maintained effectively over many years and this encouraged the conduct of similar studies on a larger scale and all children born in one week in 1958 (Pringle et al., 1966) and in one week in 1970 (Golding et al., 1990) are also now being followed.

Retrospective cohort studies

Spread of tuberculosis in families

Retrospective cohort studies have almost as long a history as the prospective studies, for one was described by Frost in 1933 (Frost, 1933), based on the black population of a small town in Tennessee. Interviews identified 556 persons living in 132 families, practically all of whom were examined clinically and radiographically, and 238 ex-members of the families, who were alive but had left the village or had died since the head of the household came into that position. From the information thus obtained, nearly 10000 person-years under observation were assembled and divided in five year age groups (though not apparently separately by sex) counting each person who entered the household in any given year or left in a given year as being under observation for half a year. Annual age-specific death rates from all causes and from tuberculosis were then compared with those for the black population of Tennessee and found to be closely similar, except at ages 20 to 49 years when the rates in the population under study were somewhat lower. The population was then divided according to whether there was a history of family contact with pulmonary tuberculosis and the annual attack rates of tuberculosis in the two groups were compared. In the presence of family contact the attack rate, standardised for age, was found to be about double that in the absence of such contact (12.9 per 1000 against 6.8 per 1000). Remarkably for that period, the attack rates were qualified by their standard deviations (respectively 1.7 and 0.64 per 1000).

Frost described this study not so much to provide evidence of the importance of family contacts in the spread of tuberculosis, for he realised that the number of persons involved was small, but as an illustration of the way records of past events could be used for the study of public health. The study is particularly notable for the clear description of the way person-years at risk can be calculated and for its success in gaining the co-operation of almost an entire population, for only three out of 135 known families were unwilling to be examined and consequently omitted from the study.

Nickel refiners' study

This technique of a retrospective cohort study is peculiarly well suited to the study of long-term occupational hazards and was, as far as I have been able to find out, first applied by Bradford Hill in a study of nickel refinery workers, which was not, however, reported publicly until he described it in the eighth edition of his textbook in 1966 (Hill, 1966). About 1000 nickel refinery workers and pensioners combined were identified from company records and followed for 10 years from 1929 to 1938. Sixteen were found to have died from lung cancer against one expected from national rates, 11 to have died from nasal cancer against less than one expected, and 67 to have died from other causes against 72 expected. The study was not published, as it had been carried out at the request of the local nickel refining industry for their information; but it was subsequently reported in brief as an example of how consistency in the results of different studies, though a useful characteristic in helping to conclude that an epidemiological association reflects causality, is not necessary for such a conclusion to be reached. Having described his findings, Hill continued in his text:

> "In 1923, long before any special hazard had been recognised, certain changes in the refinery had taken place. No case of cancer of the nose was observed in any man who first entered the works after that year, and in these men there was no excess of cancer of the lung. In other words, the excess in both sites is uniquely a feature in men who entered the refinery in, roughly, the first 23 years of the present century. No causal agent of these neoplasms has been identified. Until recently no animal experimentation had given any clue or any support to this wholly statistical evidence. Thus we have (or certainly had) to make up our minds on a unique event; and there is no difficulty in doing so. This situation very clearly makes nonsense of the assertion that if the evidence is 'only statistical' we cannot accept it for action." (Hill, 1966, p. 309).

Gas-workers' study

The first published application of the technique appeared in 1952, in a study of the mortality of men employed in the manufacture of coal gas (Doll, 1952). This had been undertaken to test a hypothesis formulated five years earlier by Kennaway and Kennaway (1947) who had analysed the occupations of men recorded on death certificates as having died from lung cancer in England and Wales over the period 1921–38 and compared the numbers in different occupations with the numbers of men classified in the same occupations in the national censuses of 1921 and 1931. Fifty six occupations were studied and the number of deaths attributed to lung cancer in each of seven groups of gas workers was found to be higher than the number expected from the total experience, the standardised mortality ratios varying from 129 to 184. This was certainly suggestive of a hazard, in view of the heavy production of coal tar fumes in the industry, but it was far from conclusive.

With the help of Dr R.E.W. Fisher, the medical officer of a large London gas company, a list was consequently drawn up of all the pensioners of the company other than salaried staff, who had reached 60 years of age and were in receipt of a pension on 1 January 1939, or who began to receive a pension in the succeeding 10 years. The date of birth, the date of entering the pension scheme, and, when applicable, the date and cause of death were recorded for each pensioner and the numbers of men at risk in each five-year age group were counted separately for each of the years 1939 to 1948, in the same way as Frost had counted his family members. Computers were not available at the time and the man-years at risk in each age and calendar year group for the 2000 odd pensioners were counted by hand. The term man-year, however, had not as yet come into general use and what would now be called a man-year (and had been called a man-year by Frost nearly 20 years before) was called simply a "unit". The units in each five year age group in each calendar year were then multiplied by the corresponding national sex- and age-specific mortality rates for all causes and for 18 specific causes or groups of causes and the numbers summed for all age groups and all 10 calendar years to give the total numbers expected. As, however, mortality rates were known to differ somewhat between London and the rest of the country, the expected numbers were multiplied by factors derived from a comparison between the London and the national rates, when appropriate data were available.

The results for seven causes of death are shown in Table 2. The excess mortality from lung cancer was not paralleled by other excesses and it was concluded that gas workers did suffer a moderately increased risk of developing lung cancer; but the number was too small to enable the risks associated with different occupations within the industry to be distinguished. By the time the results came to be published, the industry had been nationalised and the responsible authorities would not allow Dr Fisher's name to be listed as an author. Fortunately his epidemiological colleague was employed by the Medical Research Council and the report was published under his name alone (Doll, 1952).

Life span study of the atomic bomb survivors

The first really large retrospective cohort study was not undertaken until 1956 when the Atom Bomb Casualty Commission (ABCC) initiated the life span study of the survivors of the atomic bomb explosions. The history of its inception is of some inter-

Table 2 – Mortality of retired gasworkers: A London Gas Company, 1939–48 (after Doll (1952))

Cause of death	No. of deaths	Observed as a % of expected [a]
Cancers of lung and pleura	25	181 [b]
Cancers of stomach and duodenum	32	139
Other cancers	99	100
Disease of cardiovascular system	322	97
Disease of respiratory system	120	94
Other diseases	222	96
Violence	20	65
All causes	840	98

[a] Expected in Greater London.
[b] $p < 0.01$.

est, as it illustrates the way epidemiological techniques came to be accepted as important research tools in the decade that followed the end of the second world war.

Following the atomic explosions, concern about the possible effects of irradiation was greatly increased. By far the greatest proportion of the approximately 180000 deaths was the direct result of blast and heat. Several thousand of the immediate survivors, however, died shortly afterwards as a result of acute radiation sickness and thousands more experienced acute symptoms and recovered. What might happen to those who recovered was unclear. It was recognised that knowledge of the long-term effects of substantial amounts of whole-body irradiation was incomplete and the joint commission of the US Army and Navy, which visited Japan shortly after the war, recommended a long-term study of the survivors to find out what they were. In January 1948, large programmes of research were consequently initiated into the genetic and somatic effects of radiation, as seen in the survivors of the two explosions.

The somatic effects programme started by conducting surveys and selecting a relatively small group of exposed survivors for regular clinical examinations; the so-called Adult Medical Survey. Survivors were identified in a radiation census in 1949 and a sample census carried out by the ABCC a year later; but there was, at the time, no prospect of obtaining estimates of individual doses. Exposed survivors were, therefore, classified according to their distance from the hypo-centre at the time of the explosion and the presence or absence of acute symptoms attributable to irradiation. The surveys quickly provided conclusive evidence that irradiation increased the risk of leukaemia (Folley et al., 1952), cataracts (Cogan et al., 1952), and mental retardation in children heavily exposed *in utero* (Plummer, 1952); but the plan for repeated clinical examinations proved to be ill-conceived. By 1954, clinicians were seeking to examine regularly some 5000 people but the study was foundering in the face of negative findings and declining participation. There was, consequently, thought of closing it down (Beebe, 1979).

Just then, however, another event occurred that altered the perspective of governments and their scientific advisers throughout the world. In June 1954, a hydrogen bomb was exploded over Eniwetok in the Pacific, which had 1000 times the power of the Hiroshima and Nagasaki bombs, and radioactive fallout was distributed worldwide. Further test explosions seemed certain to be carried out and determination of the quantitative effects of small doses of radiation became a burning issue. National committees were appointed in the UK and the USA to review the evidence. Their reports made it clear that no quantitative estimate of the risks could then be made (Medical Research Council, 1956; National Academy of Sciences, 1956) and an immense amount of research was initiated. Epidemiology by this time had been shown to be capable of contributing to knowledge of the aetiology of non-infectious disease and radioepidemiology moved from the wings to the centre of the stage.

An ad hoc committee under the chairmanship of Thomas Francis Jr recommended a plan to determine the cause specific mortality of a cohort of some 100000 persons (subsequently increased to about 120000) selected from nearly three times that number in Hiroshima or Nagasaki at the time of the national census on 1 October 1950 and whose history of exposure was known (Francis et al., 1955). This was immediately accepted and the sample, with some minor modifications (Jablon et al., 1965; Beebe et al., 1971) became the basis for the Life Span Study, which has provided the principal evidence on which our current knowledge of the long term effects of radiation is based. To it was added a mortality study of 2800 individuals exposed in utero and non-exposed controls (Kato, 1971) and the registration of all cancers, irrespective of fatality (Beebe and Hamilton, 1975) and research was begun to enable tissue doses to be estimated for each member of the cohort.

The population so defined has been followed to this day and still continues to be followed. By the late 1980s nearly 7000 deaths from cancer and over 8500 registered cases have been recorded in a population of some 76000 people with individually estimated doses. The results have shown a lifetime risk of fatal cancer of about 10% per Sv, with about a tenth of the deaths attributable to leukaemia, a dose-response relationship for leukaemia that is fitted significantly better by a linear quadratic relationship than a linear one, and a linear relationship with dose for fatal cancers other than leukaemia (United Nations, 1994). Some uncertainties remain, particularly about the trend with time in the excess relative risk for people who were irradiated in youth and the precise extent to which the findings for a Japanese population in 1945 can be generalised to other populations at later dates; but the general picture of both the qualitative and the quantitative effects of exposure to anything more than very small doses of low linear energy transfer radiation (that is gamma rays and x-rays) is clear.

Ankylosing spondylitis study

The Life Span Study is unique in the amount of effort that has been put into quantifying the extent of the exposure of individual members of the cohort to the agent of interest. With occupational hazards, which are perhaps the most common hazards that retrospective cohort studies are required to assess, retrospective investigation is seldom able to do much more than classify individuals according to whether they were process workers, and consequently regularly exposed, maintenance workers who were periodically exposed, and other staff who should not have been exposed at all, and then to divide men in each category according to the length of their employment. Rarely, detailed records exist which allow precise quantification. When they do exist, the records are likely to be complex and the task of estimating the exposure of thousands of individuals may be impossibly heavy, with the resources likely to be available.

This was the situation with which Court Brown and I were faced when, in July 1955, we were asked by the Medical Research Council to determine the nature of the relationship between exposure to ionizing radiation and the incidence of leukaemia, one year before the Life Span Study was initiated by the ABCC, and to provide the answer as quickly as possible. Patients who had received radiotherapy for ankylosing spondylitis seemed a suitable cohort to study, as they had been given a wide range of doses and spondylitis was a benign disease, so that the subsequent occurrence of leukaemia or of any other form of cancer would not be confused with a recurrence of the disease for which the treatment had been given, as might have been the case if an attempt was made to quantify the effects of radiotherapy given for a malignant disease. It was known, too, that some thousands of patients with spondylitis had been treated with radiotherapy over the previous 20 years. Such patients were consequently identified in 81 radiotherapy centres throughout the U.K. by four teams of investigators, each of which included one epidemiologist and one radiotherapist.

Detailed accounts of the doses received by each of the 14000 odd patients identified, who had been treated before the end of 1954 would have been very time consuming and patients were therefore classified according to the number of courses of treatment they had received which ranged from one (the most common) to four or more. Random samples were then selected, stratified within treatment centres and calendar periods of treatment and weighted according to the number of courses so as to ensure about equal numbers in each category, which varied from 1 in 15 for patients who had received only one course to one in two for patients who had received four courses or more or who had been treated at two or more centres. Full details of these sampled treatments were then recorded and measurements were made of the doses received by these various treatments in three places in the spinal marrow of a human model. There was not time to follow each patient individually and we had to be satisfied with information about the development of leukaemia from the reports of physicians, the follow-up records at the co-operating centres, and the names of all individuals who had died from leukaemia in the records of the national vital statistics office over the previous ten years with which the names of the members of the cohort could be matched (Court Brown and Doll, 1957). This limited procedure has subsequently been replaced by the individual follow-up of the entire cohort; but the initial crude follow-up proved adequate to discover nearly all the leukaemias that had occurred and provided a basis for concluding that the incidence of leukaemia bore a simple proportional relationship to the dose of radiation, that there was no threshold dose for the induction of the disease, and that the dose to the marrow that doubled the incidence of leukaemia was within the range of 30 to 50 r (0.3 to 0.5 Gy), at least as a working hypothesis for x-rays of the average energy used for the treatment of the disease. As it has turned out, the estimated doubling dose has proved to be only slightly higher than that now estimated from the ABCC data with a similar postulated relationship (0.26 Gy).

Like the ABCC's Life Span Study, the cohort of spondylitic patients was subsequently followed forward, turning much of it into a prospective study. In this case, the follow-up has been continued from 1954 to the end of 1991, the radiotherapy data for the sampled cases have been used to estimate the distribution of doses to all the principal organs, and estimates have been made of the excess relative risk per Gy for a European population. The estimated overall effect has not been very different from that estimated for the Japanese atomic bomb survivors (Weiss et al., 1994; Shimizu et al., 1990) but several notable differences were observed in the distribution of risk with time which may throw light on the way different aetiological agents interact with each other.

Subsequent developments

In the last 25 years several innovations have been introduced, some of which have made cohort studies more flexible and more productive.

Age-period cohort studies

Generation cohort studies have come to be analysed in a complex way in an attempt to separate the effects of changes in the risk to cohorts born at different periods, which commonly result from changes in behaviour, from changes in periods that have affected all generations simultaneously, whether due to environmental factors or, in the case of mortality rates, to new methods of treatment.

Osmond and Gardner first did this in 1982, using as examples the age-specific mortality rates in England and Wales from cancer of the bladder in men and cancer of the lung in women (Osmond and Gardner, 1982). They recognised that there could be no unique solution for the variation in two dimensional space of the effects of age,

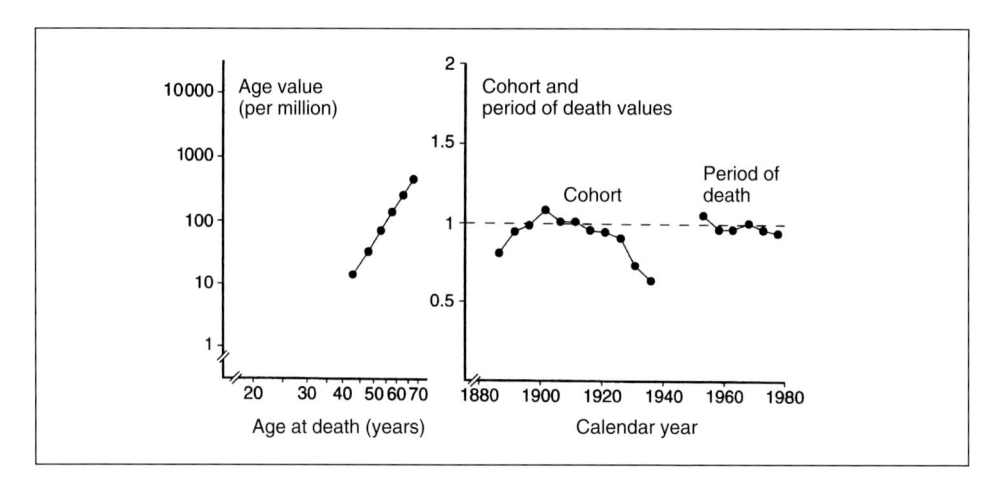

Figure 11
Mortality from bladder cancer in men in England and Wales analysed by age in years, cohort of birth, and period of death (Osmond and Gardner, 1982).

cohort, and period, but suggested a means by which the relative contributions of cohort and period could be approximated by introducing a mathematical constraint that had the effect of partitioning the drift with time between period and cohort in a ratio that depended on the relative magnitude of the non-drift effects. With this technique they obtained the results shown in Figures 11 and 12. In both cases the greater part of the trend could be explained by cohort effects with peaks of bladder cancer for men born in 1900 and for lung cancer in women born in 1920 – both of which corresponded to the generations most exposed to cigarette smoke.

In a discussion of the various methods that have been suggested, Clayton and Schifflers (Clayton and Schiffers, 1987) concluded „that the observation of incidence and mortality rates in populations over time does not provide sufficient information to ascribe smooth trends to period or cohort influences with any reliability." This is not to deny all uses for age, period, and cohort models; it is rather to stress that they must be examined and interpreted with some biological understanding of the mechanism by which the disease is being produced. As an example they cite the analysis of the trends in breast cancer mortality in Japan over the period 1955–1979. Three models fit equally well with grossly different implications regarding the separate period and cohort effects. One gives a reduction in age-specific rates above age 60 years, another gives a stabilisation of rates after the menopause, while the third gives a progressive increase in mortality to age 80 years, eliminating "Clemmesen's hook" in the increasing mortality with age which is a feature of all sets of data in relatively stable situations.

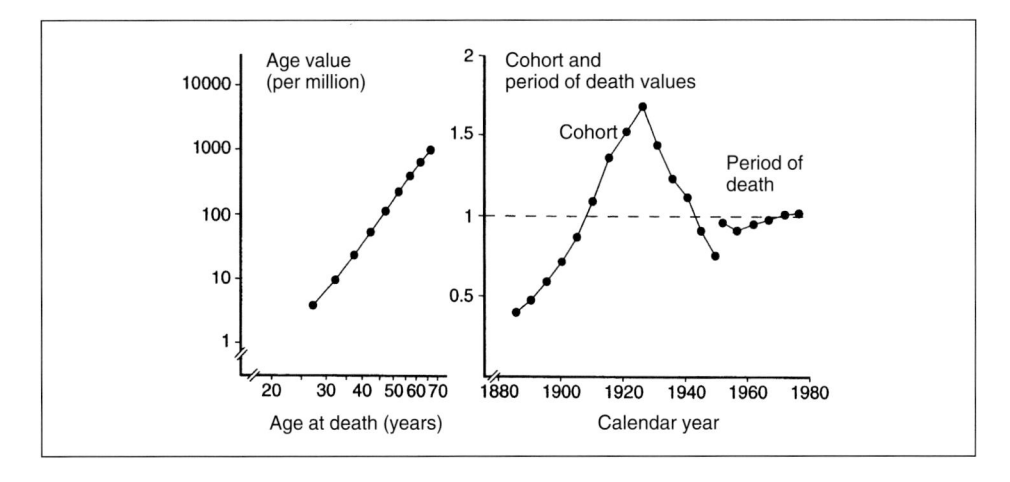

Figure 12
Mortality from lung cancer in women in England and Wales analysed by age in years, cohort of birth, and period of death (Osmond and Gardner, 1982).

Nested case-control studies

A much more important development has been the conduct of case-control studies nested within a large cohort. This is an alternative to the technique adopted by Court Brown and Doll (1957) when faced with the need to make complex estimates of the radiation dose to the bone marrow in their retrospective cohort study of the risk of leukaemia in patients irradiated for ankylosing spondylitis, to which I have referred, and it is usually simpler. To be efficient the technique requires the whole cohort to have been followed up with minimal lapse rate. The cohort can then be used as a population from which truly representative controls can be drawn at random, without risk of bias, for comparison with the members of the cohort who have developed the disease of interest. With a relatively small number of subjects, intensive efforts can then be made to quantify the exposure that cases and controls have experienced. Controls are chosen to match each case by surviving to the year when the affected member developed the disease of interest and by year of birth (the more exact the better) but they should not be required to match the affected member by year of entry to the cohort, as has sometimes been done, because this results in loss of important information relating duration of employment to the risk of developing disease. How many controls should be chosen to match each case, depends on the rarity of the cases and the complexity of the measures of exposure, but the more that are chosen the better, as greater numbers reduce the probability that any discovered differences could be due to chance.

Table 3 – Employment in occupations heavily exposed to coal tar fumes among gas retort house workers (after Doll et al., 1972)

	Men dying from	
	Occupational cancers[a]	Other causes
Number	137	137
No. employed as topmen or hydraulics mains attendants	16	9
Mean years employed as above	18.2	10.4

[a] Cancers of lung (122), bladder (12), and scrotum (3).

In retrospect, it is surprising that so many years were to pass before this method came to be commonly used. A primitive form of it was described in 1972 in the study of the occupational hazards of gas-workers (Doll et al., 1972) when it was used to define the type of occupation within gas retort houses that was most likely to give rise to the specific hazards of cancers of the lung, bladder, and scrotum. Men were not easy to classify by type of occupation as they commonly changed from one to another and different names were given to the same jobs in different works. Two occupations, however, stood out as liable to result in much heavier exposure to tar fumes than others; namely, those of topman and hydraulic mains attendant. Information was consequently obtained about the length of time spent in these occupations for men who had died of one of the three types of cancer that had been shown to occur in excess in retort house workers and from controls who died of some non-occupational cause and were matched one to one for employer and age at death within the same five-year age group. The results are summarised in Table 3.

According to Liddell (1988), the method became common only after about 1977. Two early examples of which I have personal knowledge were published in 1980. One is described later, when I consider the use of biomarkers. In the other, Peto (1980) sought to relate the risk of lung cancer in an asbestos textile factory to cumulative exposure to asbestos dust measured in the modern terms of fibres ml^{-1} years. A cohort of 679 male workers was identified who entered the factory in 1933 or later, that is after dust had been controlled to the standards of the Asbestos Industry Regulations of 1931, it was then followed to the end of 1978, and special attention was paid to those who entered in 1951 or later, when ambient dust measurements were regularly carried out. In these men, eight deaths from lung cancer had occurred 20 or more years after first exposure with only 1.62 expected. The cumulative exposure of the eight men who died of lung cancer was compared with that of 42 men employed over the same period and no difference in the measured exposure to asbestos dust was seen. This finding, the author thought, implied that static samples of the ambient environment are not the appropriate indicator of personal risk, which may be more closely related to high transient exposures during certain activities, and these could be measured only by personal monitoring. This, Peto (1980) noted had also been suggested from an earlier study of asbestos-related symptoms by Berry et al. (1979) and had been concluded some time earlier about the measurement of dust in mines in relation to the risk of pneumoconiosis, when Oldham and Roach (1952) introduced the concept of measuring the personal exposure each shift of randomly selected miners. That is not to say that static measurements of environmental pollution are no use – they have been shown to correlate with the incidence of lung cancer in other larger studies of the effects of exposure to asbestos (McDonald et al., 1983; Peto et al., 1985) – but to warn that they may provide only crude estimates of an individual's exposure with a consequent need for large numbers if statistically significant differences are to be detected.

Nested case-control studies within retrospective cohorts have come to be a major tool of the epidemiologist's armamentarium and have, in some cases, been adapted to allow for personal rather than static measurements, as in Thériault et al.'s (Thériault et al., 1994) study of the occupational hazards of leukaemia and brain cancer associated with exposure to 60 Hz electromagnetic fields produced by the passage of electricity. Many studies of such suspected hazards have been carried out in the last 16 years with inconclusive results, principally because of the lack of quantified information of the extent to which individuals in different occupations have actually been exposed. Faced with this problem, Thériault et al. (1994) carried out a cohort study of 223000 men employed by Electricité de France-Gaz de France, Ontario Hydro, and Hydro-Québec, who were observed during the period 1970 to 1989. Cases of cancer were ascertained in France from company medical records during employment. In Canada they were ascertained by matching the names of employees with the records of local cancer registries and, in Quebec, from company medical records and death certificates. Over 4000 men were identified as having developed cancer. To compare with them, controls were selected randomly from members of the whole population matched for the same utility, year of birth, and alive on the date the affected employee developed cancer: four for each man with one of the cancers of special interest (defined in this study as any haematopoietic cancer, brain cancer, or melanoma) and one for each man with a cancer of another type.

Full occupational histories were built up for all members of both groups from company records. Measurements of the fields to which a sample of over 2000 men currently employed were exposed were then made by means of personal dosemeters worn throughout a five-day week and jobs with similar mean exposures were collapsed into between 32 and 65 occupational groups, the number of groups varying between the different utilities. Allowance was made for procedural and power changes over the period of the men's exposures and each man's exposure was expressed in "µT years" by multiplying the mean exposure in each occupational group by the time spent in it. Odds ra-

Table 4 – Odds Ratios[a] for specific cancers among electric utility workers by cumulative exposure to magnetic fields (after Thériault et al., 1994)

Type of cancer	No. of cancers	Exposure equal to or above median	Exposure equal to or above 90th percentile
Acute non-lymphoid leukaemia	60	2.41 (1.07–5.44)[b]	2.52 (0.70–9.09)
Acute myeloid leukaemia	47	3.15 (1.20–8.27)	2.68 (0.50–14.50)
All leukaemia	140	1.54 (0.90–2.63)	1.75 (0.77–3.96)
Astrocytoma	41	0.97 (0.34–2.80)	12.29 (1.05–143.5)
Malignant brain tumour	108	1.54 (0.85–2.81)	1.95 (0.76–5.00)

[a] Compared to exposure less than median (3.1 µT years) and adjusted for socioeconomic status.
[b] 95% confidence interval.

tios, adjusted for socio-economic status, were then calculated for 31 cancer types for men with exposures equal to or above the median and exposures equal to or above the 90th percentile in comparison with men whose exposures were less than the median. Only three of the cancers showed statistically significant excesses in one or other of the more heavily exposed groups: those for acute non-lymphoid leukaemia, acute myeloid leukaemia, and astrocytoma. The results are shown in Table 4 along with those for all leukaemia and all malignant brain cancers. Though not conclusive, these findings greatly strengthen belief in the idea that 60 Hz electromagnetic fields may cause occupational hazards of these two diseases. It was a major task to compute the occupational exposures of the 11000 men selected for a nested case-control study and it would have been quite impracticable, at the same level of detail, to have done so for 20 times as many men, which a simple cohort study would have required.

Use of biomarkers

Still better measures of exposure can sometimes be obtained by measurements of biological characteristics or biomarkers, as they have come to be called. The early example of a nested case-control study that I referred to previously, which used biomarkers, was that initiated by Wald et al., in 1975 and first reported in 1980 (Wald et al., 1980). The biomarker of greatest interest at the time was the blood level of retinol and a sample of serum was consequently obtained from each member of the cohort studied at the start of the investigation and stored (in a so-called serum bank) at –40°C.

The study population consisted of 16000 men aged 35–64 years who attended for a comprehensive health screening examination between March 1975 and December

1978. Apart from giving a sample of blood, which was used for a number of blood tests and to provide the sample of serum, all the men completed a standard health questionnaire, were examined clinically, and had an ECG and a chest x-ray. The National Health Service records of the men were flagged centrally and Wald and his colleagues were notified in the event of a man's death or registration as having developed cancer. By the end of 1979, 86 men were identified who had developed cancer and these were matched with double the number of controls who were alive and without cancer, of similar age and smoking habits, and whose blood was taken at approximately the same date (within four months). Analysis of the blood samples showed that the men who developed lung cancer had significantly low levels of blood retinol (a mean of 187 against 229 IU per dl) while men who developed other cancers did not. This seemed to confirm the relationship between low retinol intake and lung cancer that had been recorded from dietary histories and to accord with the evidence that vitamin A analogues could decrease the risk of cancer in animal experiments. It has not, however, been supported in subsequent serum studies. Later observations showed that low serum levels of beta-carotene obtained in this (Wald et al., 1987) and other cohort studies using serum banks, predicted an increased risk of cancer better than the serum level of retinol; but this must now be interpreted as due to confounding with still another agent, as a controlled trial of the prophylactic value of beta-carotene supplements continued for 12 years has shown that raising the serum level has no effect on the risk of developing either cancer of the lung or cancer of any other organ (Hennekens et al., 1996). There remains, nevertheless, consistent evidence that a high level of consumption of green and yellow vegetables protects against the development of many cancers and further serum studies and controlled trials will be required to find out what the prophylactic agents are.

The results of nested case-control studies relating to serum sex hormones promise to be more productive. After years of conflicting reports, a relatively large study based on 130 cases of breast cancer and 251 matched controls, larger numbers than have been included in all the previous studies combined, supports the idea that high levels of available oestradiol (free and albumin bound) increase the risk of breast cancer as much as three-fold (Toniolo et al., 1996).

Urine banks have also been used. One was used in conjunction with a serum bank to test the importance of the combination of infection with the hepatitis B virus and the consumption of food contaminated with the fungal metabolite aflatoxin in the production of liver cancer in tropical climates (Ross et al., 1992). The cohort consisted of a little over 18000 men 45 to 64 years of age resident in four parts of Shanghai who volunteered to participate. Each man completed a standard questionnaire and gave samples of blood and urine, both of which were stored. After one to four years of follow up, liver cancer had been diagnosed in 22 men, and 120 controls were selected, matched within one year of age, within one month of sample collection, and for neighbourhood of residence, but otherwise at random. The results are summarised in Table 5. With blood positive for hepatitis B antigen and aflatoxin in the

Table 5 – Interaction of hepatitis B and aflatoxin in the production of liver cancer (after Ross et al., 1992).

Exposure to HBV[a]	Aflatoxin[b]	No. of cases/controls	Relative risk (95% Confidence interval)
–	–	4/74	1.0
–	+	6/51	1.9 (0.5, 7.5)
+	–	5/13	4.8 (1.2, 19.7)
+	+	7/2	60.1 (6.4, 561.8)

[a] HBs Ag in blood.
[b] Metabolite of aflatoxin in urine.

urine the relative risk of liver cancer was very much greater than when either marker was present alone and 60 times greater than when neither was present. These results are based on very small numbers and are preliminary and the study is being continued; but they provide the first objective evidence from observations on individuals of a synergism that has long been suspected from ecological observations, but has proved difficult to confirm by food frequency questionnaires.

Conclusion

What then of the future? Cohort studies in the original sense of the generation studies (Andvord, 1930) helped our understanding of the spread of tuberculosis and the aetiology of several cancers, but they are now of limited application and I doubt if they have much more to teach us. Cohort studies in the modern sense, both prospective and retrospective, have established themselves as essential tools for epidemiological research. The nested case-control study and the use of biomarkers, which will in the course of time involve the techniques of molecular biology, provide us with powerful weapons for testing hypotheses about both the genetic and environmental causes of disease and cohort studies have, I suspect, an even more important part to play in the future of medical research than they have had in the past.

Acknowledgement

I am grateful to the BMJ Publishing Group for permission to reproduce Figures 7, 8, and 9 from the British Medical Journal.

Issues of causality in the history of occupational epidemiology

Steven D. Stellman

Department of Epidemiology, Mailman School of Public Health, 722 West 168th Street, New York, NY 10032, USA

Summary

Occupational epidemiology has its roots in classical medicine. However, it became a quantitative discipline only in the 20th century, through the pioneering work of individuals such as Case, Lloyd, and Selikoff and organizations such as the Division of Occupational Health of the U.S. Public Health Service. Studies of chemical dye workers, bituminous coal miners, smelting workers, and uranium miners have been especially important sources of innovations in methodology and in development of logical reasoning leading to acceptance of causal relationships of occupational exposures that lead to respiratory diseases and cancer. The cooperation of labor unions, such as those of steel and asbestos workers, has often been a crucial factor in providing essential data.

Occupational epidemiology traces its origins at least as far back as the 1753 treatise of James Lind on his intervention trial of citrus fruits to cure scurvy among sailors in the British Navy (Lind, 1753). However, the application of scientific methods to recognition and amelioration of conditions in industry has occurred only in recent times. Before about 1950, research into causes of occupational diseases generally used methods that were little more than quantitative extensions of clinical medicine, and relied largely on cross-sectional observations at various points in time. As hazards associated with long-term exposure to carcinogens and other causes of chronic disease came under investigation, new research methods were developed.

In this paper I draw on a number of studies – some well-known, others relatively obscure – that I regard as milestones in the development of concepts and tools of occupational epidemiology. The studies cover a variety of workplaces including the chemical industry, mining, and asbestos insulation work. The methods involved either were invented because there was no existing methodology to handle the unique workplace situations, or were innovative adaptations of existing methods which were inadequate in their current forms. The developers of these methods have often had to show great resourcefulness and creativity, for the work environment is frequently inhospitable (and more than occasionally hostile) to the needs of the epidemiologist.

The birth of occupational cohort studies

The study by R.A.M. Case of the Institute of Cancer Research at the Royal Cancer Hospital, London, on causes of bladder cancer in the British chemical industry is widely regarded as the "prototype of historical cohort studies" (Case et al., 1954; Case and Pearson, 1954; Breslow and Day, 1987). Reports of bladder cancer among chemical dye workers had appeared in the 19th century (Rehn, 1895), and in a 1921 report the International Labour Office (ILO) listed benzidine and β-naphthylamine as likely causes (Averill and Samuels, 1992). The goal of Case's study was to determine "whether the manufacture or use of aniline, benzidine, α-naphthylamine, or β-naphthylamine could be shown to produce tumours of the urinary bladder in men so engaged". Case prepared a list of all men who had been employed by 21 cooperating chemical firms for at least six months between 1920 and 1952, and for whom exposure to one of the target chemical compounds could be documented. He then searched British death certificates for any that mentioned bladder cancer, and determined which belonged to men in their list. From known death rates from bladder cancer he calculated the "expected" number of deaths for bladder cancer workers. The observed number of bladder cancer deaths far exceeded the number expected on the basis of prevailing rates. An important methodological innovation was the examination of expected deaths in relation to the number of years since first employment, the so-called "latency" period. This concept has by now become a central feature of cancer epidemiology.

In 1955 Case and Lea reported a two-fold increase in deaths from lung cancer among men who suffered from mustard gas poisoning in World War I (Table 1) (Case and Lea, 1955). Their cohort study contains several innovative points. First, they asserted that the circumstances and dates of the mustard gas release were so well established and the affected population so well characterized through military and veteran records that they offered an analogy to "a carefully planned animal experiment." Secondly, they used two different non-exposed groups for comparison (men pensioned with bronchitis but who had never been exposed to mustard gas and unexposed amputees). Third, nine years before publication of the US Surgeon-General's Report on Smoking and Health, the authors recognized and demonstrated possible confounding by cigarette smoking.

Predicting that their work might be a prototype for a new genre of "environmental cancer studies", Case and Lea (1955) provided many details of their analytic method, which they termed a "comparative composite cohort analysis" to distinguish it from the cross-sectional analyses of mortality by occupation regularly published by the UK Registrar-General (1938). Their exposition of the use of age-strati-

Table 1 – Mortality in 1267 World War I veterans followed up 1930–1952 by wartime exposure to mustard gas (Case and Lea, 1955)

Cause of death	Exposed to mustard gas			Not exposed to mustard gas					
				Bronchitis			Amputation		
	Exp[1]	Obs[2]	SMR	Exp[1]	Obs[2]	SMR	Exp[1]	Obs[2]	SMR
All causes	357.3	547	153[c]	673.8	932	138[c]	365.7	383	105
All cancers	60.8	79	130[a]	95.0	104	109	72.2	72	100
Lung cancer	14.0	29	207[b]	14.4	29	201[b]	15.5	13	84
Cancers other than lung	46.8	50	107	80.6	75	93	56.7	59	104

[a] $P < 0.05$; [b] $P < 0.01$; [c] $P < 0.0001$.
[1] Expected; [2] Observed.

fied person-years is a model of clarity. This pathbreaking study was one of the earliest to make use of the standardized mortality ratio, a measure that is now one of the most common ways of expressing the magnitude of a health outcome in cohort studies (Stellman et al., 1998).

Mining, smelting, and coke-ovens: spawning ground for epidemiologic methods

The health hazards of mining have been known since antiquity. Pliny the Elder (23-79 AD) described devices used by metal refiners to prevent the inhalation of fatal dust (Plinius Secundus, Tr1929) (he himself died of asphyxiation while investigating the eruption of Vesuvius). In his 1556 treatise on mining and metallurgy "*De Re Metallica*" the German physician and mineralogist Georgius Agricola noted that "the evils which affect miners" included shortness of breath and premature death (Agricola Tr1950). Ramazzini, the father of occupational medicine, also provided clinical descriptions of diseases of miners (Tr1940).

Pneumoconiosis – a mine worker's disease

In the mid-19th century physicians began to systematically distinguish among the many forms of mining related illnesses (Pendergrass et al., 1972). In 1837 Thomson noted that British coal miners frequently had black deposits in their lungs at death (Lainhart et al., 1969). The term "pneumoconiosis" was coined by Zenker (1867), and "silicosis" by Visconti (1870). However, over half a century elapsed before epidemiological studies of miners were carried out:

> "Although the medical literature of the 19th century contained frequent warnings that coal miners suffered from an unusual chest disease, the first investigation was not made until 1928. In that year, Collins and Gilchrist (1928) in the UK published a paper that precipitated a long and detailed investigation of chest diseases among bituminous coal workers in Great Britain. Studies were initiated in 1936 by the Committee on Industrial Pulmonary Diseases of the Medical Research Council ..."
>
> "Although coal pneumoconiosis was recognized on the European continent about 1935, it was the establishment of the European Coal and Steel Community in 1952 that brought about a coordinated effort to study and prevent the disease. ... Over the next ten years, coal pneumoconiosis was recognized as a compensable disease in each of the European coal producing countries. ... Many research laboratories contributed to fundamental knowledge of the pathology and physiology of dust-induced diseases, with emphasis on coal pneumoconiosis. Environmental controls were developed, tested, and implemented, based on the principles of dust suppression at the coal face by water infusing and spray, ventilation, and respirators. Workplace dust monitoring and medical surveillance programs were instituted." (Doyle, 1969).

No comparable body of knowledge or programs then existed in the United States, where it was believed that bituminous coal did not produce a disabling pneumoconiosis, even though anthracosilicosis was well known in anthracite miners. Not until 1952 did the Division of Occupational Health of the USPHS (United States Public Health Service) conclude that a major cause of morbidity among bituminous coal miners was chronic diseases of the respiratory system. In the early 1960s, studies in Western Pennsylvania showed that 4% of working miners under age 45, 15% of working miners age 45 year or older, and 29% of retired miners had the disease. However, the sample size was small and lacked consistency between X-ray findings and symptom reports. Other studies suffered from flaws of subject selection, exclusion of retirees who might have left employment because of job-related illness, and consideration of the social environment within the extremely impoverished mining areas of Appalachia.

In 1963 the USPHS initiated The Appalachian Bituminous Coal Miners Study in the region where the majority of American coal miners live and work. The study drew a sample of 2000 working and 1000 nonworking miners, using a two-stage random selection of mines with stratification by and control for subsample size. The sample was drawn in stages from working miners in 97 counties grouped in 17 strata which averaged 6000 miners each, so as to select workers in small and large mines. To overcome the lack of a national roster of nonworking miners, the cooperation of the United Mine Workers of America was obtained. The study could not have been carried out without this collaboration. A total of 2751 working miners were identified, of whom 93% were examined. The researchers examined 617 unemployed miners and 574 pensioners, or 82% and 89% of those identified, respectively. Medical histories were gathered using the standardized Medical Research Council questionnaire (Lainhart et al., 1969).

Besides a rigorous sampling scheme, two important methodological decisions characterized the study design. First, the survey was restricted to men under age 65, recognizing that severe illnesses contracted during mine work produce a biased sample of men above retirement age. Second, separate samples of working miners and "non-working" miners were drawn, in recognition that many men left the industry before age 65 because of work-related health conditions.

Ten percent of working miners and 20% of nonworking miners had objective X-ray evidence of pneumoconiosis. X-ray findings also showed a high prevalence of definite pneumoconiosis which differed by job type and location underground, e.g., 22.3% in cutting machine operators. The prevalence of X-ray evidence of pneumoconiosis was also related directly to years of underground experience. X-ray abnormalities were definitely related to coal mining; they were not found in other workers living in the same area; they were clearly related to years of work and type of exposure. The disease was clinically identical to that in bituminous coal miners in Great Britain.

Mine radiation as a cause of lung cancer

The Erz Mountains of central Europe have been mined for metals since the Middle Ages (Figure 1). In medieval times the peculiar illnesses ("Bergsucht") acquired by local miners were well known. In 1879 Härting and Hesse noted the high percentage of deaths from "Bergkrankheit" (lung cancer) among miners in Schneeberg and Joachimsthal (Härting and Hesse, 1879). In the early 1900s, arsenic and cobalt were suspected causes, but Lorenz (1944) identified radioactivity definitively as a causative agent in the Schneeberg and Joachimsthal mines, and by 1949 the daughters of radioactive decay of radon released in the lungs by inhaled particles were identified as principal causes.

In 1950 the USPHS in cooperation with other Federal and State agencies initiated a program to assess hazards of internal radiation emitters. By 1962, Archer and colleagues had shown that lung cancer risk among uranium miners was higher than in the general population of White males (Archer et al., 1962), and in 1964 Wagoner and colleagues reported a 10-fold excess of respiratory cancer among long-term underground uranium miners in the U.S. (Wagoner et al., 1964a; 1964b). Wagoner further showed that the excess was not attributable to age, smoking, nativity, heredity, urbanization, self-selection, diagnostic accuracy, prior mining experience, or silica. The mean cumulative dose of radiation of uranium miners with lung cancer was significantly higher than in matched control miners. That was not enough proof for

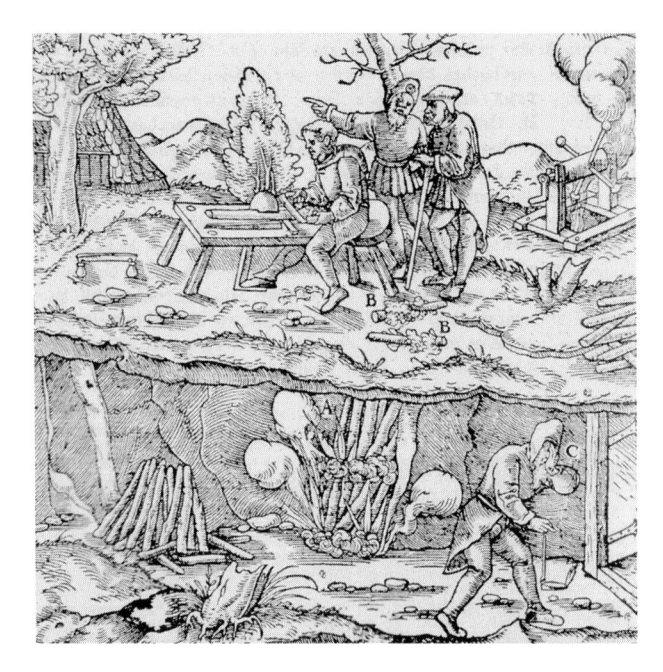

Figure 1
Mining in the Middle Ages, as depicted by Agricola 1556 (Tr1950). Fires were set to shatter rocks and break open veins of metal ore, as this man has done who is obviously on his way out. Agricola wrote, "While the heated veins and rock are giving forth a foetid vapor and the shafts or tunnels are emitting fumes, the miners and other workmen do not go down in the mines lest the stench affect their health or actually kill them."

some. The 1964 Surgeon-General's Report on Smoking and Health stated "although the induction of lung cancer by radionuclides is probable in man, the evidence is not as firm as in animals" (U.S. Public Health Service, 1964).

Wagoner and colleagues, drawing on radiation studies conducted by Court Brown and Doll (1957) and others, then constructed a cohort study which utilized statistical life table methods newly developed by Cutler and Ederer (1958). They invoked the Bradford Hill principles of causality (Hill, 1953), citing six factors supporting a causal relationship (Wagoner et al., 1965):

1) Excessive respiratory cancer
2) Dose-response relation between airborne radiation and lung cancer
3) Persistence of excess risk and dose-response after accounting for confounding variables, including time since first exposure and cigarette smoking
4) Consistency with animal studies and studies of other mining populations with similar exposures

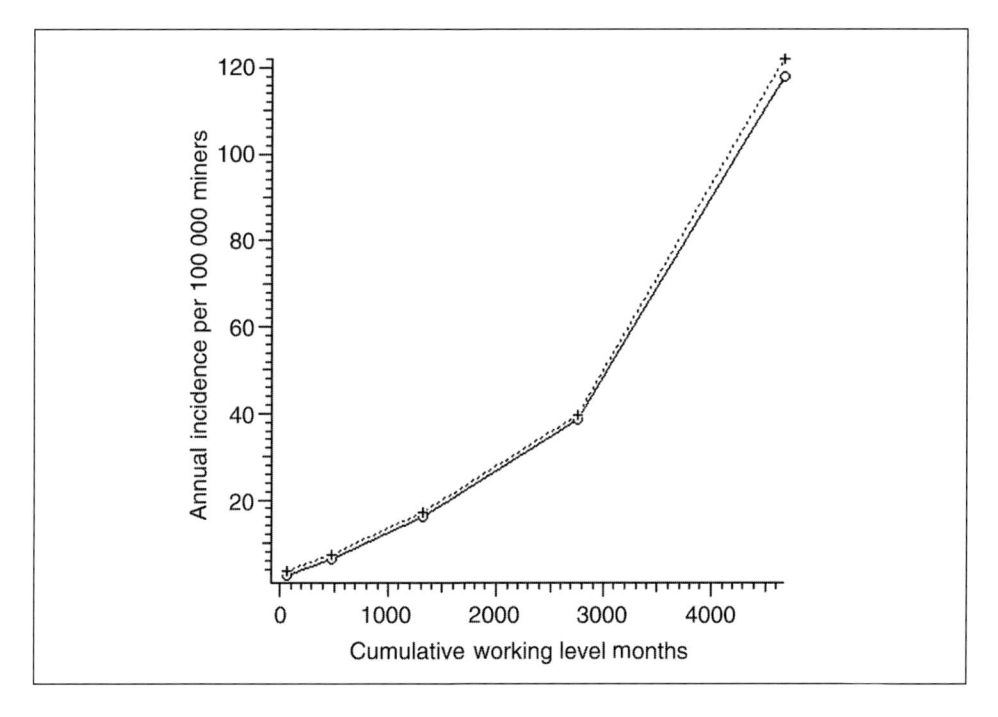

Figure 2
Incidence of lung cancer in underground uranium miners in relation to ionizing radiation dosage, expressed in "working-level months" (Wagoner et al., 1964a).

5) Specificity for the respiratory tract
6) Lung cancer pathology among miners unlike that observed among age-smoking-residence matched control group, but similar to that of factory workers exposed to mustard gas

The argument in favor of causality was bolstered by a powerful dose-response curve (Fig. 2). Use of a cumulative dose ("working-level months") of exposure to radon progeny, was one of the earliest applications of an external dosage measure in a study of occupational cancer.

Radium dial painters – another cancer hazard

Indiscriminate exposure to ionizing radiation has occurred in many industries besides mining. From 1915 to 1929 about 2 000 US women were employed to paint the faces of clocks and wristwatches with radium paint. By the early 1920s it be-

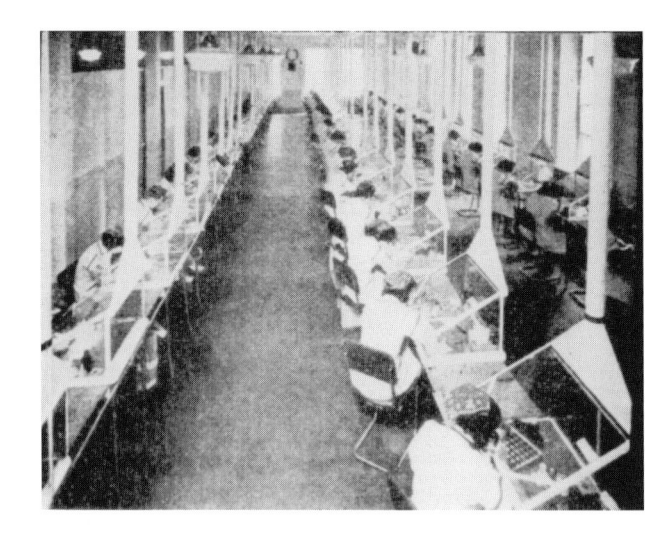

Figure 3
Radium dial painting operation after implementation of industrial hygiene measures including banning of oral "tipping" of brushes and construction of ventilated work enclosures (Hunter, 1969).

came clear that many of these women were developing a rare and disfiguring facial cancer of the paranasal sinuses. The U.S. Bureau of Labor Statistics set up a cohort of 1260 women which was later maintained by Argonne National Laboratory. In the 1950s, more than 20 years after most exposure stopped, 396 women were examined, and their body burden of radioactivity measured via a breath exhalation test. The 226 women who were first employed between 1915 and 1924 had a mean body burden of 21.19 µ Ci. Beginning in 1924 it was strictly forbidden for workers to "tip" the brushes in their mouths. This simple industrial hygiene measure reduced the exposure by over 90%, so that 170 women hired between 1925 and 1929 were eventually found to have a mean body burden of only 1.25 µ Ci. Tight control over painting operations was also exercised, with a high degree of work enclosure (Fig. 3). The reduced dosage translated to lower mortality: standard mortality ratios (SMRs), reported by Polednak et al. (1978), are shown in Table 2, subdivided into groups with cumulative radiation below 50 µ Ci (N = 302) and above 50 µ Ci (N = 58). Mortality ratios above 1.00 were observed only in the higher intake dose group. The highest SMRs were reported for bone cancer, and "other/unspecified cancer", which is thought to contain tumors in the mandibular region. Note that the body burden measurements were obtained after 1954, so that there is an unknown survival effect on initial selection into the cohort. This is probably the first occupational cohort study to employ a biomarker based upon measurement of a foreign agent in the body, and perhaps the earliest in which the favorable

Table 2 – Standardized mortality ratios (SMR) among 360 radium dial painters by radiation dose as measured after 1954 (Polednak et al., 1978)

Cause of death	< 50 µCi (N = 302) Observed/Expected	SMR	≥ 50 µCi (N = 58) Observed/Expected	SMR
All causes	46/53.3	0.86	23/12.0	1.91 [a]
Cancer	16/13.3	1.20	12/3.02	3.97 [b]
Lung	0/0.8	–	1/0.18	5.61
Breast	3/2.8	1.07	1/0.62	1.62
Bone	0/0.06	–	3/0.01	225.40 [b]
Other/unspecified	1/0.85	1.18	5/0.18	22.73 [b]
Leukemia	0/0.44	–	1/0.10	9.95

[a] $p < 0.01$; [b] $p < 0.001$.

effects of an intervention were directly measured. By the 1930s, the "luminizing" industry was mostly out of the watch business, and existed largely for military applications.

Hazards of smelting: arsenic and lung cancer

In modern industry, ores of copper, lead, and zinc are commonly smelted in order to remove impurities, chief among which is arsenic. Besides smelting, occupational exposure to arsenic occurs in production of pesticides and insecticides (including Agent Blue which was used as a defoliant by the U.S. military in Vietnam (Stellman et al., 1988; 2003)), and in agricultural workers who apply these agents (Stellman and Kabat, 1978). Heavy exposure in workers has been well documented: Pinto and McGill (1953) found high levels of urinary arsenic in 348 workers exposed to arsenic trioxide dust at ASARCO's Tacoma, Washington, smelter. By mid-20th century it had become contentious whether arsenic or its compounds were carcinogens.

Using company records, Pinto and Bennett (1963) reported an elevated proportional mortality ratio (PMR) of 174 for lung cancer among 904 active employees and 209 pensioners, a finding which Milham and Strong (1974) corroborated independently with a PMR of 222. However, proportional mortality ratios, while suggestive, are not generally regarded as being methodologically as strong as cohort data.

In the late 1960s researchers from the NCI and USPHS constructed a cohort of 8047 white male smelter workers with exposure of one year or more to arsenic trioxide between 1938 and 1963. The SMR for lung cancer was 329 (p < 0.01), and was eight-fold in workers with more than 15 years of employment and heavy exposure to arsenic (Lee and Fraumeni, 1969). The study had two innovative features. First, air measurements were used to classify various work areas as providing qualitatively light, medium, or heavy exposure. Since exposure assignments were based on job titles, this is probably one of the earliest examples of what we now call a job-exposure matrix. Secondly, the men were split into five sub-cohorts according to length of employment, so as to allow for latency and to provide stratification by calendar year. Lee and Fraumeni concluded that their findings were consistent with the "hypothesis that exposure to high levels of As_2O_3, perhaps in interaction with SO_2 or unidentified chemicals in the work environment, is responsible for the excessive number of respiratory cancer deaths among smelter workers". In 1987 IARC definitively classified both arsenic and its compounds as human carcinogens (International Agency for Research on Cancer, 1987).

Coke oven workers and lung cancer

The health hazards associated with bituminous coal do not end at the mine shaft. When bituminous coal is heated to a high temperature (350–1000°C) in the absence of air, volatile products are formed and a residue of impure carbon remains, known as coke. When the volatile products cool to ambient temperature, a portion condenses to a black viscous liquid known as coal tar, while the noncondensable gases are known as coal gas. The coke itself is used for the reduction of ores in blast furnaces, a process which is an integral part of steel manufacture (Figure 4). The by-product coke plant, designed to maximize recovery of valuable tar, oils, and chemicals from the volatiles, was the dominant type through mid-century. Many of these by-products are carcinogens or carcinogen precursors.

Until the 1960s, contradictory findings had been reported regarding lung cancer among coke-oven workers. In 1962 William Lloyd of the USPHS and Antonio Ciocco of the University of Pittsburgh School of Public Health set up a historical cohort of over 59000 steelworkers in seven plants in the Pittsburgh area. This cohort represented nearly two-thirds of all men working in basic iron and steel production in the U.S. in 1953. The study achieved an extraordinarily low rate of 0.2% loss to follow-up. Whites had lower death rates than Blacks, and both groups had favorable mortality compared with the general population, although White steelworkers had an excess of deaths due to accidents (Lloyd and Ciocco, 1969).

Shortly after this initial report, Carol Redmond joined the study team, and contributed to a series of landmark publications in the Journal of Occupational Medicine. One report assessed risk of lung cancer among coke plant workers. The by-product coke plant was a semi-continuous operation with three distinct work areas in terms of function and potential exposure to environmental hazards: (1) the coal handling area

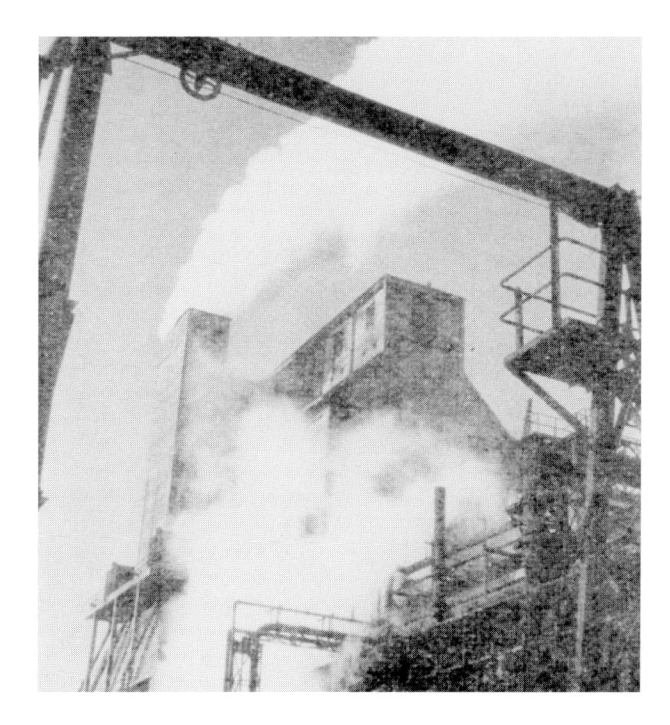

Figure 4
Coke oven plant in which bituminous coal is converted to coke for subsequent use in blast furnaces as an integral part of manufacture of steel. Workers assigned to "topside" positions closest to the top of the stack had highest rates of lung cancer (Hunter, 1969).

where coal is received by rail or barge and possibly blended with other coal types; (2) the coke ovens, grouped into one or more batteries, with equipment for charging and discharging the ovens, and for quenching; (3) a by-products plant for recovery of gas and chemical products (Lloyd, 1971).

Redmond and colleagues (1972) found the excess lung cancer limited to men employed at the ovens, with an SMR of 250. The greatest burden of risk was further borne by men working on the tops of the ovens, with an SMR of about 500, rising to 1000 for men employed at least five years. Lung cancer risk was further related to temperature of carbonization. Methodological innovations of this study thus included the use of job title (usual position on the coke oven) as a kind of dosage surrogate. Polynuclear aromatic hydrocarbons are now considered to be the major carcinogens in coke oven effluents (International Agency for Research on Cancer, 1984).

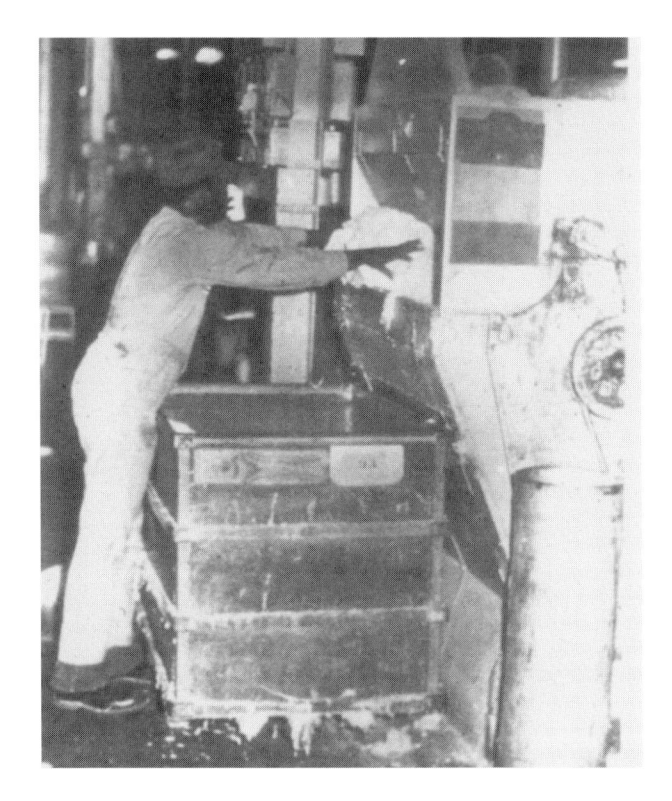

Figure 5
Worker loading chrysotile asbestos fiber by hand and without respiratory protection into the feed hopper of a carding machine at Marshville, NC, textile plant, prior to plant's acquisition and redesign by Raybestos Manhattan in 1969 (Lewinsohn et al., 1979).

Asbestos

It is impossible to discuss the development of occupational epidemiology without recognizing the extensive contributions of Irving Selikoff. Selikoff first gained fame as a developer of isoniazid for therapy of tuberculosis, but is best known for his many contributions to occupational epidemiology, done in collaboration with E. Cuyler Hammond of the American Cancer Society, which fixed asbestos as a major industrial cancer hazard. Asbestos is a highly fire-resistant mineral that has been used in construction and textiles since the late 19th century. Lack of even the most elementary industrial hygiene control (Fig. 5) has resulted in the deaths of tens of thousands of workers.

Selikoff's studies made extensive use of union (rather than employer) employment and health records. With the cooperation of the International Association of Heat

Table 3 – Deaths among 17 800 asbestos insulation workers in the U.S. and Canada, January 1, 1967 – December 31, 1976 (166 853 man-years of observation) (Selikoff et al., 1979)

Underlying cause of of death	Expected[a]	Observed (BE)	Observed (DC)	Ratio (o/e) (BE)	Ratio (o/e) (DC)
Total deaths, all causes	1658.9	2271	2271	1.37	1.37
Cancer, all sites	319.7	995	922	3.11	2.88
Deaths of less common malignant neoplasms					
Pancreas	17.5	23	49	1.32	2.81
Liver, biliary passages	7.2	5	19	0.70	2.65
Bladder	9.1	9	7	0.99	0.77
Testes	1.9	2	1	–	–
Prostate	20.4	30	28	1.47	1.37
Leukemia	13.1	15	15	1.15	1.15
Lymphoma	20.1	19	16	0.95	0.80
Skin	6.6	12	8	1.82	1.22
Brain	10.4	14	17	1.35	1.63

[a] Expected deaths are based upon white male age-specific U.S. death rates from U.S. National Center for Health Statistics, 1967–1976.
(BE) Best evidence. Number of deaths categorized after review of best available information (autopsy, surgical, clinical).
(DC) Number of deaths as recorded from death certificate information only.

and Frost Insulators and Asbestos Workers, he prepared a list of every member of two New Jersey locals as of December 31, 1942 (N = 632). The original 632 men contributed less than 9000 person-years of "exposure to risk of death," which is rather small for a modern-day cohort study. Between 1943 and 1962, 45 of the 632 insulation workers died of cancer of the lung or pleura, where only 6.6 deaths were expected. Three of the pleural cancers were mesotheliomas, and there was one death from peritoneal mesothelioma. An unexpectedly large number of men died of cancer of the stomach, colon, or rectum (29 vs. 9.4 expected), and 12 died of asbestosis, which was so rare that comparative population rates were unavailable (Selikoff et al., 1964).

Selikoff later carried out a much larger study, using the membership of 120 locals of the International Union. A total of 17800 men were enrolled as of January 1, 1967, and traced for at least 10 years, at which time over 12 000 had at least 20 years of occupational exposure to asbestos. A number of methodological explorations were

Table 4 – Deaths and death rates from pleural and peritoneal mesothelioma among 17 800 asbestos insulation workers in the U.S. and Canada, January 1, 1967 – December 31, 1976 (Selikoff et al., 1979).

Duration from onset (Years)	Number of men	Person-years of observation	Number (BE)	Number (DC)	No. per 1000 person-years of observations (BE)	Number (BE)	Number (DC)	No. per 1000 person-years of obsevations (BE)
< 10	8190	26393	0	0	0	0	0	0
10–14	9063	29003	0	0	0	0	0	0
15–19	9948	34066	2	2	0.06	3	0	0.09
20–24	8887	31268	6	4	0.19	3	2	0.10
25–29	6596	20657	13	5	0.63	19	3	0.92
30–34	3547	11598	9	3	0.78	23	6	1.98
35–39	2020	5403	15	4	2.78	19	5	3.52
40–44	1108	3160	4	3	1.27	16	3	5.06
45 +	1448	5305	14	4	2.64	29	5	5.47

(BE) Best evidence. Number of deaths categorized after review of best available information (autopsy, surgical, clinical).
(DC) Number of deaths as recorded from death certificate information only.

Table 5 – Comparison of observed cancer death rates with predictions of additive and multiplicative models, according to source of cause-of-death information (adapted from Hammond et al., 1979)

Exposure	Lung cancer death rate, based upon:	
	"Best evidence"	Death certificate
Neither smoking nor asbestos	11.3	11.3
Smoking only	122.6	122.6
Asbestos only	80.2	58.4
Both actual	693.8	601.6
Predicted from model additive model	191.5	169.7
Multiplicative (synergistic) model	870.1	633.6

made, including use of alternative control groups, different methods for taking smoking into account, and use of "best evidence" of cause of death, in place of unverified death certificate information (Hammond et al., 1979) (Table 3). In another groundbreaking study, death rates from two extremely rare cancers, pleural and peritoneal mesothelioma, were tabulated by duration of employment (Table 4). The dramatic dose-responses observed greatly reinforced the argument that asbestos insulation work was a severe cancer hazard (Selikoff et al., 1979).

Selikoff and Hammond used their data to propound the concept of synergism, in which the disease rate among persons exposed to two hazards (e.g., asbestos and smoking) is much greater than that predicted additively from the individual exposures (Hammond et al., 1979). This required identification of a suitable non-exposed "control" population socio-economically similar to the exposed insulation workers, and for whom detailed smoking data were available. Such a group was found among the half-million men enrolled in the American Cancer Society's Cancer Prevention Study (CPS-I) (Hammond, 1966). A comparison of death rates for lung cancer using additive and multiplicative (synergistic) models is shown in Table 5. The observed rates are predicted far better by the multiplicative model. This powerful demonstration of synergy was an early example of the epidemiological concept of interaction. Although initially developed for study of disease risk in relation to multiple occupational and lifestyle factors, techniques for assessing interactions are rapidly being adapted for use in studies of the joint genetic and environmental impact on disease risk (Andrieu and Goldstein, 1998). A foreseeable consequence of these methodological advances in assessing gene-environment interactions in the occupational setting is labeling the workers according to their susceptibility. The availability of such information raises ethical issues regarding the protection of workers from occupational hazards (Hemstreet, 1998).

Origins and early development of the case-control study

Nigel Paneth[1], Ezra Susser[2], Mervyn Susser[3]

[1] Department of Epidemiology, 4660 S. Hagadorn, Ste. 600, Michigan State University, East Lansing, MI 48824, USA
[2] Department of Epidemiology, Columbia University, Mailman School of Public Health, 722 West 168th Street, New York, NY 10032; and New York State Psychiatric Institute, USA
[3] School of Public Health, Sergievsky Center, 630 W. 168 St., New York, NY 10032, USA

Summary

This paper traces the origins and early development of the case-control study, focusing on its evolution in the 19th and early 20th century. As with other forms of clinical investigation, the case-control study emerged from practices that originally belonged to the realm of patient care. This form of disease investigation can be viewed as the knitting together of medical concepts (caseness, disease etiology, and a focus on the individual) – and medical procedures (anamnesis, grouping of cases into series; and comparisons of the diseased and the healthy) – that are of ancient origin, but which were seldom brought together until the 20th century. The analytic form of the case-control study can be found in 19th century medical literature, but did not appear to be viewed as a special or distinct methodology. A number of clinical investigations, and several sociological studies, in the first half of this century can be described as case-control studies. The first modern case-control study was Janet Lane-Claypon's study of breast cancer in 1926, but the design was used only sporadically in medicine and the social sciences until 1950, when four published case-control studies linked smoking and lung cancer. These 1950 studies synthesized the essential elements of the case-control comparison, produced a conceptual shift within epidemiology, and laid the foundation for the rapid development of the case-control design in the subsequent half century.

> "Judging from the manner in which the subject is usually handled, the study of the etiology of diseases is generally undertaken with great levity, even by men of high acquirement. Some slight general knowledge, supported by a little more or a little less common sense, is quite sufficient to fit its possessor for the discovery of the causes of disease, in other words, to qualify him for the most complicated problem within the whole range of pathology." (Louis, 1844: 487).

A computerised MEDLINE search did not find the term "case-control" in the title of a biomedical paper until 1967, and did not find it in the titles of more than two papers in a year until 1973. By 1980, 91 titles included the term, but in the year 2000 1795 papers had "case-control" in the title or abstract. This enormous increase is only partly a reflection of preferences in terminology, such as a shift from the term "retrospective study" to "case-control study", and of the general increase in medical publications over the last four decades. The case-control study is now firmly ensconced in epidemiology, and, because of its widespread use and the value of its results, it now rivals in importance the more straightforward cohort approach to unravelling disease etiology.

From where did this investigative tool come? The modern form of the case-control study is most easily recognised in Janet Lane-Claypon's study of breast cancer in 1926, and crystallised in the years following World War II. 1950, a year that saw the publication of four case-control studies of smoking and lung cancer, was a watershed in the acceptance of this approach to assessing disease etiology.

Each of the component practices of the case-control design, as well as each of its underlying concepts, had been used or discussed in some earlier medical setting. The embryonic development of this unique study design resulted from the knitting together of these elements for a specific purpose, namely, the uncovering of factors predisposing to disease operating at the level of the individual. Setting this as the objective for study implied a causal paradigm which was emerging but not yet fully articulated, that is, the notion that multiple causal agents may act to increase the risk of disease, particularly chronic disease. The search for risk factors would supplant the search for necessary and sufficient causes as the guiding principle of epidemiologic research.

If the period up to 1926 might be considered as the embryology of this synthetic conception, then the period after its birth in 1950 might be seen as the development of the infant into a full-fledged being. Advances in methodology since then have been particularly important in the modern era of the case-control study, but these latter advances did not require quite the same conceptual shifts as did the earlier developments.

Components of the case-control study

In our view, the case-control study is distinguished by six essential elements, each of which evolved separately in medical history. These elements include three inter-related underlying concepts:

1. The idea of the case: that is, that disease entities are specific, and are likely to have one or more specific causes.
2. An interest in disease etiology and prevention.
3. A focus on individual, as opposed to group, etiologies.

These elements of the case-control study also include three practices:

4. Anamnesis, or history taking from patients, which permits the collapse of time past without enduring its slow passage until outcomes under study evolve.
5. Grouping individual cases together into series.
6. Making comparisons of the differences between groups, in order to elicit average risk at the level of the individual.

Caseness

The case series presupposes that there is some organising principle that unites the individuals so assembled. This principle in turn depends upon the view that diseases are specific and distinguishable entities. The 17th century physician Thomas Sydenham, dubbed the English Hippocrates, was perhaps the first forceful advocate of the concept of diseases as entities distinguishable by their symptoms and signs, course and prognosis (Sydenham, 1848). This view may seem self-evident, but as late as the 19th century it was not so to many physicians (Merton, 1957). Different diseases were frequently viewed as the varying responses of individuals to differing environmental circumstances. Thomas Southwood Smith, perhaps the leading British physician-sanitarian of the first half of the 19th century argued that: "This mode of viewing fever as one great and extensive malady never differing in nature, but in every two cases differing in intensity, and giving rise by these differences in intensity to various forms of disease, thus affords a principle of arrangement, which, while it is at one simple and comprehensive, is at the same time in the highest degree practical." (Southwood Smith, 1830). In fact, this unitary concept of febrile diseases was a very powerful stimulus to sanitary reform, as it implied that all such illnesses might be prevented by environmental improvement.

Critical to the concept of caseness was the development of morbid pathology. From the time of the publication of Morgagni's classic *"De sedibus..."* or *"Seat of disease"* (Morgagni, 1761), in which the Italian physician and anatomist showed the clear relationship between local pathology and disease symptomatology, medicine began its slow but steady march towards acceptance of the distinctiveness of the several diseases. The fuller development of scientific pathology by physicians of the early 19th century – including Louis in France, Henle in Germany, Von Rokitansky in Austria and among others – gave force to the concept of unique biomedical entities with clinical manifestations linked to specific pathological findings. Louis' American student William Wood Gerhard demonstrated the concept when he first clearly separated typhoid fever from typhus fever. In making the distinction, Gerhard relied principally on the difference in intestinal pathology between the "typhus" fever he treated in Philadelphia and the "typhoid" fever he had seen with Louis in Paris (Gerhard, 1837).

Disease etiology

The conceptual basis of the case-control study is an interest in the etiology of disease, as contrasted to its prognosis or treatment. This interest is of course very ancient in medicine, but the extent of interest in etiology has varied from time to time in medical history among the ancient Greeks, the god Aesculapius presided over treatment, and another, Hygiea, over prevention. Hygiea was Aesculapius' daughter, and, paralleling the situation for daughters in ancient Greece, interest in etiology has historically been eclipsed by interest in treatment.

Interest in etiology tends to become dominant during serious epidemics, when prognosis is poor and the limitations of medical treatment are most evident. At such times, often stimulated by public alarm and political pressure, medicine has focused more intensely on etiology and prevention, and the sometimes furious investigative efforts that have surrounded epidemics in the past two centuries have often yielded major leaps in understanding. The modes of transmission of cholera (Snow, 1855), yellow fever (Reed et al., 1900) and plague (Advisory Committee, 1906) were each worked out under the pressure of epidemic disease. This perhaps explains the name of our discipline, which, in spite of its focus on the etiology of diseases of all kinds, including those that are rarely viewed as epidemic, continues to be epidemiology.

Etiology at the individual level

Not always emphasised in textbook descriptions of case-control studies is the focus of this design on causes of disease that operate at the level of the individual. Case-control studies have not generally contributed to an understanding of broad ecological risk factors such as air or water pollution, because the usual methods for choosing controls are unlikely to produce populations with differences in exposure. Optimum controls, in most definitions, are drawn from the same source population (or study base) as the cases. To obtain such controls, typical source populations are in the neighbourhood in which the case resides, or in the hospital in which the case is ascertained, the choice depending on the object of the study and the extent of ascertainment bias entering into the case diagnosis. The need to ensure the same study base for controls and cases constraints the variety of source populations that can be used to obtain controls. This constraint often eliminates any possibility of finding differences in ecological risk factors between cases and controls, because these will differ *across* rather than *within* such populations.

At least until the mid-19th century, most etiologic comparisons made in medicine were ecologic. Hippocrates contrasted the salubrity of different geographic regions, seasons of the year, and ethnic groups, but provided little description of individual behaviours as risks for disease (Hippocrates, 400a BCE). The concept of various occupations predisposing to particular diseases, as developed by Ramazzini (Trl940) and by Thackrah (1832), also viewed disease risk as a function of group membership. Comparisons of the mortality rates of counties, cities and neighbourhoods are staples of the literature of 19th century sanitarians such as Chadwick (1842), Shattuck (1850) and Farr (1852). Much rarer are comparisons of disease risk according to characteristics which, unlike water supply or weather conditions, need to be measured at the level of the individual. Nineteenth century sanitarians concerned themselves almost exclusively with broad ecological contributors to disease such as sewerage, water supply, climate and weather patterns, and poverty and crowding. The case-control study represents a very different etiologic focus.

Anamnesis

Anamnesis elicits by interview a retrospective account of events in a patient's life that the questioner, usually the physician, hypothesises may be of importance in understanding the disease process. Although the main purpose of interviewing patients in clinical practice is to establish the acute symptoms of the illness and their chronological order, the practice of asking patients about behaviours and conditions antecedent to the illness, such as places of residence, usual diet and patterns of physical activity, goes back to the Hippocratic writings of the 4th century B.C.

Epidemiology, learning from survey methods developed in the social sciences, has in recent years refined its anamnestic techniques. Although the case-control study is not in principle wedded to the interview as its only means of obtaining exposure data, to this day the bulk of case-control studies elicit most etiologic information by personal interview. This is not accidental, but rather a function of the kind of exposures that the case-control study is typically after, namely, personal exposures of long or varying duration and remote origin, rarely available from any other source than the subjects themselves. When sources other than the patient are available, as, for example, in birth and other vital statistics registers and in military or other occupational records, they are often amenable to the construction of exposure cohorts, which makes the retrospective cohort design more attractive.

In the chronic diseases that are commonly investigated in case-control studies, physical examination or laboratory testing are limited as sources of exposure to characteristics that are stable over many years, such as HLA-type, antibody status, genes, or genetic polymorphisms. Occasionally, anamnesis can be confirmed by physical examination, as in the self-report of circumcision, which has been assessed as a risk factor for cancer both by history and, with greater precision, by examination (Schrek and Lenowitz, 1947; Dunn and Buell, 1959). With the availability of banks of stored data, including especially tissue specimens, more opportunities will arise for other kinds of exposure ascertainment in nested case-control studies, including assessment of serum markers representing exposures earlier in the subject's life.

Making comparisons

The second and most essential case-control practice is the comparison of like with like in order to discern differences of interest or importance. In philosophical terms, this is exemplified in John Stuart Mill's second canon – *"the method of difference,"* – which states:

> *"In an instance in which the phenomenon under investigation occurs, and an instance in which it does not occur, have every circumstance in common save one, that one occurring only in the former; the circumstance in which alone the two instances differ, is the effect, or cause, or a necessary part of the cause, of the phenomenon."* (Mill, 1856).

In a case-control study, the instance in which the phenomenon under investigation occurs is the case-state, and the instance in which the phenomenon does not occur is the control-state. The circumstance "occurring only in the former" is the hypothesised exposure. This kind of comparison is not a new element in medicine; one can find many early attempts to elucidate Mill's method of difference to make assertions about causes of disease. But the case-control study differs from most of these historical comparisons in that the direction of the comparison runs backwards in time from caseness to etiology, rather than forward from etiology to caseness (the former being more intuitively understandable).

An elaboration of this logic was required for the development of the case-control study. In practice, the design is not used to establish a one-to-one relation between caseness and exposure. Rather, the question is whether the exposure occurs more frequently in cases than controls and the presence of this association implies that the converse will also be true, namely, that the disease occurs more often in the exposed than the unexposed. The repositing of the question in this way is essential to the causal paradigm underlying the design, which holds that many exposures can be causes of a single disease, and that each of these exposures can increase the probability of disease in an individual. It was in part for this reason that figures such as Major Greenwood and Bradford Hill (the first and second chairs of Epidemiology and Statistics at the London School of Hygiene and Tropical Medicine), who were statisticians as well as epidemiologists, played a prominent role in the early evolution of the case-control study (1925–50), as did later their statistician counterpart in the United States, Jerome Cornfield (1951).

Case series

It may seen intuitively obvious that before any useful comparisons along the lines discussed above could be made, a group of cases would need to be brought together. But the case series is largely a 19th century development. The assembly and description of cases – groups of patients with similar characteristics – was first used to study issues of practical interest to physicians – clinical presentation and prognosis. Studies gradually extended into diagnosis, pathological findings, and treatment. Etiology was less commonly of interest.

Although clinicians had occasionally assembled groups of patients and described them before the 19th century, the earliest, most systematic and most celebrated proponent of such work was the Parisian physician PCA Louis (1788–1875). A physician of great personal influence, many of whose students became leading medical figures in Britain, Germany, and the United States, Louis promulgated a belief in what he called the "numerical method", a technique whose principal tool was the tabulation of aggregated data about patients with similar pathologic and clinical findings. The disease he studied most comprehensively was tuberculosis, then usually called phthisis. Louis' interest in case series was principally designed for understanding pathology and for elaborating clinical and diagnostic observations; prognosis and treatment were his second interest; etiology, though not completely absent, took a distant third place.

19th century case-contol approaches

The 19th century provides a few interesting examples of studies that contained some or most of the essential elements of the case-control study. Below we describe three.

Louis on heredity in tuberculosis

The quote that inaugurates this chapter is taken from Louis' treatise on tuberculosis, a book of 566 pages in its English translation, which contains just one 32-page chapter entitled "Etiology" (Louis, 1844, pp. 477–508). In that chapter, Louis prefigured the case-control approach by considering the hereditary predisposition to phthisis. After first acknowledging the difficulty of obtaining good information from patients about the causes of death of their parents, he notes that in a series of phthisical patients assembled by Briquet, 36 of 101 had "phthisical parents". He then reasons thus:

> "But..if the mortality produced by phthisis at the Necker hospital during the space of three years averaged 11/37ths, or somewhat less than one third of the whole mortality; this would signify that 11/37ths of the population of Paris die phthisical, and that, consequently, whenever we proceed to the investigation of the hereditary influence in respect of any disease, we must find tuberculous parents eleven times out of thirty seven. So that if the same ratio existed in the in-

stance of the parents of tuberculous subjects, hereditary influence would be shown not to exist all." (Louis, 1844, p. 484).

Here we have perhaps the first reference to the absence of a higher rate of exposure in the diseased ("the same ratio") supporting a null hypothesis about disease etiology. Louis' insight was to recognize the insufficiency of Briquet's case series standing alone as supporting hereditary or other causes of the disease. For his theoretical comparison, therefore, he resorted to a series of deaths in a Paris hospital. Less justifiably, Louis viewed this series as a reasonable approximation of Parisian mortality overall.

Louis also developed the idea of comparison in his work on treatment. Famously, in his demonstration (widely criticised at the time) that bloodletting for acute lobar pneumonia was not especially helpful, he compared patients admitted to hospital, and hence bled, at successively longer intervals after onset. Fatalities were highest among those bled earliest (Louis, 1835). Although Louis was a pioneer in promoting the concept of fair and accurate comparison of treatments, he did not systematise the reasoning expressed in the quote above, and did not add control series to his many notable case series.

Whitehead on cholera and the Broad Street pump

John Snow, in his famous investigation of the Broad Street pump outbreak, did not systematically assess pump water exposure in individuals without cholera (Snow, 1855). But a local minister, the Reverend Henry Whitehead, did just that (Whitehead, 1855). Initially skeptical of Snow's findings, Whitehead inquired in detail (returning up to five times to the same person) as to pump water consumption among residents of Broad Street between August 30th and the removal of its handle on September 8th. He began by asking the families of cholera deaths about the habits of the decedents, and found that 45 had "decidedly" drunk from the pump, while 13 had not. Extending his inquiry to cholera survivors, he found 35 "certainly" drank pump water, while 7 did not. He then reasoned that to perform "a proper inquiry into this subject .... I must likewise examine, upon this matter, as many as possible of those who, being resident in Broad Street at the beginning of September, did not suffer at all either from Cholera or Diarrhoea." Whitehead interviewed 336 non-cholera cases, and found that 279 had not used the pump, while 57 had. He concluded that "among those attacked, the ratio of pump water drinkers to non-drinkers of the same water is 80 to 20, whilst among those who escaped the corresponding ratio is but 57 to 279". This gives an odds ratio of 19.6 for pump water use and cholera ($p < 0.001$).

This study, designed to investigate a specific exposure ascertained through interview, and using a control series of individuals, chosen from the same source population but free of the condition of interest, is, to our knowledge, the first case-control study in the medical literature. A case has been made (Lilienfeld and Lilienfeld, 1979) that William August Guy's investigation of occupation in relation to pulmonary consumption (Guy, 1843) was the first case-control study. Guy, however, while making very interesting remarks about the problems of selection bias in occupational health research, compared the proportion of deaths due to consumption in the different occupations. His outcome of interest, the relative odds of dying from consumption as compared to dying from other causes in the different occupations, though of considerable interest, was not an exposure-disease odds ratio.

Baker on breast cancer

Another pioneering use of analyses close to the modern case-control method was read to the Royal Medical and Chirurgical Society in 1862 by James Paget (of Paget's disease) but authored by W.M. Baker, entitled "Statistics of cancer" (Baker, 1862). The data source was notes on 500 cases of cancer described by Paget between 1843 and 1861. Most of the paper is a listing of typical case-series statistics, such as the age distribution and duration of survival of cases of cancer, but in two instances, the author provides a case-control type of comparison. The comparisons are of marital status and of prior pregnancy in women with breast cancer and in women with other cancers (Table 1).

Baker's study appears to be one of the first case-control approaches to the study of a chronic disease, and the numbers in the table in relation to reproductive risk fac-

Table 1 – Baker's case-control comparisons of marriage and fertility in breast cancer patients (Baker, 1862)

Social conditions, &c.
Incidence of marriage &c. – The condition of the female patient, whether single, married or widow, was noted in 260 cases of cancer of the breast, the proportion being –
Single   23.0%
Married   72.4%
Widow   4.6%
The percentage of each in fifty-four cases of cancer on other organs was
Single   20.4%
Married   68.5%
Widow   11.0%
Pregnancy
Of 163 married women suffering from cancer of the breast, 126 were fruitful, 37 barren. Of 25 cases of cancer in other organs, 22 were fruitful, 3 barren.

tors parallel current thinking, with an odds ratio for breast cancer of 1.2 for the single state, and 3.0 for marital nulliparity. But Baker was conservative, stating that "the number is too small to allow of a very fair comparison being made between them and the cancers of the breast in this respect."

Early 20th century case-control studies

A handful of studies published in the first half of the 20th century have been identified as early case-control studies by a variety of authors. These early studies appear to have lit few fires among epidemiologists and other students of disease etiology at the time, but they do clearly fall in the line of development. Not by accident, many of these studies concerned the etiology of cancer. During this period, many epidemiologists were aware of a shifting health profile in developed countries, and particularly of the increased frequency of cancer. There was some debate as to whether epidemiology should be extended from infectious to other etiologies. The position that it should be, was most fully articulated by the influential Major Greenwood, who argued that cancer was, like infectious diseases, a "crowd-sickness", and therefore within the purview of the epidemiologist (Greenwood, 1935).

Mayo clinic study of lip cancer

AC Broders of the Mayo Clinic described 537 cases (526 male) of squamous-cell epithelioma of the lip, and investigated tobacco use, including the method of use (chewing, smoking, snuff-taking or any combination of same), and among smokers, the distribution of pipe, cigar, and cigarette use. In 500 "men without epithelioma of the lip" similar smoking data were tabulated. This study, sometimes cited as an early case-control study, makes no mention of the source of the controls, nor of the method of interview, and the mean age of cases and controls differed by more than 20 years. Though seemingly not much more advanced than the work of Whitehead in 1854 or Baker in 1862, the study did suggest a role for pipe-smoking in lip cancer (78.5% in cases vs. 38.0% in controls) (Broders, 1920).

Pellagra investigations in South Carolina

Appearing almost simultaneously with the above paper, the work of Goldberger and his colleagues in South Carolina mill villages, comparing the diets in households with cases of pellagra and those without such cases, represented a signal advance in method (Goldberger et al., 1920a). The investigators first identified all active cases of pellagra in their seven study villages, in a house-to-house survey. Their method was distinguished by the use of strict clinical criteria to define a case, and by the attention paid to specifying the date of onset. Though not entirely aware of the significance of using incident versus prevalent cases, the team considered the potential differences between new, recurrent, and remitted cases, and in fact the study included mainly new and recurrent cases that were of very recent onset.

The investigators chose a two-week period in late spring (when pellagra incidence rose to its seasonal peak) to ascertain family diets, by recording purchases at company stores, and by interviewing study families. Using formulas for food consumption based on age and gender, they estimated the probable relative intake of foodstuffs within households. The authors tried to take account of what they termed "disturbing or confusing factors", for instance, by restricting both case and control households to those with the lowest incomes. The study showed a clear deficiency of fresh meat and milk products in pellagrous households. Goldberger and his colleagues appear to have designed the first case-control study in which a confounding factor (income) was taken into account.

The next case-control study to appear in the medical literature was a comprehensive study of the etiology of breast cancer by Janet Lane-Claypon.

The case-control study from Lane-Claypon to 1950

In 1926, the British Ministry of Health published a study entitled: *"A further report on cancer of the breast: reports on public health and medical subjects."* (Lane-Claypon, 1926). This detailed and sophisticated investigation (12 chapters totaling 84 pages, plus 51 pages of appendix tables) is often cited as the first case-control study (Cole, 1979). Its author was Janet Lane-Claypon, a physician employed by the British Medical Research Council, and an excellent laboratory investigator as well as an epidemiologist, who had previously been principally engaged in studies of child health, including nutrition (Lane-Claypon, 1916) and stillbirth (Lane-Claypon, 1926a). Lane-Claypon's investigation contended with issues that have come to be seen as central to the modern case-control study.

Lane-Claypon selected 500 hospitalised cases and 500 controls with non-cancerous illnesses from both inpatient and outpatient settings in London and Glasgow. The women were not matched on any characteristic, but proved quite similar in age and social class. Interviews were "obtained by a small number of competent and accurate observers, following uniform methods which had been discussed with Dr. Lane-Claypon."

The higher prevalence of the single state in breast cancer cases was noted, as well as the lower fertility of married cases. Recall bias was weighed in assessing histories of past "breast troubles":

> " ... in the event of any divergence between the two series showing a higher incidence among the cancer series, objections might fairly be raised on psychological grounds. It is evident that a woman who has suffered from a trouble so serious as to require the removal of the breast and the surrounding tissues will be likely to search in her memory for some antecedent causative agent, or event."
> (Lane-Claypon, 1926).

This paper deserves its landmark status in the history of the case-control study, even aside from providing the first solid evidence that low fertility raises the risk of breast cancer, a conclusion based on an interesting analysis, carried out by Major Greenwood, the project statistician. A regression equation, based on age at marriage and duration of marriage, was developed to describe fertility in the case series, and was then applied to the control series. The analysis was further refined by excluding cases who had pre-menopausal breast cancer, and whose fertility might therefore have been interrupted by their disease. The analysis showed 22% lower fertility in the case group.

Less well-known than the Lane-Claypon study, but in some ways similarly sophisticated, was the work of Lombard and Doering (1928) on cancer etiology in Massachusetts. This paper provides a rationale for the use of controls in words hard to improve upon:

> "We feel that any study of the habits of individuals with cancer is of little value without a similar study of individuals without cancer. To know that a large percentage of patients with cancer have certain habits is of little value for inference unless we know what percentage of the community at large has the same habit."

They analysed cases of cancer cared for by the Visiting Nurse Association in Massachusetts. In fulfilling their self-stated desire for a control group, they arranged to have:

> "*the same investigator who collected the record of the patient with cancer fill out a similar record for an individual without cancer, of the same sex and approximately the same age.*"

This is the first use we have been able to find in the medical literature of sex and age matching in a case-control study, and also the first to concern itself with the need to have the same interviewer (unblinded, however) for cases and controls. Interestingly, "several of the nurses used themselves as controls", a practice which modern epidemiologists would no doubt discourage.

We have not located another US medical case-control study until a study of penile carcinoma published 20 years later (Schrek and Lenowitz, 1947). This study too was distinguished by an attention to the control population, with the authors stating that an objective of their study was:

"... to illustrate the use of control groups in a statistical study. The use of controls is routine in experimental work and every experimental group is checked by one or more controls. In statistical studies on cancer, however, control groups are not as frequently used. This paper exemplifies several types of control groups and considers the necessity and advantages in the use of controls in statistical work."

Cases were all 139 cases of penile carcinoma admitted to the Hines, Il VA Hospital from 1931 to 1944. No less than six different control groups were initially proposed, all from among admissions to the hospital, but distinguished from each other in sample size, years of admission, cancer/disease diagnosis and ethnic composition. Each control group was considered as a series; no matching was performed. Ultimately, however, only three groups were used for comparison of the prevalence of circumcision. For comparison to the 100 white cases, the authors assembled a series of white men admitted for any cancer in 1944 who had been interviewed for another study (minus two Jewish men and four men with penile cancer). To obtain controls for the 39 "coloured" cases, the authors interviewed all "coloured" men who were in the hospital on a single day in July 1945, which yielded a control group of 55 men with "tumor", and another of 113 men with "other diseases". While between 12.8% and 24% of the three control groups had been circumcised by the age of three, none of the 139 cases had been circumcised at that age.

Case-control studies in social sciences prior to 1950

A number of investigations in sociology and psychology in the first half of this century were case-control in design. Ernest Greenwood (1945) summarised five such studies from sociology and three from psychology. Accurately, if somewhat wordily, he named the design "ex-post facto effect-to-cause experiments". In six of the eight examples, the cases were juvenile delinquents. Although one might have expected social and psychological factors to be emphasised, four of the studies focused on birth order as the major causal variable of interest. In discussing methodologic issues in such studies, Ernest Greenwood noted, as the central problem, that cases remote in time from the exposure must be a selected set of all cases because of death and other losses, a concern echoed in contemporary discussion of case-control studies in epidemiology (Kelsey et al., 1986).

In survey research it is apparent that there can be a close relationship between the case-control and cross-sectional designs. Indeed, if a cross-sectional survey simultaneously ascertains caseness and interviews individuals about their historical experiences, the raw materials of a case-control study are present, albeit with prevalent cases, and, depending upon the specific exposure and disease, perhaps without a clear sense of directionality from outcome to exposure (Kramer and Boivin, 1989). Before the modern refinements in case-control methodology, the difference between the two approaches would have been primarily in feasibility and efficiency; a cross-sectional design would greatly oversample controls, and it is hard to imagine that a cross-sectional design could be used to demonstrate the etiology of a disease as rare as lung cancer.

The "ex-post facto effect-to-cause experiment" has, however, not taken hold in sociology and psychology to anything near the extent it has in epidemiology. The central role of caseness in medicine and epidemiology certainly favors the case-control design. In addition, the design is not readily applied when the outcome variable of interest is continuous, as it so often is in the social sciences.

Lung cancer, smoking and the case-control study

A leap forward in the use and acceptance of the case-control study came with the studies that implicated cigarette smoking in cancer of the lung published in 1950 in the United States (Levin et al., 1950; Wynder and Graham, 1950; Schrek et al., 1950) and in Britain (Doll and Hill, 1950), the latter study more fully developed in the authors' 1952 publication. These 1950 studies established several features of the modern form of the case-control study, and therefore deserve detailed examination. The success of the four case-control studies in implicating smoking as a major risk factor for lung cancer led, in just over a decade, to major pronouncements on the health hazards of smoking from authorities on both sides of the Atlantic.

Before discussing the 1950 studies, we must note that the German literature includes at least one case-control study of smoking and lung cancer (Müller, 1939). Franz Müller, about whom little is known other than his membership in the Nazi party, was in conformity with Hitler's abhorrence of smoking when he mailed a questionnaire to family members of lung cancer victims requesting information about smoking history, including type (cigar, cigarette, pipe), daily consumption, and whether the victim had stopped or reduced smoking. A control group, of the same number, gender and approximate age as the series of 86 lung cancer cases for whom questionnaires had been returned, was similarly surveyed. While only 3.5% of cases were non-smokers, 16% of controls did not smoke, and heavy smoking was six times as common in lung cancer patients as in controls. This paper was cited by Wynder and Graham (1950), by the Surgeon General's 1964 report on Smoking on Health, and in more recent discussions of historical epidemiology (Susser, 1985; Smith et al., 1994), but it otherwise seems to have been widely ignored.

Schrek et al. – 1950

The Hines, IL VA hospital was again featured in the annals of case-control history as the source of the January 1950 publication of the first of the US case-control studies of lung cancer and smoking (Schrek et al., 1950). The population source was 5003

```
         FORM USED IN TAKING THE HISTORIES
           OF THE SMOKING HABITS OF PATIENTS

                     SMOKING HABITS

                 Light         Moderate    Heavy           Duration
     Cigarette   10 or less    10–20       More than 20
     Cigar       2 or less     2–4         More than 4
     Pipe        3 or less     3–6         More than 6
     None
```

Figure 1
Survey instrument used to ascertain smoking history (in Schrek et al., 1950).

male admissions to the Hines, IL VA hospital from 1941–1948, all of whom had been surveyed upon admission for smoking history using a standard form (see Fig. 1).

This data set permitted comparison of smoking histories in several case groups (lung cancer, other respiratory cancers, upper digestive cancers) and in different control groups (all other diseases, all other cancers). The authors noted that other cancers were a better comparison group, because cancer patients differed from other patients in that they were often referred from other VA hospitals. Cigarette smoking, defined as smoking more than 10 cigarettes/day, was found in 71.2% of 82 lung cancer patients, 69.7% of 73 patients with cancer of the pharynx or larynx, 62.9% of 116 lip cancer patients, 54.8% of all 5003 admissions, and 48.8% of 522 cancers of sites other than the respiratory and upper gastrointestinal tract. Neither duration nor age of onset of smoking differed across the several case and control groups. Race, age and geographic origin of patients were assessed as potential confounders (or, in the terminology of the authors, "secondary factors"), and smoking rates were examined within strata of age and race. Schrek et al. (1950) concluded: "When age and race were equalized in the control and clinical groups, there still remained a statistically significant correlation between smoking and cancer of the lung and of the larynx and pharynx."

Levin – 1950

Smoking histories had been obtained routinely upon admission to Roswell Park Memorial Institute, Buffalo, NY, since 1938. Levin et al. emphasised that "Special attention with respect to the history of smoking has not been paid to any single group of conditions, so that these records may be presumed to be free from bias which might result from preconceived ideas as to relation between smoking and a particular form of cancer." Levin et al. controlled for age by age-standardising the smoking prevalences to the age distribution of all 1650 men in the study. No women were studied. Levin et al. (1950) showed *both* the prevalence of smoking in cases and controls, and the proportion of lung cancer cases among smokers and non-smokers, the latter essentially a proportional morbidity analysis, since all study subjects were hospital admissions. 54.1% of lung cancer patients had smoked for > 25 years, compared to 34.9% of other cancer controls and 29.8% of non-cancer controls. The age-standardised proportion of lung cancer diagnoses among non-smokers (as defined at hospital admission) was 8.6%, and among cigarette smokers of > 25 years, 20.7%.

It is notable that both of these early case-control studies of lung cancer (Schrek et al., 1950; Levin et al., 1950) were in fact nested case-control studies, since the smoking interviews had been obtained in the entire population from which cases and controls were selected.

Wynder and Graham – 1950

Wynder and Graham's study, published in the same issue of JAMA as the Levin et al. paper, designed a survey instrument specifically for their study (see Fig. 2) and used it to interview cases of lung cancer of both genders (but predominantly men) from hospitals in St. Louis and elsewhere, and from several private practices around the country. Controls were similarly heterogeneous. Recruited in several hospitals in St. Louis and in other parts of the country, they constituted a population different in age and geographic origin from the cases.

The number of cases of lung cancer (685) was considerably larger than in either the Levin et al. study (236) or the Schrek et al. study (82). An interesting feature of this study is that one subset of cases and controls (in two St. Louis hospitals) were interviewed prior to the diagnosis being established. As in the Levin et al. study, the smoking habits of controls were age-standardised. The commoner type of bronchogenic carcinoma (squamous, epidermoid or undifferentiated) was analysed separately from adenocarcinomas, and smoking history was graded from 0–5 based on a duration-intensity measure similar to pack-years, based mostly on cigarette consumption, but augmented by information on cigar and pipe-smoking. Cases of lung cancer consistently showed fewer non-smokers and more class 4 and 5 smokers (> 20/cigarettes/day for ≥ 20 years) than did controls, whether from chest services or other hospital services, whether interviewed blind to diagnosis or not.

Although there were few adenocarcinomas (52 cases), their relationship to smoking in men was similar to that of other bronchogenic cancers. In women, although heavy smoking was common in most bronchogenic cancers, it was found in only 2 of 13 adenocarcinomas.

```
Name:..............................................................................................    Age:..........................
 1. Have you ever had a lung disease? If so, state time, duration and site of disease:
    Pneumonia         Asthma              Tuberculosis          Bronchiectasis
    Influenza         Lung Abscess        Chest Injuries        Others
 2. Do you or did you ever smoke?                     Yes [  ]      No [  ]
 3. At what age did you begin to smoke?
 4. At what age did you stop smoking?
 5. How much tobacco did you average per day during the past 20 years of your smoking?
    Cigarettes..................................... Cigars ....................................... Pipes .......................
 6. Do you inhale the smoke?                          Yes [  ]      No [  ]
 7. Do you have a chronic cough which you attribute to your smoking, especially upon first smoking in the
    morning? If so, for how long?
    Yes [  ]      No [  ]
    Duration..........................................
 8. Do you smoke before or after breakfast?           Before [  ]   After [  ]
 9. Name the brand or brands, and dates, if any given brand has been smoked exclusively for more than five years.
    Change frequently? [  ]
    First brand – from 19 .... to 19 ....
    Second brand – from 19 .... to 19 ....
10. What kind of jobs have you held? Have you been exposed to dust or fumes while working there? (Use back
    of page for detailed description of possible exposure)
        From            To              Position         Dust or Fumes

11. Have you ever been exposed to irritative dusts or fumes outside of your job? In particular have you ever used
    insecticide spray excessively? If so, state time and duration.
        Yes [  ]   No [  ]   Type.........................................   Duration ...............................
12. How much alcohol do you or have you averaged per day? State time and
    duration in years.
        Whiskey................. Beer ................. Wine...........................
13. Where were you born and where have you lived most of your life? State the approximate time span you have
    lived in a certain locality. Up to what grade did you attend school?
    Birthplace ............   Home .....................   Educational Level ...........
14. State the cause of death of your parents, and of brothers and sisters, if any.
15. Site of Lesion       Microscopic Diagnosis       Papanicolaou Class       Etiological Class
Interviewer .........................................................................................................
```

Figure 2
Survey instrument used to ascertain smoking history (in Wynder and Graham, 1950).

Doll and Hill – 1950

This classic study has come to be viewed as a model case-control investigation. Notifications of cancer cases (lung, colon, stomach, rectum) were received from 20 London hospitals, with the latter three cancers used as "contrasting groups". Each case was interviewed by a research almoner (social worker) who was also "instructed to interview a patient of the same sex, within the same five-year age group, and in the same hospital at or about the same time" who did not have cancer. As in Wynder and Graham (1950), attention was paid to the duration of smoking, to histories of starting and stopping smoking, and to the amount smoked. This study devised the convention of setting the lower threshold or lifetime smoking at one cigarette per day for a year. A six-month re-interview of a subset of subjects showed remarkable consistency in self-reported smoking histories.

Contrasts were made between cases of lung cancer and matched controls in overall smoking, in amount smoked most recently, in maximum ever smoked, in age of onset of smoking and in duration of smoking. Pipe smoking was shown to have a weaker relationship to lung cancer than cigarette smoking. Stratified analyses were used to deal with potential confounders, including urban/rural residence, cancer diagnosis of controls and potential interviewer bias. Unlike any other case-control study of the period, Doll and Hill (1950) used the distribution of smoking in lung cancer patients to develop "ratios" for lung cancer risk in London smokers, assuming a smoking distribution that paralleled that of the control population. This yielded estimates of relative risks for lung cancer from smoking 10, 20 and 60 cigarettes per day of 19, 26 and 65; odds ratios were not calculated. However, the authors concluded, considerably more firmly than in the US studies, that cigarette smoking was "a factor, and an important factor, in the production of carcinoma of the lung".

A retrospective account of the events surrounding the publications of these articles has been provided in recent papers in the American Journal of Epidemiology (Armenian and Szklo, 1996; Wynder, 1997; Terris, 1997).

Both the Royal College of Physician's 1962 report entitled *Smoking and Health*, and the US Surgeon General's Report of the same title, published in 1964, relied heavily on "retrospective studies" in their assessment of the evidence. The Royal College of Physicians Committee cited 23 retrospective studies, all of which showed a relationship of smoking to lung cancer, and the Surgeon General's Report cited 29 such studies, all but one of which (a study in women) confirmed the association. The powerful consistency of these case-control studies, and the replication of their findings in later prospective studies, impressed the committee members who authored the reports, notwithstanding the scarcity of epidemiologists among them. Jeremiah Morris in the UK and Leonard Schuman in the US were the only epidemiologists on these two important official committees examining smoking and health. Nonetheless, the smoking and health reports promoted the general acceptance of the case-control study as a scientific tool in clinical research.

Record and McKeown – 1949, 1950

The studies of smoking and lung cancer are rightly viewed as setting the stage for the modern era of the case-control study. Their influence was no doubt accentuated by the pressing and controversial question they addressed. Also, as we have seen, epidemiologic studies of cancers have been important to the development of the case-control design since the 19th century.

It would be unfair, however, to neglect the contemporaneous, though less well remembered, use of the case-control paradigm in the studies of birth defects by Record and McKeown (1949 and 1950) in Birmingham. Like the studies of lung cancer and smoking, this work was motivated by the shifting health patterns of the time, in this case, the increasing prominence of congenital malformations among infant deaths as other causes of infant mortality declined. In Record and McKeown's case-control study of risk factors for congenital malformations of the nervous system, the first of many such investigations on this topic from the Birmingham group, the design is clearly articulated.

Using vital records of Birmingham 1940–1947, this two-part study identified 930 consecutive cases of congenital nervous system malformation and selected a control group of approximately equal size. The controls were every 200th birth over the seven year period. Exposure data were obtained from vital records and from a home visit in which a maternal interview was conducted. Cases and controls were compared on numerous exposures, including maternal health during pregnancy, season of birth, birth order, and family history of congenital malformations. Though the findings were less immediately salient than those of the smoking and lung cancer studies, the Record and McKeown study stimulated further work on neural tube defects in Birmingham. As Ian Leck has emphasised, the work of another Birmingham investigator – W. H. Smithells – which strongly implicated folic acid deficiency in this disorder (Smithells et al., 1983) "can be traced back to these case-control studies" (Leck, 1996).

Arguably, the articulation and execution of this case-control design was better developed – though certainly less influential – than in some of the smoking and lung cancer studies. Indeed, it would be hard to improve upon the design even now. The selection of all cases within a region, and the use of a random sample of all births in the study base as controls, were remarkable for their time. It should be noted too that the cross-sectional and case-control design tend to intersect in this research on congenital malformations, where cases are of necessity ascertained at birth (and are therefore prevalent) rather than at conception.

The co-occurrence of this work with the case-control studies of smoking and lung cancer serves to demonstrate that the case-control design was not an accidental discovery in one field of research; it evolved from the context of the time. The timing of the breakthrough reflected several underlying and interrelated developments: the shifting health profile of the developed countries in the first half of the twentieth century; the corresponding evolution within epidemiology to consider not only infectious diseases, but also cancer and other chronic conditions as falling within its purview; the development of applied statistics; and the social conditions of the years immediately following World War II.

Conclusions

A constellation of developments in medicine had to be in place before the case-control study could be conceptualised and actualised. These include the definition of unique disease entities (cases), the assembling of case series, an interest in etiology at the individual level, and the practice of interviewing patients about past events. Most crucial has been the practice, refined over many years, of comparing cases of disease to cases of non-disease so that factors that might account for the difference might be ascertained. These desiderata were very rarely met in the 19th century, and only occasionally before 1950. As it emerged in the beginning of the 20th century, in the work of Goldberger and his colleagues, the case-control study was but one part of a broader plan of attack to reduce the burden of disease, which also included experimental studies at the individual level, and investigating causes and interventions at a broader societal level. Over the course of the twentieth century the precision and logic of the design was greatly enhanced, but its use was less clearly integrated with other public health actions.

While the first modern case-control study was performed in the 1920s, it was only at mid-century that the press of interest in the relationship of smoking to health provided a problem that could be addressed through the case-control method. A specific chronic disease (lung cancer) was hypothesised to be caused by an individual exposure of long duration (smoking) that was ascertainable through personal interview. The strong and consistent results that emerged from these early studies created confidence in the approach that was amplified when the findings were later confirmed by cohort studies. In the years since 1950, case-control studies have been greatly refined, but much of their popularity can be attributed to their initial success in linking smoking and cancer.

With the elaboration and wide application of this design over the subsequent half century, significant findings have been many. Diethylstilbestrol and vaginal adenocarcinoma (Herbst et al., 1971), aspirin and Reyes syndrome (Hurwitz et al., 1987), L-tryptophan and eosinophilia-myalgia (Martin et al., 1991), and tampon use and toxic-shock syndrome (Kehrberg et al., 1981) are examples of exposure-disease relationships widely accepted as causal that were uncovered in recent decades by case-control studies. Most importantly, because of the rarity of the diseases under investigation in these studies, and the lack of strong exposure hypotheses at the time these studies were initiated, there is no realistic possibility that these associations could have been uncovered by any other epidemiologic strategy.

Newer case-control studies have benefited from the advances in design, execution and analysis since 1950. These advances include more rigorous selection and matching of case and control populations, improved interviewing techniques, location of the design within a general framework of epidemiologic strategies for relating exposure to disease, understanding of the measures of effect, and application of increasingly sophisticated statistical procedures to findings.

We have noted that the case-control work of Goldberger et al. (1920a) on pellagra was characterised by the integration of this study form into public health action. More recently, the case-control design has been fitted squarely into the focus on individual level risk factors for noninfectious disease which became the dominant form of epidemiology from 1950 until the end of the century. This focus has been accompanied by a trend towards separating this form of research from a broader multilevel public health agenda. Hopefully, future epidemiologists will enlarge the scope and purview of this elegant and useful design and use it to focus on the improvement of health in the population.

The history of confounding

Jan P. Vandenbroucke

Clinical Epidemiology, Leiden University Medical Center, PO Box 9600, NL-2300 RC Leiden, The Netherlands

Summary

Confounding is a basic problem of comparability – and therefore has always been present in science. Originally a plain English word, it acquired more specific meanings in epidemiologic thinking about experimental and non-experimental research. The use of the word can be traced to Fisher. The concept was developed more fully in social science research, among others by Kish. Landmark developments in epidemiology in the second half of the 20th century were by Cornfield and by Miettinen. These developments emphasised that reasoning about confounding is almost entirely an a priori process that we have to impose upon the data and the data-analysis to arrive at a meaningful interpretation. The problems of confounding present their old challenges again in recent applications to genetic epidemiology.

The word "confounding" has over the past 20 years acquired almost mythical and even mystical proportions in the epidemiologic vocabulary. Originally, it was a plain English word – most probably of Norman origin, since one tends to hear some Latin in it. The Shorter Oxford English Dictionary on Historical Principles (3rd Edition, reprinted 1967) mentions that it is a medieval Latin word: "con-fundere", to pour together (mix together), that was taken over in medieval French, as "confondre". The same dictionary also mentions "to mix up in ideas, to fail to distinguish, to confuse", as meanings that are already distinct in the 16th century. From there other connotations come. Some of the oldest might go back to religion, when the help of the Lord was invoked, not only against pestilences, but also against human enemies. The Lord was asked: "Confound thy enemies", meaning: confuse them, bring them into disarray, a disarray so great that they will easily be dispersed, so that we, your loyal servants, will easily win the battle, and put the enemy to confounded shame. In this way, "confounded" also has other connotations, like doomed, hopeless, shameful etc. Since the 1700s it is regarded as a mild curse. Which should be telling to epidemiologists.

Where to start?

The history of confounding is a mirror image of the history of research design. Confounding is not a statistical or analytic concept. It is a concept that has to do with the logic of scientific reasoning. In particular the logic of inferring causality from observations. Therefore, the student of the history of confounding faces a dilemma that is common to historians: should one study the history of confounding only from the time that the word was coined in epidemiology with its specific methodological meaning? Or should one take the broader view and study the history of the underlying concept from time immemorial, i.e., all instances in which the concept might have been foreshadowed? The latter would include extremely varied sources, beginning with the Old Testament quotation that is often interpreted as "the first clinical trial", in which Daniel opposed the king of Babylon by adding a control group to verify the effects of the dietary precepts of the king upon the youths of Israel. The story is quoted in a paper on the history of the clinical trial, entitled "Ceteris paribus" ("other things being equal") (Lilienfeld, 1982). Should we say that this emphasis on a comparison "ceteris paribus" showed that Daniel understood what "confounding" meant, and should we therefore see the bible as the first historical source on the subject?

However tempting the broader view, I have limited my inquiry to the more restricted option, for two reasons. Firstly, because the task would otherwise become unwieldy: all texts in which problems of comparisons were ever mentioned – not only the bible, but also ancient philosophers, medieval thinkers up to modern times, should be scrutinised. Secondly, because professional historians convinced me that the history of a concept does not *really* exist before it is more or less securely coined by a name in a particular context. Even worse, they say: going back to the times that neither the word nor its context existed, is nothing but a re-interpretation by hindsight, and is unscientific for an historian, since the re-interpretation only exists grace to the modern concept. The above example makes it clear: to say that biblical Daniel understood "confounding", whereby we imply that he understood the same concept as we do, really seems stretching our imagination too far. There is one exception, however: professional historians like to go back to the time *immediately before* the concept was coined, since that may give insight into its gestation and give clues to its overt as well as covert meanings.

For all this reasons, I will limit my search to the history of confounding in the past decades. Furthermore, my treatment of the subject will be quite personal, and therefore subjective. This aspect of my commentary might not be to the liking of professional historians, because I will trace the development of the concept as if it were a story of continual refinement and improvement until the present. Today's historians frown upon such stories wherein the world continually improves until the present, because this is typical of medical amateur historians who only want to describe the triumphs of present-day insights over a darker past. Yet, I must avow that it is difficult for me to do otherwise, because it is impossible for me to take sufficient distance from today's debates on confounding and their historical roots. I witnessed the aftermath of the development of the concept myself, during my training in epidemiology at the Harvard School of Public Health, and I feel involved with some of the actors in the debates. Finally, there still is something to be said for a mere history of the development of an idea – be it only as a first stepping stone for a more in-depth treatment of the subject, wherein the causes of the evolution of the concept are also traced. As a consequence, my treatment of the history of confounding should be seen as a first rough sketch, to be improved upon by others. The interested reader will find a selection of reprints of several papers on causality and confounding in one volume (Greenland, 1987a); some of these, besides others, will be mentioned as specific references in my text. An authoritative treatment on the principles of confounding in epidemiology can be found in the textbook by Rothman and Greenland (1998, Chapter 8).

In this historical excursion, I will treat firstly the basic problem of comparability, as originally described by Claude Bernard and John Stuart Mill, and the way in which these thoughts are still very much alive in modern epidemiology. Thereafter, I will concentrate on the evolution of the concept, starting with "desirable confounding" as described by R.A. Fisher, following with "undesirable confounding" as described by L. Kish and taken over in epidemiology. Next I will deal with the interpretation of confounding variables, about which very beautiful pages have been written by J. Cornfield, most notably in discussions on smoking and lung cancer, and in some acerbic debates concerning the interpretation of randomised trials. Today's theory on confounding will by highlighted from the writings on case-control studies by O.S. Miettinen and others. I will end by delineating how confounding is still very much with us, even in the most recent endeavours, the epidemiologic study of the role of genetic factors in the causation of disease.

Comparisons and comparability

The crux of research design, the crux of any observation, is a comparison. It can be a real comparison with data on two or more groups of subjects, or a mental comparison (against what we expect). That the essence of scientific observation always involves a comparison was already beautifully described by Claude Bernard, in the middle of the 19th century, in his "Introduction à l étude de la médecine expérimentale", published in 1865 (Bernard, 1966). Although Bernard is mainly known for bringing physiologic experimentation to medicine, he also very clearly described his ideas about research methods in general. He explained that experimental research and observational research have one thing in common: that one thing is the comparison. In an experiment the researcher fiddles with reality to construct the comparison himself: for example, what happens to dogs with and without internal secretion of the pancreas. In observational research the researcher has to search for the comparison, he has to look and find where nature has made the data for him. Claude Bernard even gave an epidemiologic example: he wrote that, if a medical doctor observes that in a part of town, where hygienic conditions are appalling, some diseases are more prevalent, he might think that it is due to these conditions (Bernard, 1966, p. 35). That initial observation is already a comparison, since the doctor compares poorer and richer parts of towns. Bernard called this observation "passive". Such initial observations are the source of later hypotheses and further "active" observation. In clinical medicine, they are often communicated as case reports and case series (Vandenbroucke, 2001).

Karl Popper, who was not yet born when Bernard confined these thoughts to paper, much later remarked that anything that strikes us, always strikes us because it belies our expectations – again a comparison with the "expected". Claude Bernard made a great point in saying that any investigation always starts with some "preconceived idea" ("... une idée préconçue a toujours été et sera toujours le premier élan d'un esprit investigateur") (Bernard, 1966, p. 59). The initial comparison that led to a new idea may have been made *passively*. Thereafter this new preconceived idea, e.g., the possibility of a greater disease incidence in the poorer parts of town, can be turned into an *active* observation. Claude Bernard wrote that to prove the point, the doctor starts to travel (he will probably mount his horse or carriage – we are still in the middle of the previous century), and that he will travel to another town, to see whether in similar conditions there are similar diseases. The doctor now makes an active observation, he actively seeks another comparison, still without being able to fiddle with reality – it is still non-experimental – but nevertheless he actively checks whether his initial impression is right (Bernard, 1966, p. 35).

How comparisons should be made, be them experimental or observational, was described by J.S. Mill, in his 1856 canons on causality, as quoted in the relatively recent epidemiologic literature (MacMahon and Pugh, 1970; Susser, 1973, p. 70):

"Second Canon: If an instance in which the phenomenon under investigation occurs, and an instance in which it does not occur, have every circumstance in common save one, that one occurring only in the former; the circumstance in which alone the two instances differ, is the effect or cause, or a necessary part of the cause, of the phenomenon." (Mill, 1856).

This "method of difference" appeals most to us in medicine and epidemiology. We would wrong the genius of writers like Mill, however, to assume that this was the only way which he conceived to arrive at causal judgements. He described several others, like the "method of agreement", which says that if several circumstances in which a phenomenon occurs are completely different, except in one aspect, then the latter aspect is a likely cause. That is a type of reasoning that we also use in epidemiology: for example, we note that several different types of study in different circumstances all find the same association, which therefore strengthens our ideas about a causal interpretation. Then there is the "method of variation", which sounds very much like a dose-response argument. One might well say that these canons foreshadow Austin Bradford Hill's ideas about causality (Hill, 1965).

However, let me keep with the second canon: the idea of "ceteris paribus" that is present in that canon, applies equally well to observation as to experiment – and it applies even to thought experiments. Whenever the condition of "all other things being equal" is *not* met, the comparison might be wrong. Wrong information confuses, wrong information brings one into disarray, wrong information is confounded information.

Very crudely put: any departure from J.S. Mill's second canon, any departure of the "ceteris paribus" principle can lead to confounding. This is the essence of confounding. Nowadays, epidemiology has developed distinctions between several reasons why comparisons go wrong (the generally accepted terminology says that the comparison or the study is "biased") – of which confounding is only one.

Desirable confounding

The very first, at least to my knowledge, to apply the word confounding in thinking and writing about research designs was R.A. Fisher. He treated confounding at great length in his 1937 book on *"The design of experiments"* (Fisher, 1937). However, in his treatise, confounding was *not* something that he always sought to avoid. On the contrary, he proposed to exploit confounding, by deliberately introducing confounding in agricultural experiments. He proposed to ignore higher order interactions between treatments by deliberately confounding the higher order interactions with some of the main effects in the design of the experiment. Of course, he presupposed that the investigator was certain that she was not interested in these higher order interactions, and also that she knew in advance that they would not add important effects over and beyond the main effects. Fisher seemed to have been very fond of this invention, which is quite complicated to read and understand. No less than 40 pages of the 260 pages of his book are devoted to "confounded designs". The book is not chiefly remembered for it. However, let me retain the notion that R.A. Fisher used the word confounding as a nuisance which he tried to turn into a benefit.

Undesirable confounding

The next important use of the word confounding, which we come across is by Leslie Kish, who devoted himself to methodological theory in sociologic research. His 1959 paper about *"Some statistical problems in research design"* is still worth reading, and a great source of contemporary references (Kish, 1959) – it is indeed the time period in which the current use of the term confounding was born. In thinking about research designs, he discerned the following four variables:

I. *Explanatory* variables, or "experimental" variables: the object or research, both "dependent and independent".
II. Extraneous variables which are *controlled* (in selection and estimation).
III. Extraneous uncontrolled variables, which are *confounded* with the Class I variables.
IV. Extraneous uncontrolled variables which are either actually *randomised*, or treated as if randomised. (Randomisation is a substitution of experimental control).

Kish's use of the word confounding derived from Fisher's: a confusion of two effects. The big difference, however, is his categorisation of the different variables that might influence the outcome of a study. Although not very explicit, he seems to make already a distinction between confounding and other types of bias: his second type of controlled variables have to do with measurement and selection. Nowadays, the word confounding is indeed used for one particular form of the confusion of two effects: the confusion due to extraneous causes, i.e., other factors that really do influence disease incidence, e.g., age, sex, habits, or living circumstances. The word confounding is not used to describe the problems that arrive by differences in measurement or selection. The latter we call nowadays "information bias" and "selection bias". They are artefacts of the design of the study. The separation of confounding from selection bias and information bias is in practice not always very clear-cut – the reasoning sometimes becomes difficult.

I am not certain how Kish's use of the word confounding entered epidemiology. Kish's views obviously were very influential, and it is possible that he influenced epidemiology via the writings of other social science methodologists like H.M. Blalock (1964) or via Campbell's writings on quasi-experimentation (Campbell and Stanley, 1963).

The interpretation of a confounding variable

Two leaps in the history of confounding are linked to the name of Jerome Cornfield. One is the epochal paper of 1959 in which he discusses, together with Haenszel, Hammond, Lilienfeld, Shimkin and Wynder, whether the 10-fold increase in lung cancer observed among cigarette smokers might be due to confounding with some other effect (Cornfield et al., 1959). The paper was written against one of the major initial objections to the idea that smoking would cause lung cancer. That objection was championed, amongst others by R.A. Fisher: his proposition was that there was some "underlying constitution" which caused both lung cancer and a propensity to smoke. Thus, the association between smoking and lung cancer would not be causal, but simply due to this underlying constitution which caused both. Cornfield and his colleagues who jumped to defend the causality of the association, did not use the word confounding in their paper; they spoke about a "non-causal agent" and a "causal agent". Today, we would call the underlying truly causal agent the confounder and the non-causal agent, with the apparent association that is non-causal, the confounded variable. Cornfield and colleagues demonstrated that a confounding variable, if any, would in itself need to have an even greater effect on the occurrence of lung cancer than a 10-fold increase to explain the association of smoking with lung cancer. They challenged the non-believers to come forward with such an agent. In general, epidemiologic reasoning admits that there might be differences between smokers and non-smokers, e.g., smokers drink more coffee. The crux of the question is, however, that to deny that smoking is a potential cause of lung cancer, one has to come forward with proof that something associated with smoking, e.g., coffee drinking, is a true cause of lung cancer. Moreover, it should even be a much stronger cause than the apparent association between smoking and lung cancer – otherwise it will never suffice to explain the association. What this historical example demonstrates, is that one has to *reason* about potential confounders, and that one should not take them as mythical or uncontrollable phantoms that destroy studies. People who propose that a certain study is confounded have to make clear why and how, and have to do so in logical and credible terms. Only if they do so, a meaningful discussion becomes possible (Vandenbroucke and de Craen, 2001).

Quite recently, Cornfield's reasoning was perverted into its inverse. In the famous Science article on *"Epidemiology faces its limits"*, (Taubes, 1995), it is quoted, completely out of context that a relative risk should at least be elevated two or threefold, or even that the lower boundary of the confidence interval should be two or three, before being credible. The beautiful reasoning by Cornfield and his associates is turned into its opposite. Sometimes there is a vested interest in not wanting to believe the results of epidemiologic studies, for example when epidemiologic studies show side effects of medicines. Some persons like to teach that the possibility of confounding is so great when relative risks are low that they do not even need to name and articulate the confounder. They think they have a right to dismiss such a study without argument (Sackett et al., 1997). Wynder (1996) recently commented about "weak associations" showing the fallacy of this reasoning. After all, a twofold increase in the risk of disease is still 100% more disease. Confounding is still with us.

Cornfield's next contribution was even more subtle. It was his discussion about the results of the University Group Diabetes study (UGDP) in 1971 (Cornfield, 1971). This discussion is very important. It showed that confounding can still exist after randomisation. After all, randomisation is only a game of chance, and it might only guarantee equality of "all other known and unknown" factors that influence the outcome of the study in the very long run or with very large sample sizes. Historically, randomisation was used principally as a means to *conceal* the allocation (Chalmers,

1999). In theory, any type of allocation would be fine, except that fixed schemes like alternation, day of birth, etc. have the drawback that the physician knows in advance what treatment the next patient will receive. To circumvent that problem, randomisation was the solution. Thus, randomisation is only a guarantee against physician bias in the allocation. From a purely theoretical point of view, it has even been argued – and again Fisher was invoked – that randomisation can *never* guarantee complete equality between groups: one can always invent "a million ways to compare two groups" and there will always be something that is different (Urbach, 1993). In modern times, this idea has new relevance when we think about genetic differences. Since humans have billions of base pairs, it is mathematically certain that randomisation will not guarantee equality. Even if you were to randomise tens of thousands of patients in an enormous randomised controlled trial, there will be tens of thousands of base pairs that will differ between the two groups. Some of these might be genetic polymorphisms that are important for prognosis. We will never know, but fortunately such unknown chance variation is taken care of by the confidence interval (Altman and Bland, 1999).

Anyway, in actual practice it is quite possible, that by the luck of the draw one of the comparison groups in a randomised trial has different baseline characteristics, and has therefore a more favourable prognosis than the other. This was the case in the UGDP study (Cornfield, 1971). In that study it was found that people who had been treated with certain oral glucose lowering tablets fared worse: they sustained more myocardial death than people treated with insulin or even with diet alone. Critics of the study, however, were quick to point out that the group that was randomised to tablets had a slightly less favourable prognosis: more people in that group had a history of angina pectoris or digitalis use, they were slightly older, with a little more males, somewhat more radiologic arterial calcification, and they were slightly more obese.

Cornfield took up the challenge (1971). In his treatment of the subject, again he did not use the word confounding; he spoke about "random and non-significant base-line inequalities". He took it up in the same spirit as in the earlier contribution, that is, that one has to reason about the strength of an alternative explanation. And he did so in a multivariate way. He constructed a multivariate prognostic model, and fitted the model on all groups with an indicator variable for the different treatments. Next he did two things. He showed how the base-line prognosis in each treatment group could be estimated, and how it differed a little, but not nearly as much as the real differences in outcome. His method of estimating overall base-line prognosis was ingenious: he had fitted an outcome model on the data with an indicator variable for the treatment groups, but thereafter he estimated the baseline prognosis of both groups after omitting the treatment indicator variable. Second, he stratified all groups according to their multivariate risks, and again showed that this stratification had little effect on the difference in outcome between the treatment categories. This foreshadowed Miettinen's multivariate confounder score (Miettinen, 1976b).

The giant leap which Cornfield made was to make confounding a matter of judgement, even *after* randomisation. Even after randomisation the credibility of the comparison between the two treatment arms should be checked, and if necessary remedied. We do not care about the possibility that there are potentially innumerable differences between two groups after randomisation; we only care about the differences that matter in a causal explanation. Thus, we have to make a double judgement, based on prior knowledge: what are true prognostic variables, and do they differ between the groups. This philosophy, however, also leads to the idea that the randomised trial is not necessarily an instrument that delivers "true comparisons" automatically, by virtue of the randomisation itself. It makes the randomised trial only one of the study designs in epidemiology, about which one has to reason in exactly the same way as about the other study designs that are observational. As Cornfield later wrote himself, he placed "… emphasis on reasonable scientific judgement and accumulation of evidence and not on dogmatic insistence on the unique validity of a particular procedure" (Cornfield, 1976).

It remains ironic that Cornfield made such great contributions to our thinking about confounding, but did not use the word. I wonder whether he avoided it on purpose. In this regard he is much like two other pioneers of epidemiology, Mantel and Haenszel, who wrote in 1959 a paper about the analysis of data from case-control studies, in which they proposed the currently very famous "Mantel-Haenszel test" as well as the "Mantel-Haenszel estimator" for the common odds ratio (Mantel and Haenszel, 1959). In the treatment of the latter subject they speak of "factor control" and not about confounding. It seems that also in the earlier teaching of epidemiology at Johns Hopkins the word confounding was not used, but that it was denoted by the word "secondary association", i.e., secondary to something else that was a known cause of disease (personal communication, Milton Terris, Annecy France 1996).

Confounding in case-control studies

The idea that confounding is a matter of credibility of comparisons, hence to a certain extent subjective, was going to play an important role in the last developments of our insights into confounding. These have to do with case-control studies.

The problem faced by case-control studies, as they emerged as important tools in research, can be delineated by comparing them with follow-up studies, and in particular with the "idealised" follow-up situation, which is the randomised controlled trial like the ones we just discussed. In such a trial, and in any follow-up study, one can actually look at the data to see whether the exposed and the unexposed are different in their prognosis, at least as far as we know prognostic factors. We can tabulate the differences, which is always done in the famous "Table 1" of any randomised trial, the table with the baseline characteristics of the different treatment groups. As shown by Cornfield, one can then make a judgement: how much the groups differ and how importantly that difference will influence the outcome.

However, in case-control studies, that is not possible. Worse, when one looks at the baseline characteristics of the cases, they always have a poorer prognosis in all respects. If they are cases of myocardial infarction, for example, they will have more hypertension, more hypercholesterolaemia, more familial heart disease, more male pattern baldness, and whatever you wish to look for. It is never possible again to see whether at baseline the exposed and the unexposed, (say, smokers and non-smokers), differed. Even looking at exposed and unexposed in the control group is only a poor substitute, because the control group is only a sample (at best) of the combined population of exposed and unexposed people. Associations in the control group might be a matter of "chance" sampling variation. So, how should one go about the decision which factor is a confounder that needs adjustment – whatever the practical means: restriction, selection, matching, or multivariate analysis. The solution proposed by some is akin to the solution proposed by Cornfield on randomised trials: only adjust for *potential* confounders, i.e., other causes of the outcome that are potentially confused with the exposure of interest. This, however, is even more judgmental than with follow-up studies, because you cannot verify the baseline characteristics (the total population of exposed and non-exposed is not known). This situation may account for part of the long history of controversy that has accompanied case-control studies. Much of the theory that in the end the judgement about confounders is an *a priori* judgement has been developed in the department of epidemiology at the Harvard School of Public Health, among others by Miettinen in the 1970s (Miettinen and Cook, 1981). Pivotal in the development of these thoughts were deeper insights in the role of "matching" in case-control studies (Miettinen, 1970), and the idea of the "confounder summarising score" (Miettinen, 1976b).

Matching was a time-honoured way of tackling confounding in case-control studies, already mentioned by Mantel and Haenszel (1959). It was originally seen as the equivalent of "blocking" in a randomised design. Blocking in a randomised design means that one first assigns the subjects to various "blocks" depending on characteristics in which they are equal. Only thereafter randomised allocation to the treatment arms is performed, separately for each block. This assures that for the characteristics of the blocks, the two treatment arms will be perfectly equal. It led to the old experimental maxim: "Block where you can and randomise where you cannot" – meaning that known prognostic factors should be used for blocking, to assure their equal distribution over the treatment groups, whereas the unknown factors should be taken care of by randomisation. Superficially, making controls alike to cases in case-control studies seemed similar: e.g., if the first case of myocardial infarction is an elderly gentleman, the first control should be a man of the same age. By doing this, however, something else also takes place: by making controls alike to cases, they will also become much more alike in the exposure that one wants to study, e.g., elderly gentlemen all tend to smoke. As a matter of fact, matching on confounding factors, which is intended to make the comparison series alike to the cases in case-control studies, introduces its own "bias" – a bias towards no association, be it in a controlled way (Miettinen, 1970). The solution is to perform a stratified analysis. Indeed, a "matched analysis" wherein each case-control pair is seen as a single stratum is the same as a Mantel-Haenszel analysis with stratification for the confounding variable (Mantel and Haenszel, 1959). A nice recent explanation can be found in Rothman's textbook (Rothman, 1986). This pivotal insight, that "matching" in a case-control study performs something totally different from blocking in a follow-up study opened the way to a deeper understanding of confounding in case-control studies.

The "confounder summarising score" was developed by Miettinen as an extension of Cornfield's analysis of the UGDP study (Miettinen, 1976a). It calculated for each individual in a study his or her "baseline probability" to get diseased, or to have been exposed (depending on whether an outcome or an exposure model was used). Thereafter, the individuals were grouped in strata with similar probability, and the analysis proceeded by simple stratification. Although the use of the confounder summarising score was abandoned later, because of the wide-spread use of the logistic model in "canned software packages", it made confounding very insightful, and was therefore again an important intermediary step in our understanding.

The reason for much of the ongoing discussions about case-control studies is that case-control studies are often about side effects, be it of drugs or of exposures of daily life (like putting babies to sleep in the prone position, or eating cookies, or being exposed to cigarette smoke). There are always parties with a strong interest to challenge such findings and dream up all possible biases and confounders. An attempt at bringing people with different views on case-control studies together was the so-called "Bermuda Peace Conference" organised in 1978, whose proceedings were published in the Journal of Chronic Diseases (Ibrahim, 1979). It still makes useful reading, especially in the light of ongoing debates about confounding and selection in case-control research.

Causal pathways

Arguments what constitutes a "proper" confounder have even become more difficult because of the added complexity of "causal pathways". Causal pathways were described by Wold (1956) and Blalock (1964), and brought into epidemiology by Susser (1973, pp. 111–135).

When we want to study the relation between some exposure and some disease, a true confounder has an association with the exposure that we want to study, and is at the same time a determinant of the disease. (Thereby it confounds the relation between the exposure and the disease.) However, any "intermediary causal variable", in between exposure and disease also answers that definition. Nevertheless, it is wrong to control for this intermediary or "intervening" variable. If one does, it will take away some legitimate association of the exposure with the disease, because the intermediary variable is always linked somewhat closer to the disease than an exposure that is more remote in the causal chain. What variable is the original exposure (and ultimate cause), and what variable is only intermediary, are matters of judgement. Which is which is a decision by the investigator. No statistical model can discriminate between true confounding, spurious associations or variables that are intermediary in causal pathways. Again, the a priori reasoning predominates.

Confounding and genetic markers

Let me end with today's fashion in clinical epidemiology, which is the advent of genetics in epidemiology and the resulting problems posed by confounding.

Two decades ago, the study of genetic traits looked simple: there was no confounding involved. There is a classic example, dating from the early 1970s, that is often used for teaching. The teacher asks the students: "If you study the influence of ABO blood group on the occurrence of venous thrombosis in middle aged women, can you use new-born male babies as controls" (Hardy and White, 1971). Students more or less immediately answer: "Of course not". Then the teacher explains that the true answer is: "Yes, you can, because ABO blood group is not linked to age, nor sex". The distribution of blood groups in new-born boys is the null distribution (or the expected distribution) among middle aged women; new-born boys will serve very well for a blood group comparison.

Life has become more difficult. Take the example of a case-control study demonstrating that homozygotes for the angiotensin T235 variant are at increased risk for cardiovascular disease (Katsuya et al., 1995). The argument hinges on two odds ratios: firstly the simple age and sex adjusted odds ratio for homozygosity for T235 was 1.6, but the odds ratio increased to 2.6 after adjustment for multiple risk factors (besides age and sex, multivariate adjustment was carried out for smoking, diabetes, cholesterol, systolic and diastolic blood pressure, body mass index, current alcohol consumption, treatment for hypercholesterolaemia or hypertension, and the other genotypes studied in the same study). The increased odds ratio upon multivariate adjustment is emphasised since it seems to strengthen the conclusion of an independent causal role for T235 homozygosity.

How can we understand this result? Like in the classic blood group example, it seems evident that T235 is not linked to sex, nor age-linked, nor linked to any of the other things for which the authors adjusted. For example, it is highly unlikely that in the population at large this genetic marker is linked to smoking, or to cholesterol or to blood pressure. Thus, age and sex matching in the study design, or any other adjustment during the analysis is in principle not necessary. If adjustment has any effect on the odds ratio, that must be a result of some association with age and sex *within the data* which is not present in the population at large. Such an association can be completely spurious, but if it is in the data, that might either be like a randomisation that ends with baseline imbalances (smokers or hypertensives or alcoholics are over-represented among the people with the mutation), or be due to a sampling accident of the controls of the study. Then we are back to Cornfield: should we adjust, given that we cannot check the base-line imbalance? There are no easy solutions.

In principle, at least in a genetically reasonably homogeneous population, we expect no associations between genetic polymorphisms and environmental variables. The next point of discussion is: what constitutes a genetically reasonably homogeneous population? Population geneticists and epidemiologists seem often slightly at odds about this issue. Population geneticists maintain that even within populations that look genetically homogeneous when considered superficially, there might be genetic substrata. If these genetic substrata are also associated with personal or environmental characteristics, this might lead to confounding when studying gene-disease associations. However, epidemiologists have argued that this will only happen in extreme situations. By actual examples and simulations it has been shown that even in situations where high genetic diversity was expected, like among Caucasians of European origin in the US, the assumption that there is no confounding by admixture of genetic subgroups is quite tenable (Wacholder et al., 2000). The study of risk factors at the DNA-level brings back all old discussions and controversies about the nature of confounding in epidemiology. Confounding is still very much with us.

History of bias

Paolo Vineis

Unit of Clinical Epidemiology, Ospedale s. Giovanni Battista, University of Torino and JSJ Foundation, Via Santena 7, 10216 Torino, Italy

Summary

Epidemiologists have always been conscious of the importance of controlling for distortions, although the definition itself of bias has changed over time. Central to this discussions in the past was the relative vulnerability of different study designs to bias and uncontrollable confounding (confounding being clearly distinguishable from bias, as a problem of inter-mixed causal effects due to the non-random distribution of risk factors within the study population). In particular, controversy arose over aspects of case-control study design. Also a formulation of "typologies of bias" during the 1970s helped to define some of the most important sources of distortion in the design, analysis and interpretation of epidemiological studies. The subsequent period – until now – has been characterised by more formal and systematic definitions.

The idea of bias has been associated historically with three main meanings: a) prejudice of the observer (including the influence of a theory upon observation); b) bias as systematic error of an instrument; c) bias as a consequence of an erroneous study design.

Erroneous explanations, based on "fashionable" theories, have been rather common in medicine; e.g., a parasytic or infectious agent was sought for beri-beri and other diseases which turned out to be due to completely different aetiologies. For example, there were jails in Java where prisoners ate refined rice, and others where prisoners ate raw rice: the prevalence of beri-beri was 1/39 in the first group and 1/10000 in the second. This epidemiologic design showed that the cause of beri-beri had to be sought in dietary habits. However, Eijkman's theory on the dietary origin of beri-beri was accepted only after a long time; many researchers in the second half of the 19th century looked for infectious causes of beri-beri and, in fact, of all diseases. A second example – among many others – of the influence of general theories over disease understanding is represented by New Guinea's kuru, which still in 1958 was considered to be psychogenic.

Theoretical models are very influential in clinical medicine. In the 17th century vomiting and diarrhoea were considered as signs of effectiveness of *digitalis* treatment, while now they are considered signs of intoxication (excessive dose). This different interpretation is due to different underlying paradigms of heart failure: in the 17th century *digitalis* was thought to work because it caused a release of liquids, with a typical inversion of cause and effect.

A short history of the concept of "meter"

The classical distinction between *bias* (as a distortion, or lack of correspondence between observation and putative truth) and *imprecision* (random fluctuation) has been introduced in physics and technology first.

A considerable discussion about measurement took place during the French revolution, in particular about the definition of the "meter". Originally the meter was conceived as an absolute and "objective" measure (40×10^{-6} of the earth's meridian). However, it was soon clear that it was too difficult to measure. The platinum standard that was kept at the National Archives, in fact, was found to be biased (i.e., it did not correspond to the quantity originally meant). In addition, measurements of different "meters" in comparison with this standard were imprecise (subject to small variations, irreproducible). Nevertheless, the standard was kept as an "arbitrary" exemplar. Precision was improved by using platinun-iridium and a different shape. Only in 1952 a natural standard unit was introduced, as 1650763.73 times the wavelength of the radiation released by crypton 86. This decision improved precision and allowed an "objective" (natural) standard.

In general *absolute* measures tend to be imprecise but more valid (unbiased). They are more difficult to obtain. *Relative* measures, on the opposite, are frequently precise but may be biased if they are referred to a "natural" standard. The platinum standard was biased but it served as an arbitrary model (the unit of length).

The history of bias in epidemiology

The awareness of bias in medical observation has a long history. For example, William Augustus Guy, a student of Louis and professor of forensic medicine and hygiene, studied the relationship between occupation and health. He found that the ratio between "pulmonary consumption" and other diseases was 1:3.47 in compositors and 1:5.12 in pressmen. The hypothesis that was put forward at the time to explain these observations was that the lack of physical exercise (in compositors) lead to a greater risk of pulmonary consumption. Guy hypothesised that, in fact, the association could be explained by self-selection of workers: the weakest and sick ones were supposed to choose more sedentary works. He interviewed 503 workers and found that only 11 had been influenced by strength or health in their choice of the job. So, selection bias was ruled out (Guy, 1843).

Important discussions on bias took place when the concept of study design in epidemiology was refined. In the 1950s, the introduction of the randomised clinical trial into practice and its role as a "gold standard" for medical research lead to the idea that bias could be avoided by randomisation. However, Cornfield already in 1954 stated that the RCT was "one of various inferential instruments" (1954).

In the 1970s, intense discussion started on the merits and limitations of different study designs, in particular the case-control study (which has been considered as a powerful but dangerous tool for a long time). In particular, controversy arose over being the case-control study simply a cohort study seen from the bottom end (the "trohoc" design); over the choice of controls (population vs hospital-based studies); over the criteria for inclusion/exclusion of cases and controls; over criteria for matching, and so on.

In addition to general discussions on the sources of bias, also a *taxonomy* of bias was proposed by Murphy (1976) and Sackett (1979) among others. Murphy (1976) suggested the following examples of bias:

1. Uncontrolled studies
2. Fundamental differences in method of measurement
3. Controlled studies in treatment of "spontaneous" disease (e.g., the growth hormone has profound effects in adolescent boys, while it is not effective in middle-aged dwarfs)
4. Non-simultaneous comparisons
5. Bias of estimation
6. Bias in the assumptions underlying the analysis
7. Bias in hypothesis testing
8. Bias of reporting.

Although "selection" bias is not clearly defined as such by Murphy, he gives an example which can be classified as selection bias: Wood in 1950, in a series of 233 cases of congenital heart disease treated in London found that 5% had a specific disorder, ventricular septal defect (Wood, 1950). Estimates of 35% and 37% were reported from provincial centres. The explanation given by Wood is that ventricular septal defect is easy to recognise, also at the local level, while difficult diagnoses were referred to London. Therefore, the two series (London vs provincial centres) were not comparable.

The catalogue of 35 types of bias proposed by Sackett (1979) is very detailed, but in fact can be simplified into six categories:

1. in "reading-up" on the field
2. in specifying and selecting the study sample

Table 1 – Effect of nine biases upon observed relative risks in case-control studies (increase or decrease) (from Sackett, 1979)

Biases	Observed relative risks increase (+) decrease (−)
Prevalence-incidence bias	+ or −
Admission rate bias	+ or −
Unmasking bias	+
Non-respondent bias	+ or −
Membership bias	+ or −
Diagnostic suspicion bias	+
Exposure suspicion bias	+
Recall bias	+
Family information bias	+

3. in executing the experimental manoeuvre
4. in measuring exposures and outcomes
5. in analysing the data
6. in interpreting the analysis.

Of the 35 biases, nine are discussed more in detail (Sackett, 1979). These deserve some discussion, since they are particularly relevant to the history of epidemiology. The first is the *prevalence-incidence bias*: "a late look at those exposed (or affected) early will miss fatal and other short episodes, plus mild or silent cases and cases in which evidence of exposure disappears with disease onset". *Admission rate bias* refers to the fact that exposed and unexposed cases have different hospital admission rates, so that their relative odds of exposure to the putative cause will be distorted in hospital-based studies. *Unmasking bias* means that "an innocent exposure may become suspect if, rather than causing a disease, it causes a sign or symptom which precipitates a search for the disease". *Non-respondent bias* (i.e.: "non-respondents from a specified sample may exhibit exposures or outcomes which differ from those of respondents") is obviously crucial for all social research. Selection bias seems to be considered as a subgroup of *membership bias*, i.e. "membership in a group may imply a degree of health which differs systematically from that of the general population" (Sacket, 1979). *Diagnostic suspicion bias* is described as follows: "a knowledge of the subject's prior exposure to a putative cause may influence both the intensity and the outcome of the diagnostic process". *Exposure suspicion bias* is defined in this way: "a knowledge of the patient's disease status may influence both the intensity and outcome of a search for exposure". In more modern definitions, exposure suspicion bias and recall bias ("questions about specific exposures may be asked several times of cases but only once of controls") are considered within the same category of information bias. *Family information bias* is a special type of information bias which occurs when families are investigated about both disease status and exposure of their members. Table 1 indicates tries to evaluate the implications of the nine more important biases in terms of distortion of relative risk estimates. The most powerful in distorting measures are diagnostic suspicion bias and different categories of information bias.

The period of bias "catalogues" has been helpful in defining some of the most important and frequent distortions in the design, analysis, and interpretation of epidemiological studies. The following period is characterised by more formal and systematic definitions.

Modern formal definitions of bias

According to O.S. Miettinen (1985), bias refers to the validity of contrasts we make within epidemiologic studies: "the key to successful design of a non-experimental study in this area, as in general, is the emulation of experimentation". The validity of a randomised clinical trial, considered as the gold standard, rests on three main features:

1. the use of a placebo, i.e. *comparability of effects*
2. the use of randomisation, i.e. *comparability of populations*
3. the use of blinding, i.e. *comparability of information*.

Hence, Miettinen (1985) suggests a classification of bias into comparison, selection and information bias (according to the prevailing type of design error). Such classification is present in other texts of epidemiology, (e.g., Rothman, 1986; Hennekens and Buring, 1987). The characteristic of more modern definitions is that they are formal: selection bias is "a distortion of the effect measured, resulting from procedures used to select subjects that lead to an effect estimate among subjects included in the study different from the estimate obtainable from the entire population theoretically targeted for the study" (Rothman, 1986). *Selection bias*, in fact, depends on selection of the exposed/unexposed subjects on the basis (i.e., not independently) of the outcome, or on the selection of the diseased/healthy subjects on the basis of exposure status. Similarly, we have *information bias* when the error of classification on one axis (exposure or outcome) is not independent of the classification on the other axis.

What seems to be common to all types of bias is the fact that the main aspects of study design (selection of subjects, collection of information) are not independent of the *a priori* hypothesis: instead of a factual "truth" we incur in a "logically true" relationship. In statistical terms:

(a) $p(d \mid e \& d) > p(d \mid \bar{e})$
(b) $p(d \mid e) > p(d \mid \bar{e} \& \bar{d})$

where e = exposure ($\bar{e}$ = lack of)
        d = disease ($\bar{d}$ = lack of).

Both (a) and (b) are examples of selection bias: in (a) the exposed group is selected among ill people, like when we start a cohort study by recruiting in the exposed group a "cluster" of exposed cases; in (b) the unexposed group is recruited among healthy people. In both examples an association between exposure and disease is found as a logical, not an empirical truth (i.e., it is necessary, not contingent).

Some historical examples and controversies

Berkson's bias

In 1946, Joseph Berkson published a paper (Berkson, 1946) in which he raised doubts about the validity of epidemiologic research within hospital settings. The underlying idea was that the relative frequency of disease in a group of patients who are hospitalised is inherently biased when compared to the population served by the hospital. This phenomenon is attributable to the way in which the probabilities of hospitalisation combine in patients with more than one disease (if you have two diseases, your probability of being hospitalised is greater than the probability associated with either disease separately). Berkson's argument applies in particular to hospital-based case-control studies in which one or more risk factors are studied in relation to the risk of a specific disease. If, for example, obese people who have hypertension have a higher probability of being hospitalised than people with hypertension alone, a spurious association between obesity and anti-hypertensive drugs can be found. People with multiple diseases or conditions become over-represented in the hospital population, and this over-representation affects the distribution of risk factors as well.

Berkson's bias has been considered as an epidemiologic curiosity for a long time, until its reality was empirically demonstrated (Roberts et al., 1978). They re-analysed household surveys designed to capture health utilisation information. Information was gathered for eight clinical conditions and six medications from both hospitalised and non-hospitalised patients. All possible pairs of association were examined in the two groups, and statistically significant differences in relative risks were identified, showing that associations between drug use and specific diseases changed from community-based to hospital-based settings. Examples of associations that might have been distorted by such phenomenon are diabetes mellitus and Bell's palsy, gout and idiopathic heart block, or hypertension and peptic ulcer.

Detection bias: the example of benign breast disease vs breast cancer

When the first studies on the relationship between mammographic patterns and the risk of breast cancer appeared, suggesting that benign breast disease could predispose to cancer, the objection was raised that the observed association could be attributed to "detection bias", i.e., the greater probability that women with benign breast cancer had to undergo detailed examinations, including repeated mammograms, and to have an earlier diagnosis of cancer. This bias was empirically demonstrated in a case-control study (Silber and Horwitz, 1986). They showed that the crude odds ratio for the association between benign breast disease and breast cancer was 2.6 (statistically significant). However, when inequalities in detection of disease were considered by sampling patients according to diagnostic procedures, the association disappeared (OR = 0.9 for mammography patients, 0.8 for biopsy patients).

"Detection bias" is likely to be a common problem in case-control studies in which the risk factor investigated leads to special diagnostic procedures and thus increases the probability that the disease is identified (in contrast to unexposed subjects). Other historical examples are represented by the discussions (1) on the association between the use of reserpine (an anti-hypertensive drug) and the risk of breast cancer and (2) on the risks of women taking sex steroids. A thorough discussion on the methodological aspects of case-control studies on both issues was published in the Journal of Chronic Diseases in 1979. The same issue contained the classification of biases (Sackett, 1979) and a methodological appraisal of detection bias (Feinstein, 1979).

Detection bias can be considered within the general category of information bias in that the probability of identifying the diseased people is conditional on the clinical information collected, which is different in the categories of the risk factor.

Healthy worker effect

William Ogle, when studying death rates in different industries (1885), described two difficulties he encountered: the first was "the considerable standard of muscular strength and vigour to be maintained" in order to keep on performing many tasks in the industry. If the individual's health or strength fell below this standard, he was compelled to move to a more suitable activity, or even retire. The second difficulty was that "some occupations may repel, while others attract, the unfit at the age of starting work and, conversely, some occupations may be of necessity recruited from men of supernormal physical condition" (Ogle, 1885).

Nearly 100 years after Ogle, Fox and Collier (1976) examined the same phenomenon in terms of standardised mortality ratios with a general population referent. The overall mortality experience of an employed population is known to be more favourable than that of the general population, at least in western countries. The unemployed section of the general population includes people with serious health conditions that hamper their ability to work (this is not necessarily true in the Third World, where manual workers may undergo more superficial pre-hiring visits and may suffer from more severe consequences of workplace exposures). For example, in a study described by Richard Monson, the mortality rate per 1000 per year was 9.1 among white steelworkers, and 15.8 in the general population (non-white: 9.9 and 18.8, respectively) (Monson, 1980).

The most widely accepted explanation for the so-called healthy worker effect (HWE), that has been empirically described many times, is selection of the workforce, either as a result of self-selection by the employee or selection by the employer. For this reason the HWE has been considered to be a kind of selection bias by some of the early papers. However, Monson (1980) has claimed that it is not a selection bias, which would occur only if persons with disease were selectively entered into the study cohort. According to Monson, the HWE is a particular type of confounding, since good health status is a determinant of the outcome and is associated with the exposure (employment in industry) (this is the canonical definition of confounding). However, one can argue that selection is based on unknown variables and leads to confounding that cannot be adjusted for. More recently, Arrighi and Hertz-Picciotto (1993) have clarified that the HWE comprises two complementary processes: (1) an initial selection process whereby healthy people are more likely to seek and gain employment in a specific industry; and (2) a continuing selection process such that those who remain employed will tend to be healthier than those who leave employment. Therefore, modern definitions of the HWE include both of the "difficulties" originally encountered by Ogle.

Bias in clinical research: the Will Rogers phenomenon and "survivor treatment selection bias"

Will Rogers was a humorist-philosopher who described a geographic migration during the American economic depression of the 1930s. He said: "when the Okies (the inhabitants of Oklahoma) left Oklahoma and moved to California, they raised the average intellectual level in both states" (citation from Feinstein et al., 1985). Although the comment is slightly racist, it refers to a general phenomenon: for example, migration of an average soccer player from a very good to a poorly performing team will improve the performances of both. In medicine, the Will Rogers phenomenon refers to better classification of disease stages: if diagnostic sensitivity increases, metastases are recognised earlier, so that the distinction between early and late stages of cancer will improve. Because the prognosis of those who migrated, although worse than that for other members of the good-stage group, is better than that for other members of the bad-stage group, survival rates rise in each group without any change in individual outcomes (Feinstein et al., 1985). The Will Rogers phenomenon has been empirically demonstrated several times.

The *survivor treatment selection bias* is a potentially very serious problem that has been clearly described in AIDS research. In contrast with Berkson's bias, which was described on theoretical grounds decades ago and then empirically demonstrated, this bias has not been identified until recently. The underlying idea is that in an observational study (not in randomised trials), patients who live longer have more opportunities to select treatment, while those who die earlier may be untreated by default. The effect of the bias is to lead erroneously to the conclusion that an ineffective treatment prolongs survival (Glesby and Hoover, 1996).

Bias in screening practices

In 1928 two independent investigators, Papanicolaou in the United States and Babes in Rumania, reported that cancer of the cervix could be diagnosed by examining exfoliated cells from the cervical epithelium. Only after the war, however, their technique was systematically introduced in order to detect cervical cancer at early stages and improve survival of the patients. X-ray examination of the breast in asymptomatic women was already advocated in the 1930s by Gershon-Cohen as a means to reduce breast cancer mortality. The first mammography technique was introduced by Egan in the 1960s, and in the same period the first randomised trial (HIP) was started. Among the different methodological issues that were raised concerning mass cancer screening, two peculiar types of bias have been described in early seminal papers by Hutchinson and Shapiro (1968) and Feinleib and Zelen (1969). *Length bias sampling* concerns the fact that individuals who develop a rapidly progressive disease and who are thus more likely to die than the majority of individuals with disease, are unlikely to be found in a population that presents for screening. In other words, the screening programme is likely to select subjects with long-lasting diseases, so that the effectiveness of screening in terms of survival is overstated. Bailar (1978) has indicated how the length bias effect in the US Breast Cancer Detection Demonstration Projects may have loaded the series with individuals who were unlikely to have had much benefit from screening.

A second peculiar kind of bias in screening is the lead time effect. Lead time is defined as the interval between the time of detection by screening and the time at which the disease would have been diagnosed in the absence of screening. It is the time by which screening advances diagnosis of the disease, which does not correspond to the time by which death is postponed.

Screening is affected also by selection bias, since those who participate in screening programmes are not a random sample of the target population, but may be individuals with particularly high or low incidence rates for the disease at issue. For example, participants in screening programmes for cervical cancer are often women with lower risk than the average (high socio-economic status), thus lowering the detection rate of cancer.

Conclusions

Epidemiology is a non-experimental discipline. Although this has been mainly perceived as a weakness, it can also be seen as a strength. In fact, the lack of experiments (except for randomised clinical trials) has lead to a very critical and sophisticated (formal) attitude towards different types and sources of error. The fact that such an attitude was less developed in the social sciences is probably related to the reason that epidemiology has a very practical goal, the identification of single agents for preventive purposes, while social sciences deal with complex realities and do not aim to disentangle simple causal pathways.

Causality in epidemiology

Paolo Vineis

Unit of Clinical Epidemiology, Ospedale s. Giovanni Battista, University of Torino and JSJ Foundation, Via Santena 7, 10216 Torino, Italy

Summary

Epidemiology represents an interesting and unique example of cross-fertilization between social and natural sciences. Epidemiology has evolved from a monocausal to a multicausal concept of the "web of causation", thus mimicking a similar and much earlier shift in the social sciences. However, in comparison with the social sciences epidemiology is both more sensitive to underlying biological models (which condition the interpretation of population findings), and more prone to a simplification of the causal pathways. Paradoxically, epidemiology has developed more sophisticated theoretical models for bias and confounding than the social sciences did, but for the practical purpose of identifying single preventable risk factors. Epidemiology makes use more often of study designs that simulate experimentation, than of surveys in the general population.

Causality in medicine can be viewed from at least three perspectives. One refers to the classical epistemological question of how causes are discovered and which is the most effective model of explanation. This perspective includes for example the concept of the "arc of knowledge", i.e., the respective roles of hypothesis generation and hypothesis testing (Odlroyd, 1986). The second perspective refers to the "burden of proof" which is needed to consider an agent as a cause of disease, i.e., how much evidence should be collected before practical action is justified. The story of Semmelweis is exemplar from both perspectives: from the epistemological point of view, the work of Semmelweis, which is summarised below, has been considered as paradigmatic by Carl Hempel (1966). In the meantime, according to a popular (but inaccurate) reading of his life, the resistance to accept the practical implications of that work has been considered as an example of the conflict between academic interests, scientific standards and ethical obligations of the profession. In fact, a romantic interpretation of the relationships between Semmelweis' genius and the obtuseness of his time's academic community is mainly the invention of the writer Ferdinand Céline and is not supported by scholarly work (see e.g., Nuland, 1989).

The third perspective is related to how we interpret the relationship between cause and effect, for example according to a probabilistic or a deterministic model (the latter implying that the effect is predictable from the cause at the individual level).

Some antecedents of the modern notion of cause in medicine

The heritage of Claude Bernard

The work of Claude Bernard has played a key role in last century's medicine. I will just sketch some of his main contributions that are relevant to conceptions of causality. His well-known theory of "milieu intérieur" (internal medium) has been instrumental to the discoveries of endocrinology and, more generally, to the identification of regulatory mechanisms in physiology. The underlying idea was that the autonomy of the living being from the external world is due to the ability to regulate his internal milieu and to keep it in equilibrium in spite of environmental changes (for example, rates of glucose in the blood are kept constant in spite of variable dietary intake). This idea of "homeostatic" mechanisms, based on a feed-back between the environment and the living being, has been applied to several aspects of physiology and pathology, and is a key issue in causality. For example, the current theory of carcinogenesis is based on the central role played by DNA (see below) and the related hypothesis of a "homeostatic" mechanism of DNA repair: cancer arises because the balance between carcinogenic "hits" and DNA repair is overcome.

But Bernard's work is important also from the epistemological point of view. According to his book "*Introduction to experimental medicine*" (Bernard, 1957), theories are not built on the basis of cumulation of observations, like in the empiricist account of knowledge. Rather, there is a feedback mechanism between facts and theories, a "tension" between the proliferation of new observations and their ability to fit existing theories (like in a homeostatic model).

Virchow's school

Because of its relevance to the questions we are discussing, a debate which took place in medicine around 1900 is worth describing. I refer to the controversy between Rudolf Virchow's cellular pathology on one side and bacteriology on the other side, also referred to as the controversy between *aetiology* and *pathology* (von Engelhardt, 1993). Klebs, a student of Virchow, denied "the autonomy of the cell as a principle of disease" (i.e., the internal origin of diseases), and insisted on external causes of human pathology. Later, he refined his theory by claiming that infectious diseases can be explained neither solely from the viewpoint of the bacteriologist, nor from that of the cellular pathologist; rather, diseases represented a battle between bacteria and cells (von Engelhardt, 1993).

Subsequently, several authors, in particular Martius and Hueppe, insisted that man has to free himself from a one-sided etiological view of thinking, which aims to recognise a single and necessary cause for each event. Following the functionalist philosophy of Mach, Martius interpreted "disposition" (internal cause) and "stimulus" (external cause) as variables subject to mathematical treatment (von Engelhardt, 1993).

According to the more radical school of "conditionalists", the word "cause" should be completely substituted by the concept of "determining condition", where "all the conditions of a process or state are equally important", i.e., a hierarchy cannot be established. In the opinion of von Hasemann, the monocausal viewpoint has been promoted in medicine because of a practical interest in therapy, but from a scientific perspective monocausality must be opposed. Conditionalism stimulated the idea of a multiplicity of etiological factors and insisted on the strict relationship between external determinants and internal reaction to the stimulus. From a practical point of view, conditionalism was not able to ascribe relative importance to the determinants, and it failed in the court and in insurance decisions.

The relevance of this debate to contemporary epidemiology is rather clear. For example, O.S. Miettinen has proposed to treat causal relationships in medicine according to the concept of "occurrence function" (Miettinen, 1985); such approach is very similar to the mathematical treatment by Martius. The occurrence function is

$$\text{disease} = a + \text{determinant(s)} + \text{confounder(s)} + \text{effect modifier(s)}$$

i.e., the probability of disease is explained by the conjunction of one or more determinants, after allowing for confounding variables and for other exposures that "modify the effect" of the determinant. For example, cigarette smoking is a determinant of lung cancer, after allowing for occupational exposure as a potential confounder and considering consumption of Vitamin C as an effect modifier.

Hempel on Semmelweis

Carl Gustav Hempel, in one of his more important texts on science philosophy (Hempel, 1966), describes the work of Ignaz Semmelweis as an example of correct scientific procedure based on trial and error. Semmelweis described the occurrence of "puerperal fever" in the course of time and in two different obstetric clinics of the Vienna General Hospital: in the first period (1833–1858) mortality from puerperal fever was very similar in the two clinics, while in the second (1840–1846) it was remarkably different: in fact, 1989 deaths occurred among 20042 women in the first clinic vs. 691 among 17791 in the second. The only element that could differentiate the two time periods was that in 1840–1846 the students attending the first clinic were involved in autopsies as a part of their training. This suggested to Semmelweis the idea that the cause of puerperal fever could be related to some "particle" transmitted from the corpses; this idea was reinforced by the death of Kolletschka, a professor of pathology and friend of Semmelweis, who apparently died from a disease very similar to puerperal fever after hurting his finger accidentally during an autopsy (but the distinction between reality and legend is not clear-cut). After 1846, Semmelweis made an experiment, by introducing the very simple practice of washing hands after autopsies and before visiting the women in the obstetric department. Mortality from puerperal fever declined abruptly to 3% or less in both clinics.

Hempel (1966) describes the inferential procedures used by Semmelweis as an example of "trial and error": after the early epidemiological observations suggesting transmission of "particles" from corpses, he looked for falsifying evidence and alternative explanations. For example, he ruled out that the disease was contracted before hospitalisation for causes related to the women's living conditions. He also ruled out, partly by conducting experiments, several other potential confounders or sources of bias. Therefore, the work of Semmelweis can be described according to the idea of the *"arc of knowledge"*, i.e., research can be summarised into four phases:

1. hypothesis generation from clinical observations
2. reinforcement of the hypothesis on the basis of planned epidemiological observation
3. testing of the hypothesis with a formal study design (in clinical research the gold standard for this phase is represented by the randomised clinical trial)
4. intervention, i.e., deliberate change of exposure circumstances in order to prevent disease occurrence.

Phase 1 and 2 belong to the ascending part of the arc of knowledge (induction), while parts 3 and 4 belong to the descending arc (deduction).

The logical reconstruction of Semmelweis' work proposed by Hempel (1966) is a nice introduction to causal thinking in a non-experimental science like epidemiology, though one may not completely agree with the "trial-and-error" model he proposes. In contrast e.g., with Popper, Hempel does not stress the limitations of the observational (non-experimental) nature of epidemiology. (Incidentally, the description of Semmelweis' work cannot be separated from his biography, and in particular from his mental illness and tendencies to self-destruction; see Nuland, 1989).

From monocausality to multiple causation

Three eras in the recent history of medical causality

In a rather simplified way, causation involves the relationship between at least two entities, an agent and a disease. Both can be easy to define and identify, or, on the opposite, they can be "fuzzy sets", i.e., have blurred bounds. From this point of view, we can describe three eras in the history of medical causality in the last two centuries. The first era corresponds to the microbiological revolution, i.e., the triumph of a linear mono-causal (Aristotelian) concept of cause. After the work of Pasteur and Koch, the agent of a disease was conceived as a single *necessary* cause (e.g., *Mycobacterium tuberculosis*). The concept of necessary cause means that the disease does not develop in the absence of exposure to the agent. Such a view implies: (a) that the cause is defined univocally and is easily identifiable; (b) that the disease can be also defined univocally, i.e., it is not a complex and variable constellation of symptoms. Sometimes such conditions clearly occur and the relationship between a (necessary) cause and the corresponding disease is evident: for example, smallpox is a clear-cut disease entity, easy to define and diagnose; it is due to a single necessary virus (no smallpox develops in the absence of the specific virus); and clear proof of the causal link has come from the disappearance of smallpox after large scale vaccination. On other occasions, the disease itself is at least partly defined on the basis of its cause: for example, from the symptomatologic point of view tuberculosis is a complex constellation, and the only unifying element has been the ability to identify Mycobacterium directly (microscopically in the lesions) or indirectly (immunologically). In the case of smallpox the symptomatology of the disease is so characteristic, and specificity of the relationship between cause and effect is so high that referring to the poxvirus as a necessary cause seems natural. In the case of tuberculosis, instead, the necessary character of the cause is weaker, since it comes from grouping part of the disease manifestations on the basis of the cause.

Situations like smallpox are a minority; more frequently, in the "Pasteur-Koch" paradigm we find a clearly defined agent (usually a bacterium, a parasite or a virus) which is used as the "unifying element" of a constellation of symptoms, i.e., the disease itself is largely defined and recognised on the basis of the agent. The popularity of the "Pasteur-Koch" approach to causality has not decreased, and the concept of a necessary cause of disease has been proposed still very recently as a universal paradigm in medicine (Sutter, 1996).

The second era refers to chronic affections like cancer or cardiovascular disease. In this case the concept of "necessary" is not applicable on the basis of current knowledge. No "necessary" cause of cancer is known; rather, the idea of a "causal web" has been introduced and largely applied. The idea of a causal web implies that to induce the disease, the concurrence of different "exposures" or conditions is required, none of which is necessary. For example, lung cancer can be induced by a causal web including tobacco smoking and individual predisposition based on the CYP1A1 genotype. Another causal web may be represented by asbestos exposure and low consumption of raw fruits and vegetables in the occurrence of mesothelioma. The idea of the web implies that, while the disease is usually well defined from a clinical point of view (e.g., lung cancer or mesothelioma), causal agents are classified according to a "polythetic" classification: cases of lung cancer are not characterised all by the same exposure, but they share partially overlapping constellations of causes. The idea of "polythetic" classification corresponds to Wittgenstein's definition of "a long rope twisted together out of many shorter fibres".

The concept of causal web was already introduced in philosophy of causality by the British philosopher John Mackie, who coined the definition of INUS (Insufficient non-redundant component of unnecessary sufficient complex) (Mackie, 1965). For example, in explaining why a fire burned down the house, one can identify several components of a causal complex, like the strong wind, the fact that the electric oven was turned on, and the fact that the alarm system did not work. In such a complex, which was sufficient to start the fire, at least one component is non-redundant (i.e., it is an INUS condition), for example the failure of the alarm system (on the contrary, the strong wind is not an INUS). The definition of INUS corresponds to the logic of *"conditional counterfactuals"*, i.e., to asking for each component of the causal complex whether in its absence the effect would have developed anyway. Clearly, the idea of INUS still corresponds to the conception of causes as *necessary* events, although in the context of causal complexes.

In chronic disease epidemiology we have causal complexes without single necessary components. However, this is true only if we consider causality at the *individual level*: it is impossible to identify the necessary cause that explains the occurrence of a single case of cancer, while it is possible to identify a non-redundant component in the causal web that has lead to the fire. If we shift from the individual to the *population*, then the idea of "non-redundant" component makes sense. If we consider this century's epidemic of lung cancer, there is no doubt that it is attributable to the diffusion of the habit of smoking: although we cannot attribute each single case of lung cancer to the individual's smoking habits, we are sure that on a population level the epidemic would not have occurred without cigarette smoking (*conditional counterfactual*). The risk of cancer in those who stop smoking decreases considerably in comparison with continuing smokers, and reaches after a few years the risk of non-smokers. Apparently, therefore, we have to apply different criteria of causation if we consider the individual level or the population level. We can say that for chronic diseases the INUS model is valid at the population level.

The third era is even more complicated than that. In the case of diseases like schizophrenia, bulimia or anorexia, both disease and agent have blurred bounds. The disease cannot be easily distinguished from other similar symptomatological constellations (for example, bulimia from other conditions characterised by obesity and "binge eating"), and the causal complexes are rather ill-defined and vague. In this

Table 1 – *Diseases can be classified according to the nature of causal agents and to the appearance of signs/symptoms: in both cases monothetic or polythetic definitions are possible*

	Disease	
	Monothetic definition[a]	Polythetic definition[a]
Agent (s)		
Monothetic definition	Smallpox (group 1)	Tuberculosis (group 2)
Polythetic definition	lung cancer (group 3)	bulimia and anorexia (group 4)

[a] On the basis of clinical signs and symptoms only.

case we shift from the classical scientific paradigm of "explanation" to a more evasive and slippery paradigm of "understanding" (Von Wright, 1957) as used by psycho-social sciences.

What should be clear is that there is a continuum between the three categories in Tab. 1, and diseases like smallpox are only one extreme of the spectrum, the other extreme being represented for example by several psychic disorders.

The importance of interactions: Helicobacter Pylori and gastric lymphomas

The example I wish to describe in this paragraph is relevant from several points of view. First of all, it refers to a causal relationship in which both exposure and disease are "polythetic" (group 4 in Table 1). In fact, H. pylori is likely to be causally associated with gastric lymphomas, but it is not the only risk factor and it is certainly not a sufficient cause. Secondly, it is an example of the complex role an infectious agent can play (far from being the necessary and sufficient cause of a specific disease). Third, the example illustrates both the difficulties of identifying risk factors by simple geographic correlations, and the importance of "modifying factors" (or susceptibility factors) in carcinogenesis.

Non-Hodgkin's lymphomas (to which gastric lymphomas belong) are an extremely heterogeneous category of affections: some of them have a mild clinical course, others very rapid; histologically, they show a wide range of manifestations, and even their cells of origin are disparate (B- or T-lymphocytes). In fact there is not a simple, univocal and agreed upon classification: the recent REAL classification seems to be an operational tool rather than a new interpretation based on scientific evidence. Non-Hodgkin's lymphomas (including gastric lymphomas) are on the rise in all the Western world at a rate of 3–4% per year, but the reasons for such an increase are unknown. Better and earlier diagnosis is not an explanation.

Table 2 – Effect of genetic relatedness on host response to M. tuberculosis in families with an index case (from Evans, 1993)

Relation of family member to index case	% of exposed and susceptibles showing clinical manifestations of TB
Marriage partner	7.1
Half-sibling	11.9
Dyzigotic twin	25.5
Monozigotic twin	83.3

As far as the alleged "cause" of gastric lymphomas (H. pylori) is concerned, things are no simpler. There are several different antigenic varieties of H. pylori, apparently with different biological activities. A disease which is certainly due to H. pylori is peptic ulcer. The relationship between H. Pylori and lymphoma would *not* be demonstrated on the basis of "geographic pathology". In fact, H. pylori infection is extremely frequent (it affects around 50% of the population), and shows wide geographic variability, while non-Hodgkin's lymphomas are rare and show more limited geographic variation. There is very little overlapping of the distributions of these two conditions: 85% of the Indian population, for example, is infected with H. pylori, but the rate of lymphomas, including those of the stomach, is lower than in Western populations. In the United States, the prevalence of H. pylori infection and the mortality rate for peptic ulcer have steadily decreased during the past 50 years, but Non-Hodgkin's lymphomas are increasing. So, on the basis of geographic or time correlations, one would *not* conclude that H. pylori is a cause of gastric lymphomas. However, we have much more stringent data. Epidemiological prospective studies from distinct populations have reported that the risk of gastric lymphoma in patients with antibodies against H. pylori is about six times higher that in normal subjects, while there is no association with non-gastric lymphomas. More interestingly, eradication of H. pylori with antibiotics lead to regression of low-grade gastric lymphomas; the latter is a kind of experimental "galilean" evidence which strongly supports the causal hypothesis. Incidentally, even in the absence of such experimental evidence it would not be easy to argue against epidemiological proof. To explain away a relative risk of six, in fact, one has to suppose that an alternative exposure exists, which has a *stronger* association with both the disease and H. pylori: it is possible, but very unlikely (International Agency for Research on Cancer, 1994).

Therefore, one has to admit that a very common infection is responsible for a very rare disease. This is equivalent to admitting that something else interacts with H. pylori in order to explain its causal role. This idea of interaction is not new. Table 2 shows that also in the case of a disease belonging to group 2 in Table 1 (tuberculosis), host response is crucial: the risk of developing tuberculosis is in fact much higher in strict relatives of cases. In addition to genetic susceptibility, there are several other types of "acquired" interactions. For example, interaction occurs between cigarette smoke and asbestos in modifying the risk of lung cancer (Tomatis, 1990).

The biological background of epidemiological observations

The DNA dogma in carcinogenesis

I already anticipated that in the current interpretation of carcinogenesis and of cause-effect relationships in cancer epidemiology, inferences are made against a background represented by the idea of a "homeostatic" or feedback mechanism involving genotoxic "hits" from the environment, on one side, and DNA repair on the other side. Discussions on causality are not in a vacuum, but are strictly conditioned on the current models of disease.

Centrality of DNA in modern biology has reached the status of a "dogma". Contemporary, DNA-centred molecular biology was born from a strict interaction with physics. Seminal work was represented in 1994 by Erwin Schroedinger's book "What is life?" (Schroedinger, 1994), where he suggested very clearly that life phenomena could be explained by the properties of molecules, i.e., by their "memory". Schroedinger, a well-known quantum physicist with biological interests, was responsible for creating a bridge between the two disciplines and for the role that was attributed to DNA subsequently. In addition, he had views that were very similar to those already expressed (one century before) by Claude Bernard, updated with a reference to the theory of information: the mechanism by which an organism is kept stable consists, according to Schroedinger, in "absorbing order from the environment". In other words, Schroedinger interpreted homeostasis mainly as an exchange of information between internal and external molecules.

As far as the central role of DNA in contemporary biology is concerned, the relationship between "cause" and "mechanisms" sometimes is misunderstood. Molecular biologists tend to consider relevant changes at the molecular level as the "cause" of cancer, while epidemiologists usually refer to external agents as genuine causes. Perhaps it is not irrelevant to refer to Aristotle's four categories of cause: *material* (the cells in which cancer arises), *final* (i.e., the scope of malignant transformation, which can be described – although improperly – as a selective advantage of cancer cells, conferring them the ability to overcome the host's defences), *formal* (the morphological characteristics of cancer and the corresponding functional changes), and *efficient* (the events that trigger the mechanistic steps which lead to malignancy). Molecular changes at the DNA level refer to the "formal" cause, the molecular and functional changes that occur in a normal cell, while external agents refer to the "efficient" cause.

In spite of such distinctions, similar criteria for "causality" assessment can be applied to both external causes and mechanisms. The so called "Henle-Koch postulates" have been used for a long time to describe causality assessment in medicine. They were derived from the discoveries of the microbiological era and stated that an agent is a cause of disease if it is present in all the affected persons ("necessary" cause), it is absent in healthy subjects ("sufficient" cause) and can be inoculated into an animal to induce the same disease that it causes in humans. In fact, the long-used definition of "Henle-Koch postulates" is wrong, both because they are not postulates, and because they were changed considerably between the original formulation by Henle and the one due to Koch.

Recent developments in molecular biology seem to fit rather well with Henle-Koch's rules, for example in the case of oncogenes. Oncogenes are mutated genes that, in their normal (wild) form exert crucial functions in the cell's metabolism, and are highly conserved on the evolutionary scale. Mutated oncogenes have been found in a high proportion of malignancies and some of them have marked similarities with viral DNA sequences that are able to induce malignancies. Though the criterion of "necessary" cause does not seem to be met (since not all malignancies show oncogene mutations), this could be attributed to limited knowledge of relevant genes and limited sensitivity of tests. Both the criterion of "sufficient" cause, and the criterion of experimental reproducibility (at least in particular circumstances) are met, in that "transfection" of NIH 3T3 cells (which already underwent partial transformation) with a mutated oncogene confers malignant properties.

The nature of medical theories and conditionalized realism

What is the nature of an observational medical theory, such as "tobacco smoking causes lung cancer"? It can hardly be claimed that such theories represent universal laws of nature, comparable to the laws of thermodynamics or molecular genetics. In the meantime, they cannot be dismissed as simple empirical generalisations. We believe that the statement "smoking causes lung cancer" is clearly related to some natural phenomenon. The feeling that it reflects something more than an empirical generalisation does not mean that we are ready to accept that such statement is comparable to laws describing basic natural phenomena like the genetic code.

According to Schaffner (1993), biology is characterised by "middle range" theories, i.e., laws that are intermediate between the simple observation of empirical regularities and universal statements about nature. Such middle range theories have the peculiarity of being strongly based on mutual reinforcement between different types of evidence, at different levels of reality and including some reference to basic laws of nature. The two main features of middle range theories are their being *temporal* models (i.e., they refer to phenomena that undergo a process, like carcinogenesis) and their being "overlapping inter-level models" (i.e., they serve to connect different levels of reality).

Let us consider the relationship between tobacco and cancer (Vineis and Caporaso, 1995). Even after the publication of persuasive evidence linking lung cancer to tobacco smoking, some investigators questioned whether the epidemiologic evidence incriminated smoking as a cause of cancer in humans. In particular, R.A. Fisher, an eminent statistician of this century, claimed that the early epidemiological observations could not be interpreted as a proof of cause-effect relationship, arguing that one could not rule out that a genetic factor both increased the propensity to smoke and the risk of lung cancer. A key criticism was that exact knowledge of the mechanisms of tobacco carcinogenesis was necessary to establish a cause-effect relationship. Such criticism was at the root of scepticism towards epidemiological evidence and its applications in public health.

In fact, in addition to the (redundant) epidemiological observations linking tobacco to lung cancer in humans, we have several types of evidence at different levels. Tobacco smoke contains many mutagenic and carcinogenic substances. Both tobacco smoke and extracts induced tumours in experimental animals. A general trend in molecular studies is the increasing evidence that point mutations in tumour suppresser genes (i.e., p. 53) and oncogenes (i.e., *ras*) may be specific both for the type of tumour and for the critical environmental exposure; this is true also for tobacco.

Furthermore, Fisher's hypothesis that genetic predisposition both induces smoking habits and increases the risk of lung cancer has been refuted on the basis of twin studies (Vineis and Caporaso, 1995).

To admit that smoking causes lung cancer one need not be either a *realist* or an *empiricist*, to refer to a long-lasting debate in medicine. The realist postulates that empirical observations do refer to some reality in the external world (independently of theoretical models); the empiricist strictly sticks to observable entities, avoiding any judgement about the essence of reality. For example, realists in medicine tend to believe that basic biochemical or molecular mechanisms explain the effectiveness of therapies; while empiricists strongly advocate empirical evidence coming from randomised controlled trials. Wide areas of observational medicine, and particularly epidemiology, clearly belong to the empiricist field. As a third alternative, Schaffner (1993) proposes a *"conditionalized realism"*. This means that a "middle range" theory is held to be true if two conditions are met: (1) that also "auxiliary hypotheses" are true; (2) that no valid alternative explanation can be put forward. The second condition is well known to epidemiologists, since it corresponds to the concept of "confounding". The first condition is also easily understandable: examples of auxiliary hypotheses are that the design of a particular study did not introduce bias; that the evidence collected from animal experiments can be extrapolated to humans; that tobacco-related mutations in specific genes (oncogenes) actually are relevant to the carcinogenic process.

Which type of message does the "tobacco and cancer" example convey? *First*, we believe that smoking causes cancer not only on the basis of empirical observations in humans (which are limited by their non-experimental nature), but also because we have independent proof referring to different levels of reality. Such proof includes reference to some of our most profound beliefs concerning nature, such as the crucial role played by DNA damage in carcinogenesis. Therefore, prior beliefs in nature are essential in the interpretation of empirical observations.

Secondly, the model of causality which is valid in observational medicine is compatible with the models that have been proposed for physics (such as the INUS model), particularly if we refer not to the individual (human or molecule), but to populations. *Third*, as in other fields of science, also in observational medicine the truth of a theory is conditionalised on auxiliary hypotheses and the lack of alternative explanations. This conditionalised nature of biologic realism (Schaffner, 1993) is an example of the interplay between direct evidence and interpretation, in that even an experiment – such as a randomised trial – will be interpretable only in the context of background knowledge concerning auxiliary hypotheses (although a randomised experimental trial needs *less* auxiliary hypotheses than observational medicine).

How strictly interpretation and prior belief can be intertwined with the scientific practice of observational medicine is shown by the role of "model selection" in causal inference. According to Robins and Greenland (1986), "all modelling strategies contain implicit prior beliefs about nature". When we choose which "explanatory" variables, confounders or effect modifiers to include into the occurrence function, we anticipate which of them make biological sense and are compatible with a reasonable interpretation of the data. "[...] a statistical model is a mathematical expression for a set of assumed restrictions on the possible states of nature [...]. For example, a linear [...] logistic model for the dependence of subsequent fertility on dibromochloropropane exposure and parity implies the following restrictions about nature: (1) an exponential dependence of the fertility odds ratio on DBCP and parity; (2) a constant odds ratio across DBCP for the association of any parity level [...] with subsequent fertility; and (3) a constant odds ratio across parity for the association of any DBCP level with subsequent fertility" (Robins and Greenland, 1986). The choice of the model, in fact, is a trade-off between different and potentially conflicting goals, such as "saving variance" in the model by introducing *few* assumptions about nature, decreasing bias by introducing *correct* assumptions, and increasing bias by introducing *incorrect* assumptions. In fact, an occurrence function based on a "highly-saturated" model will have small bias provided that no confounding remains, but may have large statistical variance.

Therefore, any opposition between scientific knowledge (based on the observation of facts within an "occurrence function"), and non-scientific prior beliefs would be misleading, since prior belief is clearly necessary for a correct building and interpretation of causal models.

Conclusions

Knowledge of the causes of a disease allows therapeutic and preventive interventions in humans. Due to such practical implications (the well-being of the patient or the population), medicine is not entirely a natural science. Rather, both medicine and epidemiology are at the cross-roads of natural sciences and human sciences.

Epidemiology has evolved from a mono-causal to a multi-causal concept of the "web of causation", thus mimicking a similar and much earlier shift in the social sciences. However, in comparison with the social sciences epidemiology is both more sensitive to *underlying biological models* (which condition the interpretation of population findings), aone to a *simplification* of the causal pathways. For example, epidemiology has developed more sophisticated theoretical models for bias and confounding than the social sciences did, thus revealing the practical purpose of identifying single preventable risk factors. Epidemiology makes use more often of study designs that simulate experimentation, than of surveys in the general population. Epidemiology, therefore, represents an interesting and unique example of cross-fertilisation between social and natural sciences.

Evolution of epidemiologic methods and concepts in selected textbooks of the 20th century

Fang F. Zhang[1], Desireé C. Michaels[1, 3], Barun Mathema[1], Shuaib Kauchali[1], Anjan Chatterjee[1, 4], David C. Ferris[1], Tamarra M. James[1], Jennifer Knight[1], Matthew Dounel[1], Hebatullah O. Tawfik[1], Janet A. Frohlich[1], Li Kuang[1], Elena K. Hoskin[1], Frederick J. Veldman[1], Giulia Baldi[1], Koleka P. Mlisana[1], Lerole D. Mametja[1], Angela Diaz[1], Nealia L. Khan[1], Pamela Sternfels[1], Jeffery J. Sevigny[1], Asher Shamam[1], Alfredo Morabia[1, 2]

[1] Department of Epidemiology, Mailman School of Public Health, Columbia University, New York, NY 10032, USA
[2] Division of Clinical Epidemiology, University Hospital, 24 rue Micheli-du-Crest, 1211 Geneva 14, Switzerland
[3] Infectious Disease Epidemiology Unit, University of Cape Town, Cape Town, South Africa
[4] The Neurological Institute of New York and the Gertrude H. Sergievsky Center, Columbia University, New York, NY 10032, USA

Summary

Textbooks are an expression of the state of development of a discipline at a given moment in time. By reviewing eight epidemiology textbooks published over the course of a century, we have attempted to trace the evolution of five epidemiologic concepts and methods: study design (cohort studies and case-control studies), confounding, bias, interaction and causal inference. Overall, these eight textbooks can be grouped into three generations. Greenwood (1935) and Hill (first edition 1937; version reviewed 1961)'s textbooks belong to the first generation, "early epidemiology", which comprise early definitions of bias and confounding. The second generation, "classic epidemiology", represented by the textbooks of Morris (first edition, 1957; version reviewed, 1964), MacMahon and Pugh (first edition MacMahon et al., 1960; version reviewed MacMahon and Pugh, 1970), Susser (1973), and Lilienfeld and Lilienfeld (first edition Lilienfeld, 1976; version reviewed Lilienfeld and Lilienfeld, 1980), clarifies the properties of cohort and case-control study designs and the theory of disease causation. Miettinen (1985) and Rothman (1986)'s textbooks belong to a third generation, "modern epidemiology", presenting an integrated perspective on study designs and their measures of outcome, as well as distinguishing and formalizing the concepts of confounding and interaction. Our review demonstrates that epidemiol-

ogy, as a scientific discipline, is in constant evolution and transformation. It is likely that new methodological tools, able to assess the complexity of the causes of human health, will be proposed in future generations of textbooks.

Current courses of epidemiology teach students the tools to discover causal associations relevant to human health. These tools consist of: study designs (cohort studies and case-control studies) with their specific measures of outcomes and effects, and theories supporting the concepts of bias, confounding, interaction and causal inference. In this paper, we attempt to trace the origin of these five elements in selected textbooks published in the 20th century.

Comparing the content of textbooks of epidemiology published over the last century is therefore also a way of retracing the history of the discipline. Our objective here is to describe the evolution of the corpus of methods and concepts that are used by epidemiologists rather than reviewing the health issues that epidemiologists have been tackling over the years. This is the history of the methods and not of the scourges they helped to fight.

For this purpose, we have selected eight textbooks. The authors of the books are Greenwood (1935), Hill (1961), Morris (1964), MacMahon and Pugh (1970), Susser (1973), Lilienfeld and Lilienfeld (1980), Miettinen (1985), Rothman (1986). These books appeared in a given chronological order, but we did not necessarily review their first editions. For example, the first edition of Hill's textbook, *Principles of medical statistics*, was in 1937, compiled from a series of papers published in Lancet; Morris's first edition of "*Uses of epidemiology*" was published in 1957 (Morris, 1957) building on ideas first introduced in a 1955 British Medical Journal paper (Morris, 1955); MacMahon and Pugh's textbook, "*Epidemiology: principles and methods*", was preceded by its 1960's version, "*Epidemiologic methods*", by MacMahon, Pugh and Ipsen (MacMahon et al., 1960); and Lilienfeld and Lilienfeld's "*Foundations of epidemiology*" by Lilienfeld alone (1976). This set of textbooks is a selection which does not include influential texts such as Kleinbaum et al. (1982), Gordis (2000), Mausner and Bahn (1974), Kelsey et al. (1996), Hennekens and Buring (1987), Rose (1994), Szklo and Nieto (2000), Rothman and Greenland (1998) or textbooks whose titles indicate that they specialize, for example, in clinical, occupational and genetic epidemiology. We do not include texts in languages other than English. This selection was guided by the objective of detecting how some concepts and methods have evolved. Therefore, some texts were deemed to belong to the same generation and therefore to reflect the same degree of achievement even if they differed by the way they explained the material. Having selected some texts and not others is therefore not a quality judgment but essentially an attempt to avoid redundancy. For example, the texts by Maussner and Bahn (1974), Gordis (2000) and Lilienfeld and Lilienfeld (1980) are considered to belong to the same generation of texts, influenced by the teaching at The Johns Hopkins School of Public Health of Abraham Lilienfeld. The selection may therefore be considered as arbitrary. We would be grateful to the readers familiar with these texts or their authors to express their disagreement if they feel that we missed some substantially innovative contribution of these other texts.

We then considered five main topics of interest: study design (cohort studies and case-control studies), confounding, bias, interaction and causal inference. Here again, the choice may be considered arbitrary as we did not include the evolution of randomized trials or of ecologic studies, for example. The technique and analysis of randomized trials are not necessarily covered in depth in the current epidemiology core courses. "Ecological designs" should have been covered as they occupied an important place in classic epidemiology texts and have been the object of a renewed interest recently.

The work was divided as follows. Each of the authors, barring the first and last who were teaching the course (Epidemiology III: principles of epidemiology) in the Department of Epidemiology at Columbia University, were asked to prepare a 15 minute presentation on an assigned combination of books and topics, that is, either to review the way the five topics have been covered in a given textbook, or to follow the treatment of a given topic across all eight texts. A series of papers were available on www.epidemiology.ch/history and on the class website, including pre 1945 publications such as Snow (1936; Vandenbroucke et al., 1991), Baker (In Delta Omega Classics), Budd (In Delta Omega Classics), Louis (1836; Lilienfeld and Lilienfeld, 1980a; Morabia, 1996), to which each one added the results of their own search.

The first and last authors then synthesized the information, drafted a manuscript that was then read and commented on by all the present authors. The journal Social and Preventive Medicine invited the authors of the reviewed texts who are still alive to review the paper and/or to write specific commentaries on it.

The main results of this research are presented in Table 1. We first perform a vertical reading of the table, that is, to track the evolutions of the topics across texts, and then a horizontal reading, which consist in comparing the relative coverage of the topics in each of the chronologically ordered texts.

1. Evolution of the specific concepts and methods (vertical reading of the table)

Bias and confounding

Bias and confounding are the only issues that we found systematically across all texts. It appears that early epidemiologists primarily concerned by the potential pitfalls of spurious associations. Greenwood and Hill refer to biases as sources of "fallacy". Bias and confounding are not really distinguished in the early textbooks, so that their history needs to be considered simultaneously.

Greenwood identifies several types of fallacies (pp. 84–86), one of which was first stated by a British statistician and friend of Greenwood, G. Udny Yule (Yule, 1903).

> **Box 1 – Greenwood's formulation of Yule's "fallacy that may be caused by the mixing of distinct records", also known as Simpson's Paradox**
>
> "Sometimes the existence of a relevant difference is obvious; two fallacies which have vitiated many published reports are easily described. One has data of the experience of inoculated and uninoculated persons collected over a wide range in space or time, and brings them together in as single statistical summary, which tells us that upon *n* inoculated persons the attack-rate was *a* per cent and upon *m* uninoculated *b* per cent. If *n* and *m* are large numbers, the kind of statistical test I have described may lead to arithmetically overwhelming odds in favour of the inoculated, yet this a priori inference might be quite wrong. It might be that in some of the experiments *neither inoculated nor uninoculated ran any serious risk at all*; if in these groups there were *a great majority of inoculated*, the final summary would show a great advantage to them. Suppose in one experiment there were 1000 uninoculated with a death-rate of 50 per cent and 100 inoculated also with a death-rate of 50 per cent, while in another experiment there were 1000 inoculated with a death-rate of 5 per cent and 100 uninoculated also with a death-rate of 5 per cent. Summarizing, we should find 1100 inoculated persons with 100 deaths, and 1100 uninoculated with 505 deaths, an enormous "advantage" to the inoculated group. No confidence should be placed in odds computed from such summaries." ((Greenwood, 1935), pp. 84–85).

This fallacy (quoted in Box 1) is referred to today as the Simpson's paradox (Simpson, 1951). It actually described the mechanism of confounding. The Yule's fallacy is also described by Hill in addition to several others.

The consequences of misclassification of exposure or disease are given increasing importance from McMahon and Pugh's texts on, and a full theory of misclassification appears in Rothman's text.

Susser's text popularizes the three-point diagram (confounding, exposure and disease) that became a classic way of depicting confounding (see Fig. 1).

Cohort and case-control design

Greenwood gives the example of a study comparing "incidence" in two cohorts but does not describe or mention the case-control design. Hill mentions the existence of prospective and retrospective designs, but does not explain their properties. In contrast, Morris does. MacMahon and Pugh and Lilienfeld and Lilienfeld dedicate separate chapters to cohort and case-control studies, describing their methodological aspects in detail. Case-control studies and cohort studies are essentially considered as distinct designs until Miettinen proposes the concept of "study base". From then on,

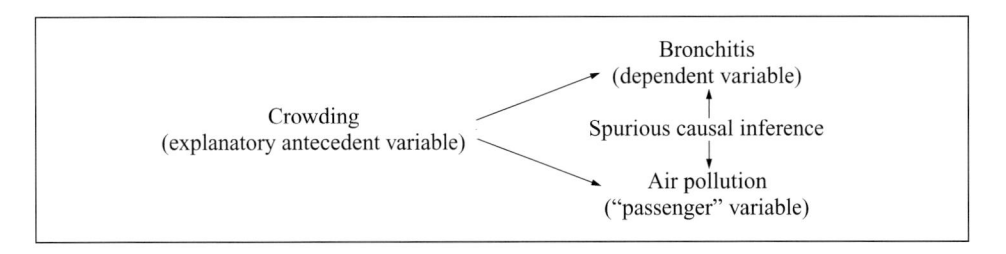

```
                                    Bronchitis
                                  (dependent variable)
                                        ↑
        Crowding              Spurious causal inference
(explanatory antecedent variable)       ↓
                                    Air pollution
                                  ("passenger" variable)
```

Figure 1
Diagram popularized by Susser to represent the potential connections between variables that may lead to confounding. Source: Susser (1973). Causal thinking in the health science, New York: Oxford University Press.

the case-control study becomes conceptualized as a specific sampling technique within cohorts or "dynamic populations". Rothman explains this with most clarity.

Causal inference

The necessary and sufficient conditions for disease occurrence are recognized in Greenwood's early textbook whereas the theory of multiple causation is first presented by Morris. The description of a specific method for causal inference in epidemiology appears in McMahon and Pugh's text. In the books of McMahon and Pugh, Susser, and Lilienfeld and Lilienfeld, we essentially find different versions of Hill's causal criteria (Hill, 1965). Susser mentions the concept of sufficient and necessary causes, and Miettinen alludes to a new approach to causality. Rothman's text has the most thorough discussion of causality. Using the now classic causal pies (Fig. 2), he relates interaction and strength of association to relation between component causes.

Interaction

The last concept to appear in this set of texts is interaction. The possibility of observing synergy and antagonism between several causes is mentioned in all texts from Greenwood to Lilienfeld and Lilienfeld, but the concept is not rigorously approached before Miettinen neatly distinguishes it from confounding (see Fig. 3) and Rothman describes it systematically. It is of note that both McMahon and Pugh and Rothman use the now classic example of the interaction between asbestos exposure, cigarette smoking and mortality from lung cancer (Hammond et al., 1979).

In summary, bias and confounding are the first modern concepts to be systematically present in the eight texts. The issue of study design has been a central concern

Table 1 – Summary of the contents of eight epidemiology textbooks with respect to the concepts of confounding, bias, cohort studies, case-control studies, causal inference and interaction. Grey background indicates that the concept is covered in the textbook

Textbook (publ. year)	Confounding	Bias	Cohort	Case-control	Causal inference	Interaction
Greenwood (1935)	• Greenwood's Fallacy (see Box 1)	• No specific mention of bias, but discusses comparability among groups and how certain differences arise	• Has an example which compares case incidence of typhoid in two cohorts of soldiers, one of which had been inoculated	• Absent	• Mentions necessary and sufficient conditions; the concept of causal inference is absent	• Mention of the interaction among innate qualities of the body, personal habits and constitutions of the atmosphere, but no theory of interaction is absent
Hill (1961)	• Emphasis on comparison groups should be the same in all relevant aspects; presents the third variable and mixing of non-comparable records but does not used the word confounding	• Has an entire chapter of selection, refers to non-representativity of the universe, self-selection and loss to follow-up as common forms of bias	• Proposes two observational forms of inquiry, one of which is prospective inquiry; however, no extensive discussion on cohort designs	• Proposes two observational forms of inquiry, one of which is the retrospective inquiry; compares the pros and cons of these two approaches; no mention on odds ratio	• Distinguishes association from causation; the concept of causal inference is absent	• Absent
Morris (1964)	• The concept is embedded in the presentation of selection problem; provides the first suggestion of stratification	• No terms of selection bias, recall bias and interviewer bias, but provides examples on all; concepts on reproducibility, validity, false positives and false negatives are developed	• Provides the first formal description of a cohort study design termed as longitudinal and forward looking	• The first mention of the term case-control studies, comparing it with prospective studies, no mention of odds ratio	• Elaborates multiple causes model	• Absent; interaction is used as meaning interrelation, not synergy or antagonism
MacMahon & Pugh (1970)	• Presented as non causal statistical associations or secondary associations; develops the criteria for potential confounders; suggests two possible solutions: matching and stratification	• No formal or systematic definition of bias, but selection bias, recall bias and interviewer bias are all described. The first theory of misclassification bias, sensitivity, specificity and predictive value are defined	• Gives a systematic treatment of cohort studies and coins the name cohort study	• Entire chapter devoted to case-control study, including control selection; case-control study is presented as inferior to the cohort study; theory of relative odds as an estimate of relative risk	• Illustrates web of causation mechanism, distinguishes causal and non-causal association, direct and indirect causal association; five criteria to evaluate causal association	• Interaction is presented as synergistic effect, corresponding to current additive interaction but proposed mode of evaluation is in the multiple scale

356

Table 1 – (continued)

Textbook (publ. year)	Confounding	Bias	Cohort	Case-control	Causal inference	Interaction
Susser (1973)	• Original contribution to confounding, introduces the now widely-used three arrows diagram; confounding can be handled in both study design and analysis	• States that randomization removes two kinds of bias: bias inherent in selecting subjects and bias inherent in foreknowledge of the outcome	• No conceptual refinements	• Indicates relative odds or cross-products ratio could stand on its own as a measure of association	• Defines necessary and sufficient cause; entire chapter on causal inference; introduces Mil's canons to identify causes	• Defines moderator variables
Lilienfeld & Lilienfeld (1980a)	• Refers to artificial association or indirect association	• Contains a more elaborated theory of selection bias; introduces Berkson's bias	• Distinguishes concurrent prospective and non-concurrent prospective studies	• Dedicates one entire chapter to retrospective and cross-sectional studies; states odds ratio	• Criteria for causal inference modified from Evans's criteria	• Calls interaction as interrelationship between risk factors, and the theory is still not fully developed
Miettinen (1985)	• Indicates that confounding belongs to conditional relations; first formalizes distinction between confounding and effect modification; introduces the method of controlling confounding in regression analysis	• Definition of bias, a classification of biases into three categories: comparability of effects, comparability of populations and comparability of information	• Introduces the concepts of study base: the population experience manifesting the occurrence under study	• Introduces the concepts of study base and case-referent study; provides a detailed mathematical discussion on odds ratio and confidence intervals	• No mention of causal inference	• Refers to interaction as interdependence in coaction, defines synergism and antagonism
Rothman (1986)	• Defines confounding as a mixing of effect; entire chapter on matching; both weak and strong criteria for confounding	• Definition of validity as lack of systematic error; distinguishes between internal and external validity; internal validity relates to selection bias, information bias and confounding	• Clarifies measures of disease occurrence in cohort studies	• Relates sampling of cases and controls independently of exposure status to removal of the sampling fractions in the odds ratio.	• Improved definition of cause; develop causal pies' and sufficient-component causes model • Elaborates on Hill's criteria as well as caveats when using these criteria as a hard and fast rule posed for causal inference	• Distinction between additive and multiplicative interaction; concepts of statistical, biological and public health interactions, applies sufficient component causes model to interpret interaction

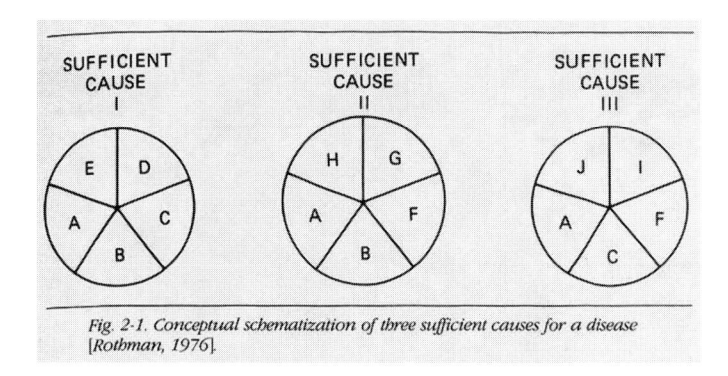

Fig. 2-1. Conceptual schematization of three sufficient causes for a disease [Rothman, 1976].

Figure 2
The causal pies popularization by Rothman to describe sufficient and component causes. Source: Rothman (1986). Modern epidemiology, Boston: Little, Brown and Company.

only since Morris. The concept of causal inference appears somewhat later and interaction is the latest concept to be formalized.

2. Evolution of the specific texts (horizontal reading of the table)

The evolution of the texts themselves, suggests that they can be grouped into three generations: the generation of early epidemiology, of classic epidemiology and of modern epidemiology.

Early epidemiology

Greenwood and Hill belong to the first generation. From the standpoint that we have chosen, they can be considered as statisticians or as epidemiologists. Their texts really insist on the issue of bias or fallacy, and for Hill on analytical methods. Interestingly, the differences between study designs do not appear to be a major concern. These designs were only starting to appear at the time of Greenwood. But even though Hill has been viewed as a pioneer of case-control studies and cohort studies, he never included specific chapters in his most reprinted text.

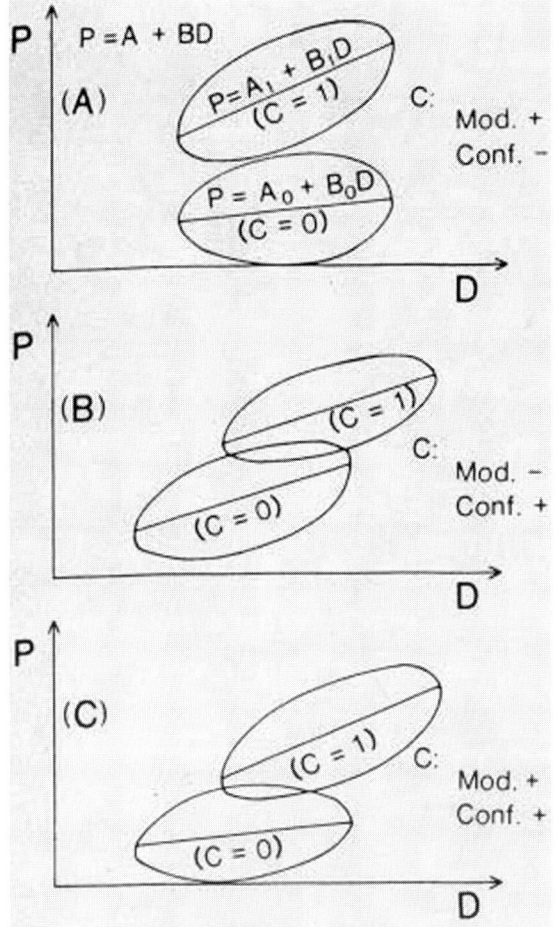

Evolution of epidemiologic methods and concepts in selected textbooks of the 20th century

Figure 1.6. Relation of occurrence parameter P to determinant D, with a view to the role of covariate C. (A) C modifies the measure of relation B but does not confound it. If C is ignored, the average (in a sense) of the conditional slopes is obtained. (B) No modification, but confounding. (C) Modification and confounding.

Figure 3
Schematic distinction between confounding and interaction (i.e., effect modification) by Miettinen. Source: Miettinen (1985). Theoretical epidemiology, New York: John Wiley & Sons.

Classic epidemiology

The senior authors of the second generation of textbooks are mostly physicians (Jerry Morris, Brian McMahon, Abraham Lilienfeld and Mervyn Susser) interested in public health. They put great emphasis on clarifying the qualities and properties of study designs, and in particular what distinguishes case-control studies from cohort studies. The texts also deal much more seriously with the issue of causal inference. This emphasis on study designs and causal inference may reflect the context in which these papers were written. These were the times when the scientific and political community met with a lot of skepticism on the epidemiological results showing that tobacco smoking had deleterious health effects. The interpretation of studies having different designs and the rationale for synthesizing the evidence demonstrating causality played a central role in the preparation of the US Surgeon General's Report on the health risk associated with smoking.

Modern epidemiology

Miettinen appears as the founder of this last generation. His innovative concepts, such as study-base, dynamic population, etc., revolutionize the way study designs and measures of effect are conceived. The theory of epidemiologic methods and concepts becomes one level more complex. Actually, Miettinen acknowledged this in the preface of his text by saying that epidemiology was previously "widely regarded as common sense activity, a line of research that any physician – even one without statistical education – is prepared to engage in" (Miettinen, 1985, p. VIII). We speculate that because of a convoluted style, which aggravates the complexity of the new material, the novelty of the approach was first only understood by a small circle of students, who re-expressed the new concepts and made them accessible to a wider audience. One of them is Rothman, whose text title can characterize the new generation: "modern epidemiology". In contrast to the previous generation, Miettinen and Rothman are much more inclined towards mathematics. Where classic epidemiology expressed concepts which have no necessary mathematical translations, almost all concepts, be it related to bias, confounding, interaction, etc., from Miettinen's and Rothman's texts can be written indifferently in words or in equations.

Conclusion

As a conclusion, we would like to stress some limitations, pitfalls and potential fallacious interpretations that may result from our work.

We insist that this review of eight texts be considered as an initial attempt to describe the evolution of epidemiologic concepts and methods in the material used for teaching the discipline. Much remains to be done. Within each generation there are many more texts. They may not only give different perspectives of the same concepts. Some may have been really innovative, in particular when they focus on specific issues (e.g., case-control study, randomized trial) or fields (e.g., occupational epidemiology, genetic epidemiology). They are certainly useful as their diversity matches the diversity of students of epidemiology.

Also, our starting points (i.e., currently taught epidemiological concepts) confer an advantage to the most recent texts, which of course cover more of the topics and discuss them more in depth. Textbooks are an expression of the state of development of a discipline at a given moment in time. They usually do not incorporate the latest methodological and conceptual developments, but tend to present material that has been around long enough to reach some level of consensus among scholars in the field. Texts therefore rarely reflect the innovative thinking of their authors but rather the author's ability to incorporate and synthesize other people's work. We found that the texts reviewed are not all as fair in acknowledging their theoretical debt.

Our review of specific topics could not capture the real historical impact of the texts. For example, Morris's text may well have been a model for the other classic epidemiology texts. Some books have genuine qualities that are not necessarily historically relevant. The texts could be reviewed for their literary quality. We are, for example, all seduced by the beautiful style and coherence of MacMahon and Pugh's text.

Textbooks are not simply a neutral compilation of material. The way the material is selected, assembled and presented reflects the global vision of the discipline of the author(s). As a whole the content of a textbook is not only of a scientific but also of a philosophical nature. This could be another way of revisiting epidemiology textbooks.

Finally, there is a time lag between the state of the literature and the content of textbooks. The content of the texts does not always reflect the full breadth of the contribution of their authors to the evolution of the discipline. This is most striking for Austin Bradford Hill whose text does not cover cohort and case-control studies in detail even though Doll and Hill designed and performed case-control and cohort studies that are considered as historical landmarks. Nor do we find before the eight edition of Hill's text a discussion of causal inference reflecting Hill's landmark paper (Hill, 1965). Similar considerations can be made about Jerry Morris, Brian MacMahon, Mervyn Susser and Abraham Lilienfeld.

Beyond these limitations, this survey of eight textbooks and five concepts/methods demonstrates that epidemiology, as a scientific discipline, is in constant evolution and transformation. Epidemiology students received a qualitatively different training across the 20th century and used texts that did not always cover the same material. All indicates that the process will continue and that epidemiology tomorrow will be taught differently from today. We are probably at the eve of a new qualitative change in epidemiology. Many have expressed the need to have new methodological tools able to assess the complexity of the causes of human health. The next generation of textbooks will have to address this issue and propose solutions.

Acknowledgments

We thank Prof Brian MacMahon and Jerry Morris for their review of a previous version of this manuscript.

Commentary on the paper by Zhang et al. – Interaction and evolution in epidemiology

Kenneth J. Rothmann

Department of Epidemiology and at the Division of Preventive Medicine, Department of Medicine, Boston University School of Medicine, 715 Albany Street, Boston, MA 02118, USA

Zhang et al. (2004) have traced the evolution of epidemiologic concepts through the "fossil record" of selected textbooks, one of which is my 1986 book, *Modern epidemiology* (Rothman, 1986). I would like to report that it feels better to be the author of a fossil than to be a fossil oneself, however fine that distinction may be – but some might argue with my premise.

Paradoxically, history seems to shorten as time progresses. When I began to study epidemiology at Harvard at the tail end of the 1960s, the text that we used was the 1960 book *Epidemiologic methods* by MacMahon, Pugh and Ipsen. Today this text is more than 40 years old, considerably older than Greenwood's (1935) text was in the 1960s. Although not on the list of Zhang et al. (2004), *Epidemiologic methods* was a clear and incisive compendium of cutting edge epidemiologic concepts. It was superseded in 1970 by a substantial revision, *Epidemiology: principles and methods*, authored by MacMahon and Pugh. The 1970 revision is on the list of books described by Zhang et al. (2004).

At about the time that the MacMahon and Pugh 1970 text was published, I was beginning to search for possible thesis topics for my doctoral dissertation in epidemiology. In my searching I came across a 1965 paper by Keller and Terris entitled "The association of alcohol and tobacco with cancer of the mouth and pharynx". Both alcohol and tobacco have causal effects on mouth cancer. These effects were mutually confounded because the two exposures were correlated. In their 1965 paper, Keller and Terris considered confounding between alcohol and tobacco, but did not address the question of possible interaction between the two causes. It was the issue of biologic interaction that first drew me into a concerted inquiry into epidemiologic concepts and methods.

The 1960 book by MacMahon et al. makes no mention of interaction, but by 1970, MacMahon had added a reference to Lancelot Hogben's description of the interaction between genes and environment (quoting Hogben's 1932 William Withering Memorial Lectures of the University of Birmingham, which were published in

1933 as *Nature and nurture*). Even so, the topic of interaction had barely been broached by epidemiologic teachers and writers. To conceptualize interaction, to proceed to evaluate it from epidemiologic data, and to distinguish it from other multivariable issues, required a synthesis of diverse epidemiologic topics, many of which were themselves in their early stages of development. These topics included causation, effect estimation, confounding, study design and analytic methods. Layered over these subjects was a fog of confusion caused by the fact that in statistics, the term "interaction" was often used in a sense that did not correspond to a singular, meaningful concept of biologic interaction.

Although I ultimately chose a different project for my epidemiology doctoral thesis, I did proceed to collaborate with Andrew Keller and to write a paper (Rothman and Keller, 1972) in which we proposed that interaction should be measured as a departure from additivity of effects, and in which we discussed the quantification of the risk of mouth cancer attributable to the interaction between alcohol and tobacco. My subsequent pursuit of this topic prepared me for *Modern epidemiology*, which I began to write a decade after the collaboration with Keller.

Today, knowledge of the core issues that drew me into the field of epidemiology has grown far beyond the more primitive levels of several decades ago. The field has also surged from having but a handful of textbooks to scores of useful texts. The hindsight provided by Zhang et al. (2004) in their review of selected epidemiology textbooks clarifies how many of the fundamental concepts have crystallized during the century in which epidemiology came of age.

Commentary on the paper by Zhang et al. – Lack of evolution of epidemiologic "methods and concepts"

Olli S. Miettinen

Joint Departments of Epidemiology & Biostatistics and Occupational Health, McGill University, 1020 Pine Avenue West, Montreal, Quebec H3A 1A2, Canada

Zhang et al. (2004), while writing about the "evolution of some epidemiologic methods and concepts," unwittingly illustrate the stagnancy of these. In particular, the still-prevalent commitment to "cohort study" and "case-control study" in etiologic research is evident from the very outset.

Different from what is definitional to a "cohort study" (Last, 2001), the etiologic history associated with a case identified in its follow-up of the cohort (closed population) should be defined and documented as of this outcome, not as of the beginning of the subject's follow-up. It should next be understood that for the thus-documented case series the referent is the population-time of the study cohort's follow-up. For, the case series is interpretable as the source of rate numerator inputs in reference to this population-time only; this referent of the case series therefore constitutes the study base to which the empirical occurrence relation – for the outcome's incidence density – refers. And as a final matter of liberation from "the cohort fallacy" (Miettinen, 1999) in etiologic research, it should be understood that this case series needs to be coupled with a similarly documented base series, a fair sample of the (infinite number of) person-moments constituting the study base. Given the database formed by these two series, it remains merely to fit to it the logistic-regression counterpart of the designed object of study – of the logarithm of the outcome's incidence density as a function of the etiologic history, conditionally on modifiers and non-modifier confounders, in a defined domain.

As for the "case-control study," then, it should be understood for a start that the case series again serves as the source of rate numerator inputs; that is, again, the rate numerator series. With this beginning of liberation from "the trohoc fallacy" (Miettinen 1999), the concern naturally is not to couple the case series with a "control group" but with a denominator series, a fair sample of the study base. The case series need not arise from follow-up of a directly-defined cohort. Instead, the source population may be a directly-defined dynamic (open) population; or it may be definable only indirectly – as the catchment population of the directly-defined scheme of case identification. For both series the etiologic histories are defined, again, as of the time of the outcome (case occurring or not occurring), and the rest also proceeds as above – as always in *the* etiologic study. In it, the comparison never is between a "case group" and a "control group." Instead, it always is between the index and reference segments of the study base. And it is only in reference to this contrast that the alternative to causality – confounding – can be understood.

It is of considerable note that this understanding of the etiologic study is key to understanding the intervention study as well. Cases are identified in a study base formed by a cohort's follow-up; the associated intervention histories as of case occurrence are documented; a similarly documented sample of the study base is obtained; etc. My current course compendium, the precursor of my upcoming textbook, actually goes well beyond intervention research, even. The working title now is "Scientific medicine: essence and epistemology." Its implicit overall message to my epidemiology colleagues is this:

Let us move beyond our traditional focus on the theory – concepts and principles – of merely etiologic research to concern for the theory of medicine, including the theory of the research that produces the knowledge base of scientific medicine; let us dedicate ourselves to such quintessentially "applied" research for the advancement of clinical as well as community medicine; and in it, let us be serious about object design – ultimately in terms of a regression function – before methods design, rejoicing in the consequent relevance of the research without concern for whether it still may be characterized as epidemiologic.

References

Ackerknecht EH (1967). Medicine at the Paris Hospital, 1794–1848. Baltimore: The John Hopkins Press.

Advisory Committee appointed by the Secretary of State for India, the Royal Society and the Lister Institute (1906). Reports on Plague investigations in India: part 1, experiments upon the transmission of plague by fleas. *J Hyg* VI: 425–482.

Agricola G (Tr1950). De Re Metallica [1556] Transl. Hoover HC, Hoover LH. New York: Dover.

Allchin D (2000). Of rice and man. http://www1.umn.edu/ships/modules/eijkman1.htm, 10/15/2000. Accessed 04/07/2004.

Altman DG, Bland JM (1999). Treatment allocation in controlled trials: why randomise? *BMJ* 318: 1209.

Altman LK (1987). Who goes first? The story of self-experimentation in medicine. New York: Random House.

American Thoracic Society, Committee on Revision of Diagnostic Standards (1969). Diagnostic standards and classification of tuberculosis. New York: National Tuberculosis and Respiratory Disease Association.

Anderson KM, Castelli WP, Levy D (1987). Cholesterol and mortality: 30 years of follow-up from the Framingham study. *JAMA* 257: 2176–80.

Andrieu N, Goldstein AM (1998). Epidemiologic and genetic approaches in the study of gene-environment interaction: an overview of available methods. *Epidemiol Rev* 20: 137–47.

Andvord KF (1930). Hvad kan vi laere ved a folge tuberkulosens gang fra generasjon til generasjon? Norsk Magasin Laegevidenskapen; 91: 642–60. (Engl. transl. by Gerard Wijsmuller).

Anonymous (1837a). Apothecaries' Company an anomaly – necessity for its reform and conversion into a college of pharmacy. *Br Ann Med* 1: 340–3.

Anonymous (1837b). Medical reform. Representative bodies v. the corporations. *Br Ann Med* 1: 63–6.

Anonymous (1837c). Progress of the medical profession – obstructions in the way. *Br Ann Med* 1: 29–31.

Anonymous (1861). [Editor's note] *Assurance Mag*; 9: 215.

Anonymous (1873). General report, census of England and Wales for the year 1871, B.P.P. LXII, pt 2: XXVIII.

Anonymous (1911). Mathematics and medicine [Editorial]. *BMJ* 2: 449.

Anonymous (1913). International Congress of Medicine. The Medical Officer 10: 104.

Anonymous (1921). The new epidemiology. *BMJ* 1: 432.

References

Archer VE, Magnuson HJ, Holaday DA, Lawrence PA (1962). Hazards to health in uranium mining and milling. *J Occup Med* 4: 55–60.

Armenian HK, Szklo M (1996). Morton Levin (1904-1995); history in the making (obituary) *Am J Epidemiol* 143: 648–9.

Arrighi M, Hertz-Picciotto I (1993). Definitions, sources, magnitude, effect modifiers and strategies of reduction of the Healthy Worker Effect. *JOM* 5: 890–1.

Ashton TS (1934). Economic and social investigations in Manchester, 1833–1933: a centenary history of the Manchester Statistical Society. London: Harvester Press.

Atkins E, Cherry N, Douglas JWB, Kiernan KE, Wadsworth MEJ (1981). The 1946 British cohort: an account of the origins, progress and results of the national survey of health and development. In: Medrick SA, Baert AE, eds. Prospective longitudinal research: an empirical basis for the primary prevention of psychosocial disorders. Oxford: Oxford University Press, 25–30.

Aubrey J [edited and with an introduction and notes by Anthony Powell] (1949) John Graunt – A brief life. http://www.ac.wwu.edu/~stephan/Graunt/AubreyGraunt.html#note. Accessed 04/07/2004.

Averill E, Samuels SW (1992). International occupational and environmental health. In: Rom WN, ed. Environmental and occupational medicine. 2nd ed. Boston: Little, Brown: 1357–64.

Bailar JC III (1978). Mammographic screening: a reappraisal of benefits and risks. *Clin Obstet Gynecol* 21: 1–14.

Baker WM (1862). Contribution to the statistics of cancer: a paper read to the Royal Medical and Chirurgical Society on June 24. Transactions of the Medico-Chirurgical Society of London, vol. XIV

Ballot AM (1873). Onderzoek naar de sterfte te Rotterdam en hare oorzaken. *Ned Tijdschr Geneeskd*; 2: 8–157.

Barabasi AL (2002). Linked: How Everything Is Connected to Everything Else and What It Means. Cambridge, MA: Perseus Publishing.

Barker DJP, Gluckman PD, Godfrey KM, Harding JE, Owen JA, Robinson JS (1993). Fetal nutrition and cardiovascular disease in adult life. *Lancet*; 341: 939–41.

Barker DJP, Osmond C (1986). Infant mortality, childhood nutrition and ischaemic heart disease. *Lancet*; 1: 1077–81.

Beebe GW, Hamilton HB (1975). Future research on atomic bomb survivors. *J Radiat Res*, 16 (Suppl): 149–65.

Beebe GW, Kato H, Land CE (1971). Studies of the mortality of A-bomb survivors. IV. Mortality and radiation dose 1950–1960. *Radiat Res*; 48: 613–49.

Beebe GW (1979). Reflections on the work of the Atomic Bomb Casualty Commission in Japan. *Epidemiologic Rev* 1: 184–208.

Bell G (1973). Predator-prey equations simulating an immune response. *Math Biosci* 16: 291–314.

Berkson J (1946). Limitations of the application of fourfold table analysis to hospital data. *Biometrics* 2: 47–53.

Bernal JD (1972). The extension of man : A history of physics before the quantum. Cambridge, MA: M.I.T. Press.
Bernard C (1865). Introduction à l'étude de la médecine expérimentale. Transl. Green H.G. New York: Dover, 1957.
Berrino F, Sant M, Verdecchia A, Capocaccia R, Estève J, Hakulinen T, eds. (1995). Survival of cancer patients in Europe: the EUROCARE study. Lyon: *IARC* (IARC Sci Publ; no. 132).
Berrino F, Capocaccio R, Coleman MP, Estève J, Gatta G, Hakulinen T, Micheli A, Sant M, Verdecchia A (2003). Survival of cancer patients in europe: the EUROCARE-3 study. *Ann Oncol*; 14 (suppl 5).
Berry G, Gilson JC, Holmes S, Lewinsohn HC, Roach SA (1979). Asbestosis: a study of dose-response relationships in an asbestos textile factory. *Brit J Industr Med*; 36: 98–112.
Blalock HM (1964). Causal inference in non-experimental research. Chapel Hill: University of North Carolina Press.
Bracken M (2003). The first epidemiologic text. *Am J Epidemiol 157*: 855–856.
Bradley DJ (1997). The intellectual legacies of Ronald Ross. *Indian J Malariol* 34: 73–5.
Breslow NE, Day NE (1987). Statistical methods in cancer research. Volume II: the design and analysis of cohort studies. Lyon: International Agency for Research on Cancer.
Brock TD (1988). Robert Koch, a life in medicine and bacteriology. Berlin: Springer.
Broders AC (1920). Squamous cell epithelioma of the lip: a study of five hundred and thirty-seven cases. *JAMA* 74: 656–64.
Brody H, Rip MR, Vinten-Johansen P, et al. (2000). Map-making and myth-making in Broad Street: the London cholera epidemic, 1854. *Lancet*; 356: 64–8.
Brown L, Pope EG (1904). The postdischarge mortality among the patients of the Adirondack Cottage Sanitarium. *Am Med*; 8: 879–82.
Brown PE (1964). Another look at John Snow. *Anesth Analg*; 43: 646–54.
Brown PE (1961). John Snow – the autumn loiterer. *Bull Hist Med*; 35: 519–28.
Buck C (1975). Popper's philosophy for epidemiologists. *Int J Epidemiol*; 4: 159–68.
Budd W (1849). Malignant Cholera: its cause, mode of propagation, and prevention. London: J. Churchill.
Busk T, Clemmesen J, Nielsen A (1948). Twin studies and other genetical investigation in the Danish cancer registry. *Br J Cancer* 2: 156–63.
Cameron D, Jones IG (1983). John Snow, the Broad Street pump and modern epidemiology. *Int J Epidemiol*; 12: 393–6.
Campbell DT, Stanley JS (1963). Experimental and quasi-experimental designs for research on teaching. In: Gage NL, ed. Handbook of research on teaching. Chicago: R. McNally: 171–246.
Carpenter KJ (1986). The history of scurvy and vitamin C. Cambridge: Cambridge University Press.
Carpenter KJ (2000). Beriberi, white rice, and vitamin B: A disease, a cause and a cure. Berkeley: University of California Press.
Carter KC (1983). Ignaz Semmelweis. The etiology, concept and prophylaxis of childbed fever. Madison: University of Wisconsin Press.

Case RAM, Hosker ME, McDonald DB, Pearson JT (1954). Tumours of the urinary bladder in workmen engaged in the manufacture and use of certain dyestuff intermediates in the British chemical industry. Part 1, The role of aniline, benzidine, alpha-naphthylamine and beta-naphthylamine. *Brit J Indust Med* 11: 75–104.

Case RAM, Lea AJ (1955). Mustard gas poisoning, chronic bronchitis, and lung cancer: an investigation into the possibility that poisoning by mustard gas in the 1914–18 war might be a factor in the production of neoplasia. *Brit J Prev Soc Med* 9: 62–72.

Case RAM, Pearson JT (1954). Tumours of the urinary bladder in workmen engaged in the manufacture and use of certain dyestuff intermediates in the British chemical industry. Part 2, Further considerations of the role of aniline and of the manufacture of auramine and magenta (fuchsine) as possible causative agents. *Brit J Indust Med* 11: 213–6.

Cassedy JH (1962). Charles V. Chapin and the Public Health Movement. Cambridge, MA: Harvard University Press.

Chadwick E (1842). Report of Her Majesty's Principal Secretary of State for the Home Department, from the Poor Law Commssioners, on an inquiry into the sanitary condition of the labouring population of Great Britain; with Appendices. London: Her Majesty's Stationery Office.

Chalmers I (1934) MRC Therapeutic Trials Committee's report on serum treatment of lobar pneumonia. BMJ 1934, The James Lind Library: http://www.jameslindlibrary.org/trial_records/20th_Century/1930s/MRC_trials/MRC_trials_commentary.html. Accessed 04/07/2004

Chalmers I (1999). Why transition from alternation to randomisation in clinical trials was made. *BMJ* 319: 1372.

Chave SPW (1958). Henry Whitehead and cholera in Broad Street. *Med Hist*; 2: 97–98.

Clarke R, Shipley M, Peto R, Collins R, Marmot M (1999). Underestimation of risk due to regression dilution bias in long-term follow-up of prospective studies. *Am J Epidemiol*; 150: 341–53.

Clayton D, Schifflers E (1987). Models for temporal variation in cancer rates II: age-period-cohort models. *Stats Med* 6: 469–81.

Clegg S (1913–14). Notes on an outbreak of enteric fever in Newcastle-upon-Tyne, August-October 1913. *Public Health*; 27: 235–43.

Clemmesen J (1974). Statistical studies in malignant neoplasms, vol. IV. Copenhagen: Munksgaard.

Cogan DG, Donaldson DD, Reese AB (1952). Clinical and pathological characteristics of radiation cataract. *Arch Ophthalmol*; 47: 55–70.

Cole P (1979). The evolving case-control study. *J Chron Dis* 32: 15–27.

Coleman MP, Estève J, Damiecki P, Arslan A, Renard H (1993). Trends in cancer incidence and mortality. Lyon: *IARC* (IARC IARC Sci Publ; no. 121).

Coleman W (1987). Yellow Fever in the North: the methods of early epidemiology. Madison: University of Wisconsin Press: 173.

Collins EL, Gilchrist JC (1928). Effects of dust upon coal trimmers. *J Indust Hyg* 10: 101–10.

Court Brown WM, Doll R (1957). Leukaemia and aplastic anemia in patients irradiated for ankylosing spondylitis. London: Her Majesty's Stationery Office. (Medical Research Council. Special report series; No. 295).

Comstock GW (Part II). Cohort analysis: W.H. Frost's contributions to the epidemiology of tuberculosis and chronic disease. *Soz Praventivmed* 2001; 46: 7–12.

Comstock GW (1985). Early studies of tuberculosis. National Cancer Institute Monograph 67. Selection, follow-up, and analysis in prospective studies: a workshop. Washington: U.S. Government Printing Office. (NIH Publication No. 85-2713).

Cornfield J (1951). A method of estimating comparative rates from clinical data; applications to cancer of the lung, breast, and cervix. *J Natl Cancer Inst* 11: 1269–1275.

Cornfield J (1954). Statistical relationhips and proof in medicine. *Am Statistician* 8: 19–21.

Cornfield J (1971). The University Group Diabetes Program: a further statistical analysis of the mortality findings. *JAMA* 217: 1676–87.

Cornfield J (1976). Recent methodological contributions to clinical trials. *Am J Epidemiol* 104: 408–21.

Cornfield J, Haenszel W (1960). Some aspects of retrospective studies. *J Chronic Dis* 11: 523–534.

Cornfield J, Haenszel W, Hammond EC, Lilienfeld AM, Shimkin MB, Wynder EL (1959). Smoking and lung cancer: recent evidence and a discussion of some questions. *J Natl Cancer Inst* 22: 173–203.

Correspondence (2000). Snow and the Broad Street pump: a rediscovery. *Lancet*; 356: 1688–9.

Court Brown WM, Doll R (1957). Leukaemia and aplastic anaemia in patients irradiated for ankylosing spondylitis. London: HMSO. (*Med Res Council Special Report Series*; No. 295).

Creighton Ch (1891). A history of epidemics in Britain. Cambridge: Cambridge University Press, vol II.

Creighton Ch (1894). A history of epidemics in Britian. Cambridge: Cambridge University Press, vol. II.

Crellin JK (1968). The Dawn of the germ theory: particles, infection and biology. In: Poynter FNL, ed. Medicine and science in the 1860s. Proceedings of the Sixth British Congress on the History of Medicine. London, Wellcome Institute of the History of Medicine: 57–76.

Cullen MJ (1975). The statistical movement in early Victorian Britain: the foundations of empirical social research. New York: Barnes and Noble.

Cutler SJ, Ederer F (1958). Maximum utilization of the life table method in analyzing survival. *J Chronic Dis* 8: 699–712.

Dawber TR, Meadors GF, Moore FE (1951). Epidemiological approaches to heart disease: the Framingham study. *Am J Public Health*; 41: 279–286.

De Morgan A (1860–61a). On an unfair suppression of due acknowledgment to the writings of Mr. Benjamin Gompertz. *Assurance Mag* 9: 86–89.

De Morgan A (1860–61b). On Gompertz's law of mortality. *Assurance Mag* 9: 214–215.

De Morgan A (1861–62). Mr. Edmonds: college life. *Assurance Mag* 10: 29–30.

Doll R (1952). The causes of death among gas-workers with special reference to cancers of the lung. *Brit J Industr Med* 9: 180.

Doll R (1955). Mortality from lung cancer in asbestos workers. *Br J Ind Med* 12: 81–86.
Doll R (1984). Landmark perspective: Smoking and death rates. *JAMA* 251: 2854–2857.
Doll R (1994) Austin Bradford Hill. *Biog Mem Fell Roy Soc* 40: 129–140.
Doll R (1998). The first reports on smoking and lung cancer. *Clio Med* 46: 130–140.
Doll R (Part II). Cohort studies: history of the method. I. Prospective cohort studies. *Soz Praventivmed* 2001; 46: 75–86.
Doll R (Part II). Cohort studies: history of the method. II. Retrospective cohort studies. *Soz Praventivmed* 2001; 46: 152–160.
Doll R, Hill AB (1950). Smoking and carcinoma of the lung; preliminary report. *Br Med J* 2: 739–748.
Doll R, Hill AB (1954). The mortality of doctors in relation to their smoking habits: a preliminary report. *Br Med J* 1: 1451–1455
Doll R, Hill AB (1956). Lung cancer and other causes of death in relation to smoking: a second report on the mortality of British doctors. *BMJ* 2: 1071–1081.
Doll R, Hill AB (1964). Mortality in relation to smoking: ten years' observations of British doctors. *BMJ* 1: 1399–1414, 1460–1467.
Doll R, Muir C, Waterhouse J, eds. (1970). Cancer incidence in five continents, vol. II. Berlin: Springer.
Doll R, Payne P, Waterhouse J, eds. (1966). Cancer incidence in five continents: a technical report. New York: Springer.
Doll R, Peto R (1981). The causes of cancer: quantitative estimates of avoidable risks of cancer in the United States today. *J Natl Cancer Inst* 66: 1191–1308.
Doll R, Peto R, Wheatley K, Gray R, Sutherland I (1994). Mortality in relation to smoking: 40 years' observations on male British doctors. *BMJ* 309: 901–911.
Doll R, Vessey MP, Beasley RWR, et al. (1972) The mortality of gas-workers: final report of a prospective study. *Brit J Industr Med* 29: 394–406.
Doll WR, Hill AB (1952). A study of the aetiology of cancer of the lung. Br Med J ii: 1271–1286.
Dormanns E (1936). Die vergleichende geographisch-pathologische Reichscarcinom-statistik. 11th Congrès Internationale de Lutte Scientifique et Sociale contre le Cancer. Bruxelles: Ligue Nationale Belge contre le Cancer: t. 1, 460–482.
Dorn HF (1951). Methods of measuring incidence and prevalence of disease. *Am J Public Health* 41: 271–278.
Dorn HF (1959). Some problems arising in prospective and retrospective studies of the etiology of disease. *N Engl J Med* 261: 571–579.
Dorn HF, Culter SJ (1959). Morbidity from cancer in the United States. Washington D.C.: U.S. Government Printing Office (Publ Health Monogr; vol. 56).
Downes J (1935). A study of the risk of attack among contacts in tuberculous families in a rural area. *Am J Hyg* 1935; 22: 731–742.
Doyle AC (1890a). The end of the Islander. In: Doyle AC: The complete Sherlock Holmes: The sign of four, Chapter 10, http://www.bakerstreet221b.de/canon/sign-10.htm. *Accessed 04/15/04.*

Doyle AC (1890b). The science of deduction. In: Doyle AC: The complete Sherlock Holmes: The sign of four, Chapter 1, http://www.bakerstreet221b.de/canon/sign-1.htm. *Accessed 04/15/04.*

Doyle HN (1969). Pneumoconiosis in bituminous coal miners. In: Lainhart WS, Doyle HN, Enterline PE, Henschel A, Kendrick MA, eds. Pneumoconiosis in Appalachian bituminous coal miners. Washington DC: USDHEW *Public Health Service Bureau of Occupational Safety and Health*: 3–20.

Driver CH (1929). A forgotten sociologist. *J. Adult Ed* 3: 134–154.

Ducan W (1852). Letter. *J Statist Soc Lond* 15: 183.

Dunn JE, Buell P (1959). Association of cervical cancer with circumcision of sexual partner. *J Nat Cancer Inst* 22: 749–64.

Editorial (1942). Cancer of the lung. *Br Med J* 1: 672–673.

Editorial (1950). Cigarettes and cancer. *Br Med J* 2: 767–768.

Editorial (1952). Cancer of the lung. *Lancet* ii: 667.

Edmonds TR (1828). Practical, moral and political economy, or the government, religion and institutions most conducive to individual happiness and to national power. London: E. Wilson.

Edmonds TR (1832a). An enquiry into the principles of population, exhibiting a system of regulations for the poor; Designed immediately to lessen, and finally to remove, the evils which have hitherto pressed upon the labouring classes of society. London: J. Duncan.

Edmonds TR (1832b). Life Tables founded upon the discovery of a numerical law, regulating the existence of every human being. Illustrated by a new theory of the causes producing health and longevity. London: J. Moyes.

Edmonds TR (1834–35a). On the laws of collective vitality. *Lancet* 2: 5–8.

Edmonds TR (1834–35b). On the mortality of the people of England. *Lancet* 1834–35b; 2: 310–316.

Edmonds TR (1835–36a). On the law of mortality in each county of England. *Lancet* 1: 364–371, 408–416.

Edmonds TR (1835–36b). On the laws of sickness, according to age, exhibiting a double coincidence between the laws of sickness and the laws of mortality. *Lancet* 1: 855–858.

Edmonds TR (1835–36c). On the mortality at Glasgow, and on the increasing mortality in England. *Lancet* 2: 353–359.

Edmonds TR (1835–36d). On the mortality of infants in England. *Lancet* 1: 690–694.

Edmonds TR (1835–36e). Statistics of the London Hospital, with remarks on the law of sickness. *Lancet* 2: 778–783.

Edmonds TR (1836). Laws of human mortality. *Br Med Almanack*: 104–109.

Edmonds TR (1836–37). [sic] Defense of an article in the "British Medical Almanack" entitled "National Statistics". *Lancet* 1: 590–592.

Edmonds TR (1837). Statistics of mortality in England. *Br Med Almanack* suppl: 130–137.

Edmonds TR (1855). On the laws of mortality and sickness of the labouring classes of England. *Assurance Mag* 5: 127–145.

Edmonds TR (1859). To William Farr, 6 April 1859, London School of Economics, Farr Collection I: ff. 44–45b.

References

Edmonds TR (1860). To Farr, 25 May 1860, London School of Economics, Farr Collection I: ff 46–47b.

Edmonds TR (1860–61a). On the discovery of the law of human mortality, and on the antecedent partial discoveries of Dr. Price and Mr. Gompertz. *Assurance Mag* 9: 170–184.

Edmonds TR (1860–61b). On the law of human mortality; and on Mr. Gompertz's new exposition of his law of mortality. *Assurance Mag* 9: 27–41.

Edmonds TR (1861–62). On the value of Mr. Gompertz's formula for the number living, in terms of the mortality according to age, compared with the value of a similar formula published in 1832. *Assurance Mag* 10: 104–113.

Einstein A, Imfeld L (1966). The evolution of physics. New York: Touchstone.

Elandt-Johnson R (1975). Definition of rates: some remarks on their use and misuse. *Am J Epidemiol* 102: 267–271.

Elandt-Johnson RC, Johnson NL (1980). Survival models and data analysis. New York: J. Wiley.

Elderton WP, Perry SJ (1910). Drapers' Company Research Memoirs. Studies in National Deterioration. VI: A third study of the statistics of pulmonary tuberculosis. The mortality of the tuberculous and sanatorium treatment. London: Cambridge University Press.

Elliott P, Cuzick J, English D, Stern R, eds. (1992). Geographical and environmental epidemiology: methods for small area studies. Oxford; New York; Tokyo: Oxford University Press.

Elmore JG, Feinstein AR (1994) Joseph Goldberger: An Unsung Hero of American Clinical Epidemiology. *Ann Intern Med* 121: 372–375

Epidemiological Society of London (1884). Epidemic Diseases: International Health Exhibition Conferences. London: Executive Council of the International Health Exhibition: 1.

Evans AS (1993). Causation and disease: a chronological journey. New York: *Plenum Medical Book Co.*

Eyler J (1979). Victorian social medicine: the ideas and methods of William Farr. Baltimore: The Johns Hopkins University Press.

Eyler JM (1973). William Farr on the cholera: the sanitarian's disease theory and the statistician's method. *J Hist Med* 28: 79–100.

Eyler JM (1980). The conceptual origins of William Farr's epidemiology: numerical methods and social thought in the 1830s, in Times, places, and persons: aspects of the history of epidemiology, ed. Abraham M. Lilienfeld. Baltimore: Johns Hopkins University Press, 1–21.

Eyler JM (Part IIa). The changing assessments of John Snow's and William Farr's cholera studies. *Soz Praventivmed* 2001; 46: 225–232.

Eyler JM (Part IIb). Constructing vital statistics: Thomas Rowe Edmonds and William Farr, 1835–1845. *Soz Praventivmed* 2002; 47: 6–13.

Eyler JM (2002). Edmonds, Thomas Rowe. New Dictionary of National Biography (forthcoming).

Eyler JM (Part IIc). Understanding William Farr's 1838 article "On prognosis": comment. *Soz Praventivmed* 2003; 48: 290–292.

Farr W (1835). Lecture on the history of hygiene. *Lancet* i: 773–780.

Farr W (1835–36a). Lecture introductory to a course on hygiene, or the preservation of the public health. *Lancet* 1: 240–245.
Farr W (1835–36b). Lecture on the history of hygiene. *Lancet* 1: 773–780.
Farr W (1837a). On a method of determining the danger and the duration of diseases at every period of their progress, Article I. *Br Ann Med* 1: 72–79.
Farr W (1837b). On the law of recovering and dying in small–pox, Article II. *Br Ann Med* 1.
Farr W (1837c). Statistics of insanity. *Br Ann Med* 1: 648–563, 679–683, 744-748, 811–814.
Farr W (1837d). Vital statistics. *Br Ann Med* 1: 353–360.
Farr W (1837e). Statistics of insanity. *Br Ann Med* 2: 137–140, 171–174, 204–207, 235–239, 357–361.
Farr W (1837f). Vital statistics. In: McCulloch JR, ed. A statistical account of the British Empire: exhibiting its extent, physical capacities, population, industry, and civil and religious institutions. London: C. Knight.
Farr W (Part II). On prognosis. *British Medical Almanack* Suppl: 1838: 199–216.
Farr W (1839). Diseases of towns and open country. 1st A.R.R.G., *B.P.P*; XVI: 76–81 (108–118).
Farr W (1840a). Diseases of towns and of the open country. 2nd A.R.R.G., *B.P.P.*; XVII: 9–12 (79–85).
Farr W (1840b). Progress of epidemics. Epidemic of small pox. 2nd A.R.R.G., *B.P.P.*; XVII: 16–20 (91–98).
Farr W (1840c), Letter. 2nd A.R.R.G.B.P.P.; XVII: 88 [14].
Farr W (1841a). Diseases of towns, and of the open country. 3rd A.R.R.G., *B.P.P.* Sess 2; VI: 20–22 (98–101).
Farr W (1841b). Report on the mortality of lunatics. *J Statist Soc Lond* 4: 17–33.
Farr W (1842). Letter, 4th A.R.R.G., *B.P.P.* XIX.
Farr W (1843a). Causes of the high mortality in town districts. 5th A.R.R.G., *B.P.P.*; XXI: 00–15 (406–35).
Farr W (1843b). Construction of life tables. 5th A.R.R.G., *B.P.P.*; XXI: 161–77 (342–367).
Farr W (1843c). Diseases of towns and of the open country. 5th A.R.R.G., *B.P.P.*; XXI: 194–199 (50–51, 397–405).
Farr W (1844). Letter, 6th A.R.R.G., *B.P.P.*; XIX: 290–358 (517–666).
Farr W (1852). Report on the cholera mortality in England, 1848–49. London: Her Majesty's Stationery Office.
Farr W (1852a). Influence of elevation on the fatality of cholera. *J Statist Soc Lond*; 15: 155–83.
Farr W (1856). "Letter to the Registrar General", 17th A.R.R.G. *B.P.P.*, XVIII: 74–99.
Farr W (1857–58). Testimony. Report of the commissioners appointed to inquire into the regulations affecting the sanitary condition of the army, the organization of military hospitals, and the treatment of the sick and wounded. *British parliamentary papers*, XVIII: 242–247.
Farr W (1859a). Letter. 20th A.R.R.G., *B.P.P.* Sess 2; XII: 174–176.
Farr W (1859b). On the construction of life tables. *Phil Trans* 149: 864–878.

Farr W (1862). A method of determining the effects of systems of treatment in certain diseases. *BMJ* 2: 193–195.

Farr W (1864). Letter to the Registrar General on the Causes of Death in England. 25th annual report of the Registrar General of births, deaths, and marriages in England.

Farr W (1865). Letter. Suppl. 25th A.R.R.G., *B.P.P.* XIII.

Farr W (1866). Mr. Lowe and the cattle plague. *Daily News* (London), 19 Feb.: 5–6.

Farr W (1868–69). Letter, 30th A.R.R.G., *B.P.P.* XVI.

Farr W (1875). Letter to the Registrar-General on the mortality in the registration districts of England during the years 1861–70 in Supplement to the 35th annual report of the Registrar-General of births, deaths, and marriages in England.

Farr W (1875a). Letter, suppl. 35th A.R.R.G. *B.P.P.* XVIII, Pt. 2.

Farr W (1878). Density or proximity of population: Its advantages and disadvantages. *Trans Nat Assn Prom Soc Sci*: 530–535.

Farr W (1878–79). Letter. 40th A.R.R.G., *B.P.P.*; XIX: 331–346.

Farr W (Part II) "On prognosis" by William Farr (British Medical Almanack 1838; Supplement 199–216). *Soz Praventivmed* 2003; 48: 219–224, 279–284.

Farr W (1866a). Address on public health, trans. *Natl Assn Prom Social Science*. Manchester: National Association for the Promotion of Social Science: 75–76.

Farr W (1867–68). Report of the cholera epidemic of 1866 in England, Suppl. 29th A.R.R.G. *B.P.P.*: XXXVII.

Farr W (1885). The mortality of cholera in England, 1848–49 and 17th Annual Report. In: Humphreys NA, ed. Vital statistics. A memorial volume of selections from the reports and writings of William Farr. London: *Sanitary Institute*

Fee E (1987). Disease and discovery. A history of the Johns Hopkins School of Hygiene and Public Health, 1916–1939. Baltimore: *The Johns Hopkins Press*.

Feinleib M, Zelen M (1969). Some pitfalls in the evaluation of screening programs. *Arch Environ Health* 19: 412–415.

Feinstein AR (1979). Methodologic problems and standards in case-control research. *J Chron Dis* 32: 35–41.

Feinstein AR, Sosin DM, Wells CK (1985). Stage migration and new diagnostic techniques as a source of misleading statistics for survival in cancer. *N Engl J Med* 312: 1604–1608.

Finer SE (1952). The life and times of Sir Edwin Chadwick. London: Methuen.

Fisher RA (1937). The design of experiments. London: Oliver and Boyd.

Fisher RA (1959). Smoking-the cancer controversy; Some attempts to assess the evidence. Edinburgh, Scotland: Oliver and Boyd.

Folley JH, Borges W, Yamasaki T (1952). Incidence of leukaemia in survivors of the atomic bomb in Hiroshima and Nagasaki. *Am J Med*; 13: 311–321.

Fox AJ, Collier PF (1976). Low mortality rates in industrial cohort studies due to selection for work and survival in the industry. *Br J Prev Soc Med* 30: 225–230.

Francis T Jr, Jablon S, Moore FE (1955). Report of ad hoc committee for appraisal of ABCC program. [Technical report] Hiroshima; Nagasaki: Atomic Bomb Casualty Commission: 33–59.

Freeman J, Hutchison GB (1980). Prevalence, incidence and duration. *Am J Epidemiol* 112: 707–723.

Freeman J, McGowan JE Jr (1978). Risk factors for nosocomial infection. *J Infect Dis* 138: 811–819.

Freud, KM, Belanger AJ, D'Agostino RB, Kannel WB (1993). The health risks of smoking: the Framingham study: 34 years of follow-up. *Ann Epidemiol*; 3: 417–424.

Frost WH (1923). The importance of epidemiology as a function of health departments. *Medical Officer* (London); 23: 113–4.

Frost WH (1927). Epidemiology. Nelson Loose-Leaf System, Public Health – Preventive Medicine. Volume 2, Chapter 7. New York: Thomas Nelson & Sons. [Reprinted in (Frost, 1941)].

Frost WH (1933). Risk of persons in familial contact with pulmonary tuberculosis. *Am J Public Health*; 23: 426–32.

Frost WH (1935). The outlook for the eradication of tuberculosis. *Am Rev Tuberc* 1935; 32: 644–50.

Frost WH (1937). How much control of tuberculosis? *Am J Public Health*; 27: 759–66.

Frost WH (1939). The age selection of mortality from tuberculosis in successive decades. *Am J Hyg* 30: 91–96. Reprinted in AmJ. Epidemol 1995; 141: 4–9.

Frost WH (1941). Epidemiology. In: Maxcy KF (ed): Papers of Wade Hampton Frost, M.D.: A contribution to epidemiological methods. New York: Common Wealth Fund.

Galbraith N (1966–67). A national epidemiological service. *Public Health*, 81: 224–225.

Garrison F (1929). An introduction to the history of medicine. 4th ed. Philadelphia: W.B. Saunders.

Gaynes RP, Martone WJ, Culver DH, et al. (1991). Comparison of rates of nosocomial infections in neonatal intensive care units in the United States. National Nosocomial Infections Surveillance System. *Am J Med* 91: 192S–6S.

Gerhard WW (1837). On the typhus fever, which occurred at Philadelphia in the spring and summer of 1836; illustrated by clinical observations at the Philadelphia hospital; showing the distinction between this form of disease and dothinenteritis, or the typhoid fever, with alteration of the follicles of the small intestine. *Am J Med Sci* 19: 289–322.

Gerstman BB (Part II). Comments regarding "On prognosis" by William Farr (1838), with reconstruction of his longitudinal analysis of smallpox recovery and death rates. *Soz Praventivmed* 2003; 48: 285–289.

Glesby MJ, Hoover DR (1996). Survivor treatment selection bias in observational studies: examples from the AIDS literature. *Ann Intern Med* 124: 999–1005.

Goldberger J, Wheeler GA, Sydenstricker E (1920a). A study of the relation of diet to pellagra incidence in seven textile-mill communities of South Carolina in 1916. *Public Health Rep* 35: 648–713.

Goldberger J, Wheeler GA, Sydenstricker E (1920). A study of the relation of family Income and other economic factors to pellagra incidence in seven cotton-mill villages of South Carolina in 1916. *Public Health Rep* 35: 2673–2714.

Golding J, Paterson M, Kinlen LJ (1990). Factors associated with child cancer in a national cohort study. *Br J Cancer* 62: 304–308.

Gompertz B (1825). On the nature of the function expressive of the law of human mortality, and on a new mode of determining the value of life contingencies. *Phil Trans* 115: 513–583.

Gordis L (2000). Epidemiology. Philadelphia: W.B. Saunders.

Gordon JE (1950). Epidemiology – old and new. Journal of the Michigan State Medical Society 49: 194–199.

Graunt J (1939). [1662] Natural and political observations made upon the Bills of Mortality. Baltimore: Johns Hopkins University Press. www.ac.wwu.edu/~stephan/Graunt/. Accessed 04/08/2004.

Greenland S (1987a). Evolution of epidemiologic ideas. Annotated readings on concepts and methods. Chesnut Hill, MA: *Epidemiologic Resources Inc.*

Greenland S (1987b). Joseph Berkson: Limitations of the application of fourfold table analysis to hospital data. Biometrics 1946; 2: 47-53. In: Greenland S (ed): Evolution of epidemiologic ideas. Los Angeles: *Epidemiology Resource Inc*: 86.

Greenland S, Thomas DC (1982). On the need for the rare disease assumption in case-control studies. *Am J Epidemiol* 116: 547–553.

Greenland S, Thomas DC, Morgenstern H (1986). The rare-disease assumption revisited. A critique of "estimators of relative risk for case-control studies". *Am J Epidemiol* 124: 869–883.

Greenwood E (1945). Experimental sociology: a study in method. New York: King's Crown Press.

Greenwood M (1904). A first study of the weight, variability, and correlation of human viscera, with special reference to the healthy and diseased heart. *Biometrika* 3: 63–83.

Greenwood M (1916). The application of mathematics to epidemiology. *Nature* XCVII: 243–244.

Greenwood M (1919). The epidemiological point of view. *BMJ* 2: 406.

Greenwood M (1924). Is the statistical method of any value in medical research? *Lancet* 2: 153–158.

Greenwood M (1926). A report on the natural duration of cancer. London: His Majesty's Stationery Office.

Greenwood M (1932). Epidemiology historical and experimental. Baltimore: Johns Hopkins Press.

Greenwood M (1935). Epidemics & crowd diseases: Introduction to the study of epidemiology. North Stratford: Ayer Company Publishers, Inc. or London: Williams and Norgate.

Greenwood M, Yule G (1914–15). The statistics of anti-typhoid and anti-cholera inoculations, and the interpretation of such statistics in general. *Proc Roy Soc Med*; 8: 113–194.

Greenwood M. (1944) William Whiteman Carlton Topley. *Biog Mem Fell Roy Soc*; 4: 699–712.

Guy WA (1843). Contributions to a knowledge of the influence of employment on health. *J Roy Stat Soc* 6: 197–211.

Hacking I (1975). The emergence of probability. Cambridge: Cambridge University Press.

Haley RW, Hooton TM, Culver DH et al. (1981). Nosocomial infections in U.S. hospitals, 1975–1976: estimated frequency by selected characteristics of patients. *Am J Med* 70: 947–959.

Hamer WH (1917). The epidemiology of cerebrospinal fever. *Proc R Soc Med* 10: 17–44.

Hammond EC (1966). Smoking in relation to death rates of one million men and women. *Natl Cancer Inst Monogr* 19: 127–204.

Hammond EC, Horn D (1954). The relationship between human smoking habits and death rates: a follow-up study of 187,766 men. *JAMA*; 154: 1316–1328.

Hammond EC, Horn D (1958) Smoking and death rates, Report on forty four months of follow-up of 187,783 men. *JAMA* 166: 1159–1172, 1294–1308.

Hammond EC, Selikoff IJ, Seidman H (1979). Asbestos exposure, cigarette smoking and death rates. *Ann N Y Acad Sci* 330: 473–490.

Hardy A (1998). On the cusp: Epidemiology and bacteriology at the Local Government Board, 1890–1905. *Med Hist*; 42: 328–346.

Hardy A (2000). Food, hygiene and the laboratory: a short history of food poisoning in Britain, circa 1850–1950. *Soc Hist Med*; 12: 293–311.

Hardy A (Part II). Methods of outbreak investigation in the "era of bacteriology" 1880–1920. *Soz Praventivmed* 2001; 46: 355–360.

Hardy A, Magnello ME (Part II). Statistical methods in epidemiology: Karl Pearson, Ronald Ross, Major Greenwood and Austin Bradford Hill, 1900–1945. *Soz Praventivmed* 2002; 47: 80–89.

Hardy RC, White C (1971). Matching in retrospective studies. *Am J Epidemiol* 93: 75–6.

Härting FH, Hesse W (1879). Der Lungenkrebs, die Bergkrankheit in den Schneeberger Gruben. Vierteljahreschr Gerichtl Med Offentl Gesundheitswesen 31: 102–32, 313–337.

Hempel CG (1966). Philosophy of natural science. Englewood Cliffs, NJ: Prentice-Hall.

Hemstreet GP (1998). Renal-urinary system. In: Encyclopaedia of occupational health and safety. Vol. 1. (ed: Stellman JM), Chapter 8. 4th ed. Geneva: ILO.

Hennekens CH, Buring JE (1987). *Epidemiology in medicine*. Boston: Little Brown.

Hennekens CH, Buring JE, Manson JE, et al. (1996). Lack of effect of long-term supplementation with beta-carotene on the incidence of malignant neoplasms and cardiovascular disease. *New Engl J Med*; 334: 1145–1149.

Herbst AL, Ulfelder H, Poskanzer DC (1971). Adenocarcinoma of the vagina: association of maternal stilbestrol therapy with tumor appearance in young women. *N Engl J Med* 284: 878–881.

Hill AB (1933). Some aspects of the mortality from whooping-cough (with discussion). *J R Stat Soc* 96: 240–273; 283–285.

Hill AB (1937). Principles of medical statistics. London: *The Lancet*. (Postgraduate series; vol. 3).

Hill AB (1939). Principles of medical statistics. London: The Lancet Ltd.

Hill AB (1953). Observation and experiment. *N Engl J Med* 248: 995–1001.

Hill AB (1961). Principles of medical statistics. New York: Oxford University Press.

References

Hill AB (1965). Environment and disease: association or causation? *Proc Royal Soc Med* 58: 295–300.

Hill AB (1966). Principles of medical statistics. 8th ed. London: *The Lancet Ltd*.

Hill AB (1984). A short textbook on medical statistics. 11th ed. London: Hodder & Staughton.

Hill GB (1997). RE: "P. C. A. Louis and the birth of clinical epidemiology". *J Clin Epidemiol* 50: 1187–1188.

Hippocrates (translated by Francis Adams) (400a BCE). On Airs, Waters, and Places. http://etext.library.adelaide.edu.au/h/h7w/airs_wat.html. *Accessed* 04/06/2004.

Hippocrates (translated by Francis Adams) (400b BCE). The Book of Prognostic. http://classics.mit.edu/Hippocrates/prognost.html. *Accessed* 04/06/2004.

Hippocrates (translated by Francis Adams) (400c BCE). Of the Epidemics. Book I. Sect.1. First constitution. http://etext.library.adelaide.edu.au/h/h7w/epidemic.html. *Accessed* 04/06/2004.

Hogben L (1933). Nature and nurture. London: Williams and Northgate.

Hogben L (1950–51). Major Greenwood. Obituary Notices of Fellows of the Royal Society 7: 139–54.

Hogue CJ, Gaylor DW, Schulz KF (1983). Estimators of relative risk for case-control studies.

Houston A (1904). The bacteriological examination of oysters and estuarial waters. *J Hyg* 1904; 4: 173–200.

Hrobjartsson A, Gotzsche PC, Gluud C (1998). The controlled clinical trial turns 100 years: Fibiger's trial of serum treatment of diphtheria. *BMJ* 317: 1243–1245.

Hume D (1739). A Treatise of Human Nature. Oxford, New York: Oxford University Press. 1978

Humphreys N, ed. (1885a). Vital statistics: a memorial volume of selections from the reports and writings of William Farr. London: Offices of the Sanitary Institute.

Humphreys NA (1885b). Biographical sketch of William Farr. In: Vital Statistics: a memorial volume of selections from the Reports and Writings of William Farr. London: Office of the Sanitary Institute: VII–XXIV.

Hunter D (1969). The disease of occupations. 4th ed. Boston: Little, Brown.

Hurwitz ES, Barrett MJ, Bregman D (1987). Public Health Service study of Reye's syndrome and medications: report of the main study. *JAMA* 257: 1905–1911.

Hutchinson GB, Shapiro S (1968). Lead time gained by diagnostic screening for breast cancer. *J Natl Cancer Inst* 41: 665–681.

Ibrahim MA, ed. (1979) Proceedings of symposium on the case-control study. *J Chron Dis* 32: 1–139.

Iezzoni LI (1996). 100 apples divided by 15 red herrings: a cautionary tale from the mid-19th-century on comparing hospital mortality rates. *Ann Intern Med* 124: 1079–1085.

International Agency for Research on Cancer, ed. (1984). IARC monographs on the evaluation of the carcinogenic risk of chemicals to humans. Polynuclear aromatic compounds. Part 3, Industrial exposure in aluminum production, coal gasification, coke production, and iron and steel founding. Vol. 34. Lyon: *IARC*: 133–190.

International Agency for Research on Cancer, ed. (1987). Arsenic. In: IARC monographs on the evaluation of carcinogenic risks to humans. Suppl. 7, Overall evaluations of carcinogenicity: an updating of *IARC* monographs 1 to 42. Lyon: IARC: 100–106.

International Agency for Research on Cancer (1994). IARC Monographs on the evaluation of carcinogenic risks to humans. Lyon: *IARC*. (Vol. 61).

International Agency for Research on Cancer (1995). Biennial Report 1994–95. Lyon: IARC.

Jablon S, Ishida M, Yamasaki M (1965). Studies of the mortality of A-bomb survivors. 3. Description of the sample and mortality, 1950–1960. *Radiat Res*; 25: 25–52.

Jones H (1994). Health and society in twentieth-century Britain. London: Longmans.

Kagan A, Dawber TR, Kannel WB, Revotskie N (1962). The Framingham study: a prospective study of coronary heart disease. *Federation Proc*; 21 pt. 2: 52–57.

Kannel WB, Gordon T (1970). Some characteristics related to the incidence of cardiovascular diseases and death: Framingham Study, 16-year follow-up. Washington DC: Govt Printing Office.

Kasius RV, ed. (1974). The challenge of facts. Selected public health papers of Edgar Sydenstricker. New York: Prodist.

Kato H (1971). Mortality in children exposed to A-bombs while in utero. *Am J Epidemiol*; 93: 435–442.

Katsuya T, Koike G, Yee TW, et al. (1995). Association of angiotensin gene T235 variant with increased risk of coronary heart disease. *Lancet* 345: 1600–1603.

Kehrberg MW, Latham RH, Haslam BT, et al. (1981). Risk factors for staphylococcal toxic-shock syndrome. *Am J Epidemiol* 114: 873–879.

Keller AZ, Terris M (1965). The association of alcohol and tobacco with cancer of the mouth and pharynx. *Am J Public Health* 55: 1578–1585.

Kelsey JL, Thompson WD, Evans A (1986). Methods in observational epidemiology. New York: Oxford University Press.

Kelsey JL, Whittemore AS, et al. (1996). Methods in observational epidemiology. New York: Oxford University Press.

Kennaway EL, Kennaway NM (1947). A further study of the incidence of cancer of the lung and larynx. *Brit J Cancer*; 1: 260.

Kiernan KE, Colley JRT, Douglas JWB, Reid DD (1976). Chronic cough in young adults in relation to smoking habits, childhood environment and chest illnesses. *Respiration*; 33: 236–244.

King JE (1983). Utopian or Scientific? A reconsideration of the Ricardian Socialists. *Hist Polit Econ* 15: 345–373.

Kish L (1959). Some statistical problems in research design. *Am Sociol Rev* 26: 328–338.

Kleinbaum DG, Kupper LL, Morgenstern H (1982). Epidemiologic research: Principles & quantitative methods. New York: Van Nostrand Reinhold.

Klinger D. Epidemiological observations on the antityphoid campaign in the south-west of the German empire. *JRAMC* 1910; 14: 90–101.

Korteweg R (1952). The age curve in lung cancer. *Br J Cancer* 5: 21–27.

References

Kramer MS, Boivin JF (1989). Directionality, timing and sample selection in epidemiologic research designs. *J Clin Epid* 42: 827–828.

Kraus AS (1954). The use of hospital data in studying the association between a characteristic and a disease. *Public Health Rep* 69: 1211–1214.

Kurland LT, Molgaard CA, Schoenberg BG (1982). Mayo clinic record-linkage: contribution to neuroepidemiology. *Neuroepidemiology* 1: 102–114.

Lainhart WS, Doyle HN, Enterline PE, Henschel A, Kendrick MA, eds. (1969). Pneumoconiosis in Appalachian bituminous coal miners. Washington DC: *USDHEW* Public Health Service Bureau of Occupational Safety and Health.

Lambert R (1965). Sir John Simon, 1816–1904, and English Social Administration. Bristol: McGibbon and Kee: 400–404, 432, 568–569.

Lancet (1868). 2: 223

Lane-Claypon J (1916). Milk and its hygienic relations. London. Longmans, Green and co.

Lane-Claypon J (1926). A further report on cancer of the breast: reports on public health and medical subjects. London: Ministry of Health.

Lane-Claypon J (1926a). Child life investigations: a clinical and pathological study of 1673 cases of dead-births and neo-natal deaths. London: *HMSO*. Medical Research Council. Special Report Series; no. 109.

Langmuir AD (1976). William Farr: founder of modern concepts of surveillance. *Int J Epidemiol* 5: 13–18.

Langmuir AD (1961). Epidemiology of airborne infection. *Bact Rev*; 25: 174.

Laplace P de (1814). Théorie analytique des probabilités. Paris: Courcier.

Last JM (1963). The iceberg: "Completing the clinical picture" in general practice. *Lancet* 6: 28–31.

Last JM, ed. (1988). A dictionary of epidemiology. 2nd ed. New York; Oxford; Toronto: Oxford University Press.

Last JM, ed. (2001). A dictionary of epidemiology. 4th ed. Oxford: Oxford University Press.

Laupacis A, Sackett DL, Roberts RS (1988). An assessment of clinically useful measures of the consequences of treatment. *N Engl J Med* 318: 1728–1733.

Leavitt J (1992). "Typhoid Mary" fights back. Bacteriological theory and practice in early twentieth-century public health. *Isis*; 83: 608–29.

Leck I (1996). McKeown, Record, and the epidemiology of malformations. *Paediatr Perinat Epidemiol*. 10: 2–16.

Ledermann S (1956). Alcool, alcoolisme, alcoolisation. Paris: *INED*.

Lee AM, Fraumeni JF Jr (1969). Arsenic and respiratory tract cancer in man: an occupational study. *J Natl Cancer Ins* 42: 1045–52.

Legendre A (1805). Nouvelles méthodes pour la détermination des orbites des comètes. Paris: Courcier. Cited in Stigler S (1986). The history of statistics. The measurement of uncertainty before 1900. Cambridge, Massachusetts: Harvard University Press.

Levin ML, Goldstein H, Gerhardt PR (1950) Cancer and tobacco smoking: a preliminary report. *J Am Med Assoc* 143: 336–338

Lewinsohn HC, Kennedy CA, Day JE, Cooper PH (1979). Dust control in a conventional asbestos textile factory. *Ann NY Acad Sci* 330: 225–241.

Liddell FD (1988). The development of cohort studies in epidemiology: a review. *J Clin Epidemiol* 41: 1217–1237.

Lilienfeld AM (1976). Foundations of epidemiology. New York: Oxford University Press.

Lilienfeld AM (1982). The Fielding H. Garrison Lecture: Ceteris paribus: the evolution of the clinical trial. *Bull Hist Med* 56: 1–18.

Lilienfeld AM (1983). Wade Hampton Frost: contributions to epidemiology and public health. *Am J Epidemiol* 117: 379–383.

Lilienfeld AM, Lilienfeld DE (1979). A century of case-control studies: progress? *J Chronic Dis* 32: 5–13

Lilienfeld AM, Lilienfeld DE (1980). Foundations of epidemiology. 2nd ed. New York: Oxford University Press.

Lilienfeld AM, Lilienfeld DE (1980a). The French influence on the development of epidemiology. Henry E Sigerist. *Suppl Bull Hist Med* 4: 28–42.

Lilienfeld DE (1978). "The greening of epidemiology": sanitary physicians and the London Epidemiological Society (1830–1870). *Bull Hist Med* 52: 503–528.

Lilienfeld DE (2000). John Snow: the first hired gun? *Am J Epidemiol*; 152: 4–9.

Lilienfeld DE (2003). The first epidemiology textbook, revisited. *Am J Epidemiol* 157: 856–857.

Lilienfeld DE, Lilienfeld AM (1977). Epidemiology: a retrospective study. *Am J Epidemiol* 106: 445–459.

Lind J (1753). A treatise on the scurvy in three parts, containing an inquiry in the nature, causes, and cure of that disease together with a critical and chronological view of what has been published on the subject. Edinburgh: A. Millar.

Linder FE, Grove RD (1947). Vital statistics rates in the United States, 1900–1940. Washington: U.S. Government Printing Office.

Lister J (1870a). Effects of the antiseptic system of treatment upon the salubrity of a surgical hospital. *Lancet* 1: 40–42.

Lister J (1870b). Further evidence regarding the effects of the antiseptic system of treatment upon the salubrity of a surgical hospital. *Lancet* 2: 287–289.

Lloyd JW (1971). Long-term mortality study of steelworkers. 5, Respiratory cancer in coke plant workers. *J Occup Med* 13: 53–68.

Lloyd JW, Ciocco A (1969). Long-term mortality study of steelworkers. 1, Methodology. *J Occup Med* 11: 299–310.

Lombard HL, Doering CR (1928). Cancer studies in Massachusetts. 2. Habits, characteristics and environment of individuals with and without cancer. *N Engl J Med* 195: 481–487.

London County Council (1912). Medical Officer's Annual Report. London: London County Council: 35–40.

Lorenz E (1944). Radioactivity and lung cancer: critical review of lung cancer in miners of Schneeberg and Joachimsthal. *J Natl Cancer Ins* 5: 1–15.

Louis P (1835). Recherches sur les effets de la saignée. Paris: de Mignaret.

Louis PCA (1828). Recherche sur les effets de la saignée dans plusieurs maladies inflammatoires. Archives générales de médecine 18: 321–336.

Louis PCA (1835). Recherches sur les effets de la saignee dans quelques malades inflammatoires, et sur l'action de l'emetique et des vesicatoires dans la pneumonie. Paris: J.B. Balliere.

Louis PCA (1836). Researches on the effects of bloodletting in some inflammatory diseases. Boston: Hilliard, Gray and Company.

Louis P (1837) Recherches sur l'emphysème des poumons. In: Mémoires de la Société Médicale d'Observation: 160–257.

Louis PCA (1844). Researches on phthisis, anatomical, pathological and therapeutical. Transl. by Walter Hayle Walshe. 2nd ed. considerably enlarged. London: The Sydenham Society.

Luckin W (1877). The final catastrope – cholera in London, 1866. *Med Hist* 21: 35–36.

Mackie JL (1965). Causes and conditions. *Am Philosoph Quart* 2: 245–255.

MacMahon B, Pugh TF, Ipsen J (1960). Epidemiologic methods. Boston, MA: Little, Brown & Co.

MacMahon B, Pugh TF (1970). Epidemiology: principles and methods. Boston: Little, Brown and Company.

Magnello ME (1996). Karl Pearson's Gresham Lectures: W.F.R.Weldon, speciation and the origins of Pearsonian Statistics. *Br J Hist Sci* 29: 43–64.

Magnus K, ed. (1981). Trends in cancer incidence: causes and practical implications. Washington: Hemisphere.

Mantel N (1973). Synthetic retrospective studies and related topics. Biometrics 29: 479–486.

Mantel N, Haenszel W (1959). Statistical aspects of the analysis of data from retrospective studies of disease. *J Natl Cancer Inst* 22: 719–748.

Martin RW, Duffy J, Lie JT (1991). Eosinophilic fasciitis associated with use of L-tryptophan: a case control study and comparison of clinical and histopathologic features. *Mayo Clin Proc* 66: 892–898.

Matthews JR (1995a). Quantification and the quest for medical certainty. Princeton: Princeton University Press.

Matthews JR (1995b). Major Greenwood versus Almwroth Wright: contrasting visions of "scientific" medicine in Edwardian Britain. *Bull Hist Med* 69: 30–43.

Mattmueller M (2004). Platters Pestforschung im Zusammenhang mit der zeitgenoessischen Pestpolitik der Stadt Basel. In: Troehler U (ed): Felix Platter (1536–1614) in seiner Zeit. Basel: Schwabe Verlag: pp 53–59.

Mausner JS, Bahn AK (1974). Epidemiology: an introductory text. Philadelphia: Saunders.

Maxcy KF, ed (1941). Papers of Wade Hampton Frost MD A contribution to epidemiological method. New York: The Commonwealth fund. (This is the major source of material for this article).

Mayr EE (1985). The growth of biological thought: Diversity, evolution, and inheritance. Cambridge MA: Belknap Press

McDonald AD, Fry JS, Woolley AJ, McDonald JC (1983). Dust exposure and mortality in an American chrysotile textile plant. *Brit J Industr Med*; 40: 361–367.

McGregor OR (1957). Social research and social policy in the nineteenth century. *Br J Sociol* 8: 146–157.

McNeil WH (1976) Plagues and Poeple. Doubleday.

Medical Research Council (1956). The hazards to man of nuclear and allied radiations. London: Her Majesty's Stationery Office.

Mendelsohn J (1998). How epidemics became complex after World War I. In Lawrence C, Weisz G, eds. Greater than the parts. Holism in biomedicine 1920–1950. Oxford: Oxford University Press: 309–310.

Merton RK, ed. (1957). The student physician. New York: Free Press.

Miettinen OS (1970). Matching and design efficiency in retrospective studies. *Am J Epidemiol* 91: 111–118.

Miettinen OS (1976a). Estimability and estimation in case-control studies. *Am J Epidemiol* 103: 226–235.

Miettinen OS (1976b). Stratification by a multivariate confounder score. *Am J Epidemiol* 104: 609–620.

Miettinen OS (1985). Theoretical epidemiology: principles of occurrence research in medicine. New York: John Wiley & Sons.

Miettinen OS (1999). Etiologic research: needed revisions of concepts and principles. *Scand J Work Envir Health* 25 (6, special issue): 484–490.

Miettinen OS, Cook EF (1981). Confounding, essence and detection. *Am J Epidemiol* 114: 593–603.

Milham S Jr, Strong T (1974). Human arsenic exposure in relation to a copper smelter. *Environ Res* 7: 176–182.

Mill JS (1856). A system of logic (Eight Edition 1881). In: Nagel E (ed): J.S. Mill's Philosophy of Scientific Method. New York: Hafner Publishing Co: 1950

Monson RR (1980). Occupational epidemiology. Boca Raton: CRC Press.

Morabia A (1991). On the origin of Hill's causal criteria. *Epidemiology* 2: 367–369.

Morabia A (1996). P. C. A. Louis and the birth of clinical epidemiology. *J Clin Epidemiol* 49: 1327–1333

Morabia A (2001a). Snow and Farr: a scientific duet. *Soz Praventivmed* 46: 223–224.

Morabia A (2001b). The essential tension between absolute and relative causality. *Am J Public Health* 91: 355–357.

Morabia A (2003). Ferrara 1855: Cholera without epidemiology. *Eur J Epidemiol* 18: 595–597.

Morabia A, Rochat T (2001). Reproducibility of Louis' definition of pneumonia. *Lancet* 358: 1188.

Morabia A, Ten Have T, Landis JR (1995). Empirical evaluation of the influence of control selection schemes on relative risk estimation: the Welsh nickel workers study. *Occup Environ Med* 52: 489–493.

Morabia A, Zhang FF (2004). History of medical screening: from concepts to action. *Postgrad Med J* 80: 463–469.

Morgagni JB (1761). De sedibus et causas morborum per anatomen indegitis, libre quinque. 2 vols. Venetiis, typog: Remondiniana.

Morgenstern H, Kleinbaum DG, Kupper LL (1980). Measures of disease incidence used in epidemiologic research. *Int J Epidemiol* 9: 97–104.

Morris JN (1955). Uses of epidemiology. *Br Med J*: 395–401.

Morris JN (1957). Uses of epidemiology. Edinburgh: E. & S. Livingstone.

Morris JN (1964). Uses of epidemiology. Edinburgh: E. & S. Livingstone.

Morris JN (1970). Uses of epidemiology. 2nd ed. London: E. & S. Livingston.

Muir CS, Waterhouse J, Mack T, Powell J, Whelan S, eds. (1987). Cancer incidence in five continents, vol. V. Lyon: IARC (IARC Sci Publ; no. 88).

Müller FH (1939). Tabakmissbrauch und Lungencarzinom. *Ztschr Krebforsch* 49: 57–85.

Murphy EA (1976). The logic of medicine. Baltimore: Johns Hopkins University Press.

National Academy of Sciences (1956). Biologic effects of atomic radiation. Washington, DC: National Academy of Sciences.

National Tuberculosis Association, Committee on Diagnostic Standards (1940). Diagnostic standards and classification of tuberculosis. 1940 edition. New York: National Tuberculosis Association.

Newell DJ (1962). Errors in the interpretation of errors in epidemiology. *Am J Public Health* 52: 1925–1928.

Newsholme A (1899). The elements of vital statistics. London: Swan Sonnenschein.

Newton I (translated by Cohen B, Whitman A) (1999). [1687] Mathematical principles of natural philosophy. Berkeley, CA: University of California Press.

Nuland SB (1989). Doctors: the biography of medicine. New York: Vintage Books.

Nuttall GFH (1932–35). Sir Ronald Ross. Obituary Notices of Fellows of the Royal Society, 1: 108–115.

Odlroyd D (1986). The arch of knowledge. New York: Methuen.

Ogle W (1885). Letter to the Registrar-General on the mortality in the registration districts of England and Wales during the ten years 1871–80. Supplement to the 45th Annual Report of the Registrar General of Births, Deaths, and Marriages, in England: xxiii.

Oldham PD, Roach SA (1952). A sampling procedure for measuring industrial dust exposure. *Brit J Industr Med*; 9: 112–119.

Osmond C, Gardner MJ (1982). Age, period and cohort models applied to cancer mortality rates. *Stats Med*; 1: 245–259.

Pan American Health Organization (1988) The challenge of epidemiology. Issues and selected readings. Washington: PAHO

Paneth N, Susser E, Susser M (Part II). Origins and early development of the case-control study: Part 1, Early evolution. *Soz Praventivmed* 2002; 47: 282–288.

Paneth N, Susser E, Susser M (Part II). Origins and early development of the case-control study: Part 2, The case-control study from Lane-Claypon to 1950. *Soz Praventivmed* 2002; 47: 359–365.

Paneth N, Vinten-Johansen P, Brody H, Rip M (1998). A rivalry of foulness: official and unofficial investigations of the London cholera epidemic of 1854. *Am J Public Health*; 88: 1545–1553.

Parkes EA (1864). A Manual of practical hygiene. London: J. Churchill: 57.

Parkes EA (1885). Review. *Br Foreign Med Rev*; 15: 449–463.

Parkin DM, Muir CS, Whelan SL, Gao YT, Ferlay J, Powell J, eds. (1992). Cancer incidence in five continents, vol. VI. Lyon: IARC (IARC Sci Publ; no. 120).

Parkin DM, Pisani P, Ferlay J (1993). Estimate of the worldwide incidence of eighteen major cancer in 1985. *Int J Cancer* 54: 594–606.

Parkin DM, Whelan SL, Ferlay J, Raymond L, eds. (1997). Cancer incidence in five continents, vol. VII. Lyon: IARC (IARC Sci Publ; no. 143).

Parkin DM, Whelan SL, Ferlay J, Teppo L,. Thomas DB (2003). Cancer incidence in five continents, vol. VIII. Lyon: IARC Sci Publication.

Pearson K (1900). The grammar of science. 2nd ed London: Adam and Charles Black.

Pearson K (1904). Report on certain enteric fever inoculation statistics. *Br Med J* ii: 1243–1246.

Pearson K (1922). Francis Galton 1822–1922. A centenary appreciation. London: Cambridge University Press.

Pelling M (1978). Cholera: fever and English medicine 1825–1865 Oxford: Oxford University Press.

Pendergrass EP, Lainhart WS, Bristol LJ, Felson B, Jacobson G (1972). Historical perspectives of coal workers' pneumoconiosis in the United States. *Ann NY Acad Sci* 200: 835–854.

Perelman M (1980). Edmonds, Ricardo, and what might have been. *Sci Soc* 44: 82–85.

Peterson MJ (1978). The medical profession in mid-Victorian London. Berkeley, Los Angeles, London: University of California Press.

Peto J, Doll R, Hermon C, Clayton R, Goffe T, Binns W (1985). Relationship of mortality to measures of environmental asbestos pollution in an asbestos textile factory. *Ann Occup Hyg*; 29: 305–335.

Peto J (1980). Lung cancer mortality in relation to measured dust levels in an asbestos textile factory. In: Wagner JC, Davis W, eds. Biological effects of mineral fibres: Lyon: International Agency for Research on Cancer: vol. 2, 829–836.

Piaget J (1967). Logique et connaissance scientifique. Encyclopédie de la Pléiade, Paris: Gallimard.

Piaget J (1970). Genetic Epistemology. New York: Columbia University Press.

Pinto SS, Bennett BM (1963). Effect of arsenic trioxide exposure on mortality. *Arch Environ Health* 7: 583–591.

Pinto SS, McGill CM (1953). Arsenic trioxide exposure in industry. Ind Med Surg 22: 281–287.

Plinius Secundus C (Tr1929). Naturalis historiae. Book 2. In: Bailey KC. The elder Pliny's chapters on chemical subjects. Transl. part 1. London: Arnold.

Plummer GW (1952). Anomalies occurring in children exposed in utero to the atomic bomb in Hiroshima. *Paediatrics*; 10: 687–693.

Polednak AP, Stehney AF, Rowland RE (1978). Mortality among women first employed before 1930 in the U.S. radium dial-painting industry. *Am J Epidemiol* 107: 179–195.

Population Investigation Committee (1948). Maternity in Great Britain. Oxford: Oxford University Press.

Porter D (1991). "Enemies of race": biologism, environmentalism, and public health in Edwardian England. *Vict Stud* 34: 160–177.
Pringle ML, Butler NR, Davie R (1966). 11000 seven-year-olds. London: Longman in ass. With National Children's Bureau.
Puffer RR (1946). Familial susceptibility to tuberculosis. Cambridge, MA: Harvard University Press.
Putnam P (1936). Tuberculosis incidence among white persons and negroes following exposure to the disease. *Am J Hyg*; 24: 536–551.
Ramazzini B (Tr1940). De morbis artificum [1713] Transl. Wright WC. Diseases of workers. Chicago: University of Chicago Press.
Record RG, McKeown T (1949). Congenital malformations of the central nervous system. I. *Br J Soc Med* 3: 183–219.
Record RG, McKeown T (1950). Congenital malformations of the central nervous system. II. Maternal reproductive history and familial incidence. *Br J Soc Med* 4: 26–50.
Redmond CK, Ciocco A, Lloyd JW, Rush HW (1972). Long-term mortality study of steelworkers. 6, Mortality from malignant neoplasms among coke oven workers. *J Occup Med* 14: 621–629.
Reed W, Carroll J. Agramonte A, Lazear JW (1900). The etiology of yellow fever: a preliminary note. Proceedings of the 28th annual meeting of the American Public Health Association.
Registrar-General (1938). Occupational mortality: census of England and Wales. 1931, Decennial supplement, part 2a. London: Her Majesty's Stationer's Office.
Rehn L (1895). Blasengeschwülste bei Fuchsin Arbeitern. *Arch Klin Chir* 50: 588–600.
Report of the Advisory Committee to the Surgeon General of the Public Health Service (1964). Smoking and Health. Washington, D.C.: U.S. Department of Health, Education and Welfare.
Review. Lancet 1852; 1: 268.
Riley JD (1993). Measuring morbidity and mortality. In: Kiple KF, ed. The Cambridge world history of human disease. Cambridge: Cambridge University Press: 230–238.
Roberts RS, Spitzer WO, Delmore T, Sackett DL (1978). An empirical demonstration of Berkson's bias. *J Chronic Dis* 31: 119–128.
Robins J, Greenland S (1986). The role of model selection in causal inference from nonexperimental data. *Am J Epidemiol* 123: 392–402.
Robinson WS (1950). Ecological correlations and the behavior of individuals. *Am Sociol Rev* 15: 351–357.
Roe DA (1973). "A Plague of Corn". The social history of pellagra. Ithaca: Cornell University Press.
Rose G (1981). Strategy of prevention: lessons from cardiovascular disease. *Br Med J* (Clin Res Ed) 282: 1847–1851.
Rose G (1994). The strategy of preventive medicine. New York: Oxford University Press.
Rose G, Day S (1990). The population mean predicts the number of deviant individuals [see comments]. BMJ 301: 1031–1034.
Rosen G (1958). A history of public health. New York: MD Publications, Inc.

Ross R (1911). Some quantitative studies in epidemiology. *Nature* 1911; 87: 466–467.
Ross RK, Yuan J-M, Yu MC, et al. (1992). Urinary aflatoxin biomarkers and risk of hepatocellular carcinoma. *Lancet*; 339: 943–946.
Roth D (1976). The scientific basis of epidemiology: an historical and philosophical enquiry. [Thesis]. Berkeley: University of California: 91.
Rothman KJ (1976). Causes. *Am J Epidemiol* 104: 587–592.
Rothman KJ (1986). Modern epidemiology. Boston: Little Brown and Co.
Rothman KJ (ed) (1988). Causal inference. Boston: Epidemiology Resources.
Rothman KJ (1996). Lessons from John Graunt. *Lancet* 347: 37–39.
Rothman KJ, Greenland S (1998). Modern epidemiology. 2nd ed. Philadelphia: Lippincott-Raven.
Rothman KJ, Greenland S, Walker AM (1980). Concepts of interaction. Am Epidemiol 112: 467–470.
Rothman KJ, Keller A (1972). The effect of joint exposure to alcohol and tobacco on risk of cancer of the mouth and pharynx. *J Chronic Dis* 25: 711–716.
Royal College of Physicians (1962). Smoking and Health. Summary and Report of the Royal College of Physicians of London on Smoking in Relation to Cancer of the Lung and Other Diseases. New York: Pitman.
Rusnock AA (2002). Vital accounts. Quantifying health and population in eighteenth-Century England and France. Cambridge: Cambridge University Press.
Sackett DL (1979). Bias in analytic research. *J Chron Dis* 32: 51–63.
Sackett DL, Richardson WS, Rosenberg W, Haynes RD (1997). Evidence-based medicine: how to practice and teach EBM. New York: Churchill Livingstone: 148–9.
Saltet RH (1913). Voordrachten over gezondheidsleer. Haarlem: F. Bohn.
Saltet RH (1914). Theorieën en voorbeelden uit den strijd tegen de besmetting. Haarlem: Bohn.
Sandler DP (2000). John Snow and modern-day environmental epidemiology. *Am J Epidemiol*; 152: 1–3.
Sartwell PE, ed. (1965). Section One: Methods in public health and preventive medicine 1. Epidemiology. In: Sartwell PE (ed.): Maxcy-Rosenau: preventive medicine and public health 9th ed. New York: Meredith Publishing Company.
Sartwell PE (1972). Trends in epidemiology. In: Stewart GT, ed. Trends in epidemiology: application to health services research and training. Springfield, Il.: C.C. Thomas: 3–22.
Savage W, Bruce White P (1925a). An investigation of the salmonella group, with special reference to food poisoning. *MRC Spec Rep Ser*: 91.
Savage W, Bruce White P (1925b). Food poisoning: a study of 100 recent outbreaks. *MRC Spec Rep Ser*: 92.
Savage W (1907). Recent work upon the bacteriology of typhoid fever in relation to preventive measures. *Public Health*; 20: 19.
Scapoli C, Guidi E, Angelini L et al. (2003). Sociomedical indicators in the cholera epidemic in Ferrara of 1855. *Eur J Epidemiol* 18: 617–621.

References

Schaffner KF (1993). Discovery and explanation in biology and medicine. Chicago: Chicago University Press.

Schlesselman JJ (1982). Case-control studies. Design, conduct, analysis. New York: Oxford University Press.

Schrek R, Baker LA, Ballard GP, Dolgoff S (1950). Tobacco smoking as an etiologic factor in disease. I. Cancer. *Cancer Res* 10: 49–58.

Schrek R, Lenowitz H (1947). Etiologic factors in carcinoma of the penis. *Cancer Res* 7: 180–187.

Schroedinger E (1994). What is life? Cambridge: Cambridge University Press.

Schwartz S (1994). The fallacy of the ecological fallacy: the potential misuse of a concept and the consequences. *Am J Public Health* 84: 819–824.

Selikoff IJ, Churg J, Hammond EC (1964). Asbestos exposure and neoplasia. *JAMA* 188: 22–26.

Selikoff IJ, Hammond EC, Seidman H (1979). Mortality experience of insulation workers in the United States and Canada, 1943–1976. *Ann NY Acad Med* 330: 91–116.

Shattuck L (1850). Report of a general plan for the promotion of public and personal health, devised, prepared and recommended by the Commissioners Appointed under a resolve of the legislature of Massachusetts relating to a sanitary survey of the state. Boston: Dutton and Wentworth.

Shephard DAE (1995). John Snow: anaesthetist to a Queen and epidemiologist to a nation: a biogra- phy. Cornwall: *York Point Publishing*.

Shimizu Y, Kato H, Schull WJ (1990). Studies of the mortality of A-bomb survivors. Report 9. Mortality, 1950–1985: Part 2. Cancer mortality based on the recently revised doses (DS86). *Radiat Res*: 121: 120–141.

Shryock R (1979). The development of modern medicine. An interpretation of the social and scientific factors involved. Madison, WI: The University of Wisconsin Press.

Silber ALM, Horwitz RL (1986). Detection bias and relation of benign breast disease toi breast cancer. *Lancet* i: 638–640.

Simon J (1856). Report of the last two cholera-epidemics of London, as affected by the consumption of impure water. British Parliamentary Papers (B.P.P.); LIII.

Simon J (1890). English sanitary institutions, reviewed in their course of development, and in some of their political and social relations. London: Cassell: 259–260.

Simon J (1897). English sanitary institutions, reviewed in their cause and development and in some of their political and social relations. 2nd ed. London: Smith, Edler & Co: 263.

Simpson SH (1951). The interpretation of interaction in contingency tables. *J Royal Stat Soc Ser. B* (13): 238–241.

Smith GD, Ebrahim S (2001). Epidemiology – is it time to call it a day? *Int J Epidemiol*; 30: 1–12.

Smith GD, Strobele SA, Egger M (1994). Smoking and health promotion in Nazi Germany. *J Epidemiol Community Health* 48: 220–223.

Smith PG, Rodrigues LC, Fine PE (1984). Assessment of the protective efficacy of vaccines against common diseases using case-control and cohort studies. *Int J Epidemiol* 13: 87–93.

Smithells RW, Nevin NC, Seller MJ, et al. (1983). Further experience of vitamin supplementation for prevention of neural tube defects recurrences. *Lancet* i: 1027–1031.

Snow J (1836a). On the mode of communication of cholera. 2nd ed. reprinted in: Frost WH, ed. Snow on Cholera. New York: The Commonwealth Fund.

Snow J (1836b). Snow on cholera. New York: The Commonwealth Fund. In Delta Omega Classics www.deltaomega.org/ classics.htm. delta omega classics.

Snow J (1849). On the pathology and modes of communication of cholera. *London Medical Gazette* 44: 745–752.

Snow J (1849a). On the mode of communication of cholera. London: J. Churchill: 6–9.

Snow J (1849b). On the pathology and mode of communication of cholera. *London Med Gazette* 9: 745–753 and 923–949.

Snow J (1854). On the mode of communication of cholera. London: Churchill.

Snow J (1855). On the mode of communication of cholera. 2nd edition, much enlarged. London: Churchill.

Southwood Smith T (1830). A treatise on fever. London: Longman, Rees, Orme, Brown and Green.

Sprague TB (1861–62). On the recent imputations made as to Mr. Gompertz's Accuracy. *Assurance Mag* 10: 32–44.

Stellman JM, Kabat G (1978). An assessment of the health effects of arsenic germane to low-level exposure. Report to USEPA Science Advisory Board Study Group, October. Washington DC: U.S. Environmental Protection Agency.

Stellman JM, Stellman SD, Christian R, Weber T, Tomasallo C (2003). The extent and patterns of usage of Agent Orange and other herbicides in Vietnam. *Nature* 422: 681–687.

Stellman SD (Part II). Issues of causality in the history of occupational epidemiology. *Soz Praventivmed* 2003; 48: 151–160.

Stellman SD, Demers PA, Colin D, Boffetta P (1998). Cancer mortality and wood dust exposure among American Cancer Society Cancer Prevention Study-II (CPS-II) participants. *Amer J Indust Med* 34: 229–237.

Stellman SD, Stellman JM, Sommer JF Jr (1988). Combat and herbicide exposure in Vietnam among American legionnaires. *Environ Res* 47: 112–128.

Stolley PD (1991). When genius errs: R.A. Fisher and the lung cancer controversy. *Am J Epidemiol* 133: 416–425.

Susser M (1973). Causal thinking in the health sciences: concepts and strategies of epidemiology. New York: Oxford University Press.

Susser M (1985). Epidemiology in the United States after World War II: The evolution of technique. *Epidemiologic Reviews* 7: 147–177.

Susser M, Adelstein A (1975). An introduction to the work of William Farr. *Am J Epidemiol* 101: 469–476.

Susser M, Adelstein A (1975a). Introduction. Vital statistics: a memorial volume of selections from he Reports and Writings of William Farr (1885). Metuchen, NJ: Scarecrow Press: iii–xiv.

Susser M, Susser E (1996). Choosing a future for epidemiology. II. From black box to Chinese boxes and eco-epidemiology. *Am J Pub Health* 86: 674–677.

Sutter MC (1996). Assigning causation of disease: beyond Koch's postulates. *Persp Biol Med* 39: 581–592.

Sydenham T (1848). The works of Thomas Sydenham. Transl. from the Latin by Dr. Greenhill. London: Sydenham Society.

Sydenstricker E (1926). A study of illness in a general population group. Hagerstown morbidity studies n.1: the method of study and general results. *Public Health Rep* 41: 2069–2088.

Sykes B (2002) The seven daughters of Eve. New York: W.W. Norton & Company

Szklo M, Nieto FJ (2000). Epidemiology: beyond the basics. Gaithersburg: Aspen Publishers.

Taubes G (1995). Epidemiology faces its limits. *Science* 269: 164–169.

Taylor I, Knowelden J (1964). Principles of epidemiology. Boston: Little, Brown & Co.

Terracini B, Zanetti R (Part II). A short history of pathology registries, with emphasis on cancer registries. *Soz Praventivmed* 2003; 48: 3–10.

Terris M (1964). Goldberger on Pellagra. Baton Touge: Louisiana State University.

Terris M (1997). Re: "Morton Levin (1904–1995): history in the making". *Am J Epidemiol* 146: 365.

Thackrah CT (1832). The effects of the arts, trades and profession, and of civic states and habits of living, on health and longevity. London: Longman, Rees, Orme, Brown and Green

The Committee for Scientific Inquiries. Report in relation to the cholera-epidemic of 1854. B.P.P. 1854–55; XXI: 48.

Therapeutic Trial Committee of the Medical Research Council (1934). The serum treatment of lobar pneumonia. *Lancet* 1: 290–295.

Thériault G, Goldberg M, Miller AB, et al. (1994). Cancer risks associated with occupational exposure to magnetic fields among electric utility workers in Ontario and Quebec, Canada, and France, 1970–1989. *Am J Epidemiol*; 139: 550–72.

Thorvaldren P, Kjall A, Kuulasmaak K, et al. (1995). Stroke incidence, case fatality and mortality in the WHO MONICA project. Stroke 26: 361–367.

Tomatis L, ed. (1990). Cancer: causes, occurrence and control. Lyon: IARC (IARC Sci Publ; no. 100).

Toniolo PG, Levitz M, Zeleniuch-Jacquotte A, et al. (1996). A prospective study of endogenous estrogens and breast cancer in postmenopausal women. *J Natl Cancer Inst*; 87: 190–197.

Topley W (1919). The spread of bacterial infections. *Lancet*: 2: 1–5, 45–49, 91–96.

Troehler U (1978). Quantification in British medicine and surgery, 1750–1830, with special reference to its iIntroduction into therapeutics. Thesis/Dissertation, London: University of London.

Troehler U (2000). 'To improve the evidence of medicine': The 18th Century British origins of a critical approach. Edinburgh: Royal College of Physicians.

Troehler U (2003). Cheselden's 1740 presentation of data on age-specific mortality after lithotomy. The James Lind Library: http://www.jameslindlibrary.org/trial_records/17th_18th_Century/cheselden/cheselden_commentary.html. Accessed 04-08-2004.

Tukey JW (1962). The future of data analysis. *Ann Math Stat* 33: 1–67.

Tuormilehto J, Polsc M, Rastenyta D, et al. (1996). Ten-year trends in stroke incidence and mortality in the Finmonica stroke study. Stroke 27: 825–832.

Tuyns AJ (1978). Che cos'è un registro tumori? Epidemiologia e prevenzione 4: 4–7.

U.S. Public Health Service, Division of Public Health Methods and Tuberculosis Control Division. Tuberculosis in the United States, graphic presentation. Vol 2: Proportionate mortality statistics for states and geographic divisions by age, sex and race. Washington: Medical Research Committee, National Tuberculosis Association, 1944.

U.S. Public Health Service, ed. (1964). Smoking and health: a report of the advisory committee to the Surgeon-General of the Public Health Service. Washington DC: USDHEW. *Public Health Service Publication* No 1103.

United Nations Scientific Committee on the Effects of Atomic Radiation. Sources and effects of ionizing radiation. New York: United Nations, 1994. (1994 Report to the General Assembly with scientific annexes).

Urbach P (1993). The value of randomization and control in clinical trials. *Stat Med* 12: 1421–1431.

van Loghem JJ (1935). Algemeene gezondheidsleer. Amsterdam: Kosmos.

van Loghem JJ (1955). Algemeene gezondheidsleer. 5th ed. Amsterdam: Kosmos.

Vandenbroucke JP (1985). On the rediscovery of a distinction. *Am J Epidemiol* 121: 627–628.

Vandenbroucke JP (1988a). Which John Snow should set the example for clinical epidemiology? *J Clin Epidemiol* 41: 1215–1216.

Vandenbroucke JP (1988b). Is "The causes of cancer" a miasma theory for the end of the twentieth century? *Int J Epidemiol* 17: 708–709.

Vandenbroucke JP (1992). Colon cancer and ulcerative colitis: an epidemiologic exercise revisited. *J Clin Epidemiol* 1992; 45: 923–924.

Vandenbroucke JP (2000). Invited commentary: the testimony of Dr. Snow. Am J Epidemiol; 152: 10–12.

Vandenbroucke JP (2001). In defense of case reports and case series. *Ann Intern Med* 134: 330–334.

Vandenbroucke JP (2003). The 1855 cholera epidemic in Ferrara: lessons from old data reanalyzed with modern means. *Eur J Epidemiol* 18: 599–602.

Vandenbroucke JP (Part IIa). Changing images of John Snow in the history of epidemiology. *Soz Praventivmed* 2001; 46: 288–293

Vandenbroucke JP, de Craen AJ (2001). Alternative medicine: a "mirror image" for scientific reasoning in conventional medicine. *Ann Intern Med* 135: 507–13.

Vandenbroucke JP, Eelkman Rooda HM, Beukers H (1991). Who made John Snow a hero? *Am J Epidemiol* 133: 967–973.

Vandenbroucke JP, Vandenbroucke-Grauls CMJE (1988). A note on the history of the calculation of hospital statistics. *Am J Epidemiol* 127: 699–702.

Vandenbroucke JP, Vandenbroucke-Grauls CMJE (1996). In defense of Farr and Nightingale. *Ann Intern Med* 125: 1014.

Vandenbroucke JP, Vandenbroucke-Grauls CMJE (1997). A return to Farr and Nightingale. *Ann Intern Med* 127: 170–171.
Vineis P (Part IIa). History of bias. *Soz Praventivmed* 2002; 47: 156–161.
Vineis P (Part IIb). Causality in epidemiology. *Soz Praventivmed* 2003; 48: 80–87.
Vineis P, Caporaso N (1995). Tobacco and cancer: epidemiology and the laboratory. *Environ Health Persp* 103: 156–160.
Vinten-Johansen P, Brody H, Paneth N, Rackman S, Rip M (with Zuck D) (2003). Cholera, Chloroform and the Science of Medicine: A Life of John Snow. New York: Oxford University Press.
Virchow R (1985). Collected essays on public health and epidemiology. Rather LJ, ed. Canton, MA: Science History Publications.
Visconti L (1870). Protocollo generale delle necropsie eseguite nell' Istituto Anatomo Patologico dell' Ospedale Maggiore. Milan, Ospedale Maggiore.
von Engelhardt D (1993). Causality and conditionality in medicine around 1900. In: Delkeskamp-Hayes C, Gardell Cutter MA, eds. Science, technology, and the art of medicine. Dordecht: Kluwer: 75–104.
von Pettenkofer M (1887). Zum gegenwärtigen Stand der Cholerafrage. München: von Oldenbourg.
von Wright GH (1957). Logical studies. London: Routledge and Kegan Paul.
Wacholder S, Rothman N, Caporaso N (2000). Population stratification in epidemiologic studies of common genetic variants and cancer: quantification of bias. *J Natl Cancer Inst* 92: 1151–1158.
Wagner G (1991). History of cancer registration. In: Jensen OM, MacLennan R, Muir CS, Skeet RG, eds. Cancer registration, principles and methods. Lyon: IARC (IARC Sci Publ; no. 95).
Wagoner JK, Archer VE, Carroll BE, Holaday DA, Lawrence PA (1964a). Cancer mortality patterns among U.S. uranium miners and millers, 1950 through 1962. *J Natl Cancer Ins* 32: 787–801.
Wagoner JK, Archer VE, Carroll BE, Holaday DA, Lawrence PA (1964b). Mortality patterns among United States uranium miners and millers, 1950–1962; preliminary report. In: Radiological health and safety in mining and milling of nuclear materials. Vol. 1. Vienna: International Atomic Energy Agency: 37–48.
Wagoner JK, Archer VE, Lundin FE, Holaday DA, Lloyd JW (1965). Radiation as a cause of lung cancer among uranium miners. *N Engl J Med* 273: 181–188.
Wald NJ, Idle M, Boreham J, Bailey A (1980). Low serum vitamin A and subsequent risk of cancer. *Lancet*; 2: 813–815.
Wald NJ, Thompson SG, Densem JW, Boreham J, Bailey A (1987). Serum beta-carotene and subsequent risk from cancer: results from the BUPA study. *Brit J Cancer*; 57: 428–433.
Walford C (1873). Edmonds, Thomas Rowe. Insurance Cyclopaedia London: C. & E. Llayton, vol. 2: 470–474.
Warner JH (1998). Against the spirit of system: the French impulse in nineteenth-century American medicine. Princeton: Princeton University Press.

Waterhouse J, Muir CS, Correa P, Powell J, eds. (1976). Cancer incidence in five continents, vol. III. Lyon: IARC (IARC Sci Publ; no. 15).

Waterhouse J, Muir CS, Powell J, Shanmugaratnam K, eds. (1982). Cancer incidence in five continents, vol. IV. Lyon: IARC (IARC Sci Publ; no. 42).

Weinberg W (1913). Die Kinder der Tuberkulosen. Leipzig: Hirzel.

Weingarten S (2003). Food in Daniel 1:1–16: the first controlled experiment? The James Lind Library: http://www.jameslindlibrary.org/trial_records/bc/daniel/daniel_commentary.html. Accessed 04/06/2004

Weiss HA, Darby SC, Doll R (1994). Cancer mortality following x-ray treatment for ankylosing spondylitis. *Int J Cancer*; 59: 327–338.

White C (1990). Research on smoking and lung cancer: a landmark in the history of chronic disease epidemiology. *Yale J Biol Med* 63: 29–46.

Whitehead H (1855). Mr. Whitehead's Report of his Special Investigation of Broad Street. In Cholera Inquiry Committee. Report of the Cholera Outbreak in the Parish of St. James, Westminster, during the Autumn of 1854. London: Churchill.

Wiehl D (1974). Edgar Sydenstricker: A Memoir. In: Kasius RV (ed.): The Challenge of facts. Selected public health papers of Edgar Sydenstricker. New York: Prodist

Windeler J, Lange S (1995). Events per person year – a dubious concept. BMJ 310: 454–6. (http://bmj.com/cgi/content/full/310/6977/454). (accessed May 2003).

Winkelstein W, Jr. (1995). A new perspective on John Snow's communicable disease theory. *Am J Epidemiol* 142: S3–S9.

Winkelstein W, Jr. (2002). From the editor: The first epidemiology textbook? Am J Epidemiol 156: 684.

Winkelstein W, Jr. (2003). From the editor: The first epidemiology textbook? –continued. *Am J Epidemiol* 157: 855.

Wold H (1956). Causal inference from observational data. *J Royal Stat Soc* (A) 119: 28–61.

Wood P (1950) Congenital heart disease; a review of its clinical aspects in the light of experience gained by means of modern techniques. *Br Med J*; 2: 639–645, 693–698.

Woodhead GS (1915). Preventive inoculation. *J Royal Sanit Inst* 36: 22–23.

World Health Organization (1950). WHO Rep Ser. Geneva: WHO 23: 18–27.

Wynder E, Graham E (1950). Tobacco smoking as a possible etiologic factor in bronchiogenic carcinoma: a study of six hundred and eighty-four proved cases. JAMA 143: 329–336.

Wynder EL (1996). Invited commentary: response to Science article "Epidemiology faces its limits". *Am J Epidemiol* 143: 747–749

Wynder EL (1997). Tobacco as a cause of lung cancer: some reflections. *Am J Epidemiol* 146: 687–694.

Yerushalmy J, Palmer CE (1959). On the methodology of investigations of etiologic factors in chronic diseases. *J Chronic Dis* 10: 27–40.

Yule GU (1903). Notes on the theory of association of attributes in statistics. *Biometrika* 2: 121–134.

Zeger SL (1991). Statistical reasoning in epidemiology. *Am J Epidemiol* 134: 1062–1066.

Zeidberg LD, Gass RG, Dillon A, Hutcheson RH (1963). The Williamson County Study. A twenty-four-year epidemiologic study. *Am Rev Respir Dis*; 87 (No. 3, Part 2): 1–88.

Zenker FA (1867). Über Staubinhalationskrankheiten der Lungen. *Arch Clin Med* 2: 116–171.

Zhang FF, Michaels DC, Mathema B et al. (Part II). Evolution of some epidemiologic methods and concepts in selected textbooks of the 20th Century. *Soz Präventivmed* 2004; 49: 97–104.

Index of persons

Agricola, G 277
American Cancer Society Study 62, 119
Andvord, KF 227, 245, 274
Appalachian Bituminous Coal Miners Study 278
Arbuthnot, J 84
Archimedes 91
Aristotle 91, 345

Babes, A 335
Baker, WM 299, 353
Ballard, E 203
Barry, WF 201
Beal, LS 138
Berkson, J 65, 67, 88, 332
Bernard, C 108, 180, 315, 316, 338, 345
1946 birth cohort 260
Bishop, EL 225
Blalock, HM 318, 323
Blane, G 36
Bohr, N 92
Bradford, A = Hill, AB
British doctors study 62, 119, 191, 251, 259
Broad Street 130, 131, 142, 146, 298
Broders, AC 300
Broussais, FJV 37-39
Brown, C 269, 280
Brown, L 226
Brownlee, J 211, 212, 216
Budd, W 130, 144, 200, 353

Campbell, DT 318
Case, RAM 276
Céline, F 338
Celsus 160
Chadwick, E 295
Ciocco, A 284
Claypon, JL = Lane-Claypon, J 115, 291, 301
Clemmesen, J 235
Coleman, W 201
Comte, A 109
Cornfield J 75-79, 82, 117, 120, 296, 315, 318, 324, 329
Corvisart, JN 97
Creighton, C 145, 146, 208

D'Amador, BJIR 108
Daniel 96, 314
Dawber, TR 258
Doll, R 60, 62, 118, 119, 191, 220, 308
Dormanns, E 247
Dorn, H 122, 234, 235, 242
Douglas, JWB 260
Duncan, W 135

Edmonds, TR 149, 152, 161, 180, 184, 197
Eijkman, C 111, 327
Einstein, A 92, 106

Farr, W 16, 30, 39, 40, 85, 98, 106, 107, 111, 129, 133, 134, 137, 149, 152, 154, 156, 159, 179, 183, 191, 192, 195, 200, 208, 218, 251, 295
Feinleib, M 335
Feinstein, AR 333
Fibiger, J 86
Finlaison, J 150
Fisher, RA 58, 88, 315, 317, 318, 347
Fisher, REW 263
Framingham Heart Study 25, 26, 119, 258
Frost, WH 53, 55, 59, 85, 112, 114, 116, 142, 146, 223, 244, 261, 263

Galen 68
Galilei, G 92
Galton, F 181, 207, 209
Garrison, F 145, 179
Gas-workers' study 262
Gerhard, WW 293
Goldberger, J 48-50, 52, 85, 86, 113, 116, 251, 300, 310
Gompertz, B 153, 155
Gordis, L 352
Gordon, JE 5
Graham, EA 60, 255, 304, 306
Graham, T 138

397

Index of persons

Graunt, J 10, 11, 30, 48, 83, 100, 107
Greenland, S 30, 79, 315, 348, 352
Greenwood, E 204, 303
Greenwood, M 45, 46, 68, 94, 112, 115, 116, 145, 181, 193, 205-207, 210-213, 217, 219, 296, 300, 302, 352, 353-356, 363
Guy, WA 111, 299, 328

Haenszel, W 318, 321, 322
Hamer, W 204, 214
Hammond, EC 62, 63, 69, 119, 254, 286, 318
Hempel, CG 337, 339, 340
Henle, J 293, 346
Hill, AB 19, 45, 56, 60, 62, 72, 102, 103, 113, 116, 119, 191, 206, 216, 219, 251, 253, 262, 280, 296, 308, 317, 352, 353, 356
Himsworth, H 251
Hippocrates 93, 94, 97, 159, 160, 179, 208, 293, 294
Hiroshima 265
Holmes, S 98, 101
Horn, D 62, 119, 254
Hume, D 100, 103
Hutchinson, GB 335

IARC 237, 240
Ipsen, J 352, 363

Jurin, J 84

Kelsey, J 352
Kennaway, EL 262
Kennaway, NM 262

Kish, L 315, 317
Klebs, E 338
Kleinbaum, DG 21, 352
Koch, R 102, 143, 144, 146, 203, 341, 346
Korteweg, R 246, 249
Kupper, LL 21, 352

Lane-Claypon, J 115, 291, 301
Laplace, PS 180
Ledermann, S 7
Legendre, A 180
Leishman, W 205
Levin, ML 59, 305
Liebig, J 134, 138
Life Span Study 265
Lilienfeld, AM 73, 114, 117, 314, 318, 352, 353, 357
Lilienfeld, DE 352, 357
Lind, J 33, 34, 84, 105, 275
Lister, J 108
Lloyd, W 284
London Epidemiological Society 112, 199
Louis, PCA 38, 39, 84-86, 106, 108, 109, 180, 196, 293, 297, 353

Mach, E 339
Mackie, J 342
MacMahon, B 24, 31, 117, 191, 316, 352, 356, 363
Malthus, T 151, 152
Mantel, N 79, 321, 322
Martin, C 211
Marx, K 151
Maxcy, KFK 146, 225
McCulloch, JR 154, 196
McKeown, T 308

Metchnikoff, E 144
Miettinen, OS 21, 32, 79, 121, 192, 315, 322, 331, 339, 352, 357, 359
Mill, JS 100, 296, 315, 316, 317
MONICA 233
Morgagni, JB 293
Morgenstern, H 21, 352
Morris, J 117, 308, 352, 356
Müller, F 304
Murphy, EA 329

Newman, G 205
Newsholme, A 205, 211
Newton, I 17, 92
Nickel refiner's study 262
Nightingale, F 192
Nuttall, GFH 213

Ogle, W 333, 334

Paccini, F 138
Paget, J 299
Palmer, CE 72, 102
Panum, PL 110
Papanicolaou, GN 335
Pasteur, L 138, 341
Pearl, R 221
Pearson, K 59, 86, 113, 204, 207, 209, 211, 212, 221
Peto, R 118
Petty, W 10
Piaget J 89-91, 97, 105, 124
Platter, F 11
Pliny the Elder 277
Popper, K 123, 316, 340
Price, R 153
Puffer, R 225, 226

398

Index of persons

Pugh, TF 24, 316, 352, 356, 363

Queen Victoria 147

Ramazzini, B 277, 295
Reade, WW 98
Record, RG 308
Redmond, C 284
Rickman, J 150
Rogers, W 334
Rose, G 8, 25, 32, 117, 352
Rosen, G 10
Ross, R 209, 216
Rothman, KJ 10, 28, 47, 82, 101, 315, 323, 331, 352, 357
Roux, E 208

Sackett, DL 329, 333
Sartwell, P 73
Savage, W 203, 204
Schlesselman, JJ 66
Schrek, R 305
Schroedinger, E 345
Schuman, L 308
Selikoff, I 69, 286
Semmelweis, IP 110, 337, 339
Shapiro, S 335
Shattuck, L 295

Sherlock = Holmes, S 98, 101
Shimkin, MB 318
Shryock, R 179
Simon, J 133, 145, 200
Simpson, EH 46
Smith, TS 154, 161, 293
Snow, J 14, 30, 39-41, 85, 86, 105-107, 109, 110, 114, 129, 137, 141, 147, 200, 251, 298, 353
Surveillance Epidemiology and End Results (SEER) 236, 237
Susser, M 73, 101, 117, 316, 323, 352, 355, 357
Sydenham, T 97, 208, 293
Sydenstricker, E 48, 85, 86, 113, 116, 224, 226-228, 233, 244, 310
Szklo, M 352

Terris, M 321, 363
Thackrah, CT 295
Thompson, T 202, 213
Topley, WWC 206, 215

UICC 237
University Group Diabetes study 319

US Breast Cancer Detection Demonstration Projects 335

Valkenburg, H 146
Virchow, R 146, 338
Von Pettenkofer, M 143, 146, 147
Von Rokitansky, K 293
Vonderman, A 111

Weinberg, W 251
Welch, WH 224
Weldon, WFR 207, 209
White, B 203
Whitehead, H 298
Whiteman, W 206
WHO 233, 237
Wittgenstein, L 342
Wold, H 323
Wright, A 86, 204, 212, 213, 217, 221
Wynder, EL 60, 87, 255, 304, 306, 318, 319

Yerushalmy, J 72, 102
Yule, GU 43, 44, 85, 116, 205, 214, 353

Zelen, M 335
Zeno 98

Subject index

Absolute risk 65
Affected vs. non-affected 33, 51, 87
Aflatoxin 273
Allocation 319
Analogy 74, 104
Anesthesia 130
Ankylosing spondylitis 266
Antagonism 355
Arsenic 283
Arteriosclerosis 224
Asbestos 69, 70, 220, 270, 286, 288, 342
Aspirin 310
Asthma 161
Atom bomb 263, 267
Attack rate 261
Attributable risk 25, 28, 64, 65, 71, 123, 256

Backward study 253
Bacteriology 200, 201, 203, 206, 208, 214
Belief 100, 102
Beriberi 111, 327
Bias 19, 31, 120, 123, 192, 250, 299, 305, 322, 327, 328, 353, 356, 358
  admission rate 330
  allocation 320
  Berkson's prevalence-incidence 66
  compensated 68
  detection 333
  diagnostic suspicion 330
  diagnostic 250
  exposure suspicion 330
  fallacy 19
  family information 330, 331
  follow-up 31
  information 318, 331, 333
  lead time 335
  length 335
  losses to follow-up 123
  membership 330
  misclassification 120, 354
  misclassification 123
  non-respondent 330
  prevalence-incidence 330
  recall 301, 330
  selection 65, 120, 123, 299, 318, 329, 331
  survivor treatment selection 335
  taxonomy 329
  unmasking 330
  Will Rogers 334
Bible 96
Biological gradient 74, 103
Biological plausibility 103, 104
Biology 103
Biomarkers 272
Biometry 204, 212

Bladder cancer 268, 276
Bloodletting 37, 38, 84
Blood pressure 258, 260
Breast cancer 241, 268, 291, 333
Brain cancer 271, 273
Bulimia 342

Capitalism 151
Cancer 231, 234, 238
Cases 304
  prevalent 303
Case fatality 9
  definition 9
Case-control 60, 354, 356
Case-control study 33, 59, 62, 64-66, 76, 78, 80, 82, 88, 101, 120, 122, 184, 192, 220, 250, 251, 253, 255, 269, 272, 291, 295, 299, 308, 315, 321, 324, 332, 354, 365
  bias 62
  case-base 80
  confounding 321
  first 299, 301
  hospital-based 65, 67, 332
  incidence-density 80
  nested 33, 79, 269,
  sampling fraction 66, 83
  traditional 80
Case-control 355
Case-fatality rate 180

401

Subject index

Causal inference 120, 123, 355, 356
   viewpoints 103
Causality 63, 280, 337
   absolute 63
   relative 63
Cause 28, 101, 102, 144, 345, 358
   causal inference 73
   component 28, 29, 358
   necessary 341
   of cancer 118
   rules 103
   sufficient 28, 29, 358
Census 150, 156
Cervical cancer 241
Chemical dye 276
Cholecystitis 65
Cholera 14-17, 40, 41, 85, 106, 109, 110, 114, 129, 137, 141, 143, 157, 161, 163, 164, 167, 169, 170, 176, 190, 216, 251, 294, 298
Cholerine 136, 138
Cholesterol 25, 258, 260
Cholrads 138
Clinical trials 33, 56, 57, 96-98, 106, 197, 220, 314, 329
   alternate allocation 86
   controlled 33, 58
   random allocation 86
   randomised 33, 58, 329, 331
Coal 262, 278
Coherence 74, 103, 104
Cohort 54, 69, 79, 82, 85, 119, 122, 184, 189, 223, 258, 267, 354, 356
   analysis 55, 116
   birth 54

definition 54
   effect 54, 268
Cohort study 33, 76, 79, 86, 101, 114, 119, 123, 220, 244, 276, 287, 354, 365
   occupational 282
   prospective 33, 251, 253
   retrospective 33, 119, 261, 263, 266
Coke oven 284
Comparison 315
Concepts 5, 124
   definition 5
Concurrent study 250
   See cohort study
Confounding 42, 56, 58, 85, 116, 120, 123, 280, 313, 318, 320, 323, 334, 339, 353-356, 358, 359, 364
   adjustment 52
   alternate allocations 56
   definition 42
   desirable 315
   fallacy 43, 44, 47
   first 317
   restricting 52
   Simpson's paradox 46, 48
Congenital malformations 309
Consistency 73, 103, 104, 280
Control 58, 79
   non-cases 79
   sampling 79
Coronary artery disease 64, 256, 258
Counter fact 97
Cowpox 130, 134

Cross-sectional design 304, 309
Cumulative incidence 21, 22, 32, 80, 122, 191
   definition 21

Diabetes 65
Diet 49
   pellagra 49
Diphteria 208, 220
Dose-response 104, 280
Duration 24, 31, 80, 116, 169, 173, 174, 185, 192

Ecologic studies 353
Ecologic correlations 118, 119
Effect modifier 68, 339
   See interaction
Electromagnetic fields 271
Emphysema 109, 161
Eosinophilia-myalgia 310
Epidemiology 4, 5, 107, 123
   contribution 5
   definitions 116, 120, 123, 124, 224
   High Victorian 199
   mission 4
   phases 124
Epistemology 6, 89, 124, 366
   definition 6
   genetic 89
Eugenics 212, 217
Excess deaths 63
Excess mortality 156
Excess risk 25, 32, 64, 280
Experiment 4, 41, 74, 104
Exposed vs. non-exposed 33, 51, 86

402

Fallacy 353, 365
Fatality 162
Fatality-rates 217
Fever 37
Folic adic 309
Follow-up 79, 80, 186, 192, 234, 261, 267, 321, 365
  loss to 284
Follow-up study 250, 321
Force of morbidity 21
Force of mortality 17, 18, 21, 167, 169, 170, 174, 175, 178, 180, 184, 191
Forward study 253

Gas 270, 276, 281
  mustard 276, 281
Group comparisons 6
  definition 6

Hazard 180, 185
Healthy worker effect 333, 334
Hemolytic anemia 68
Hepatitis B 273,
Heredity 218
Hippocrates 93
  hippocratic texts 93
History 214, 221, 314

Imprecision 328
Incidence 9, 23, 24, 64, 113, 116, 236, 238, 240, 250, 354
  definition 9
  prevalence 24
Incidence density 21, 22, 32, 80, 122, 365
Incidence rate 76, 77, 82, 185, 191, 192, 217, 241, 246

Individual thinking 7
  definition 7
Inoculation 204
  anti-typhoid 204
Influenza 215, 217
Insanity 165
Interaction 120, 123, 343, 355, 356, 359, 364
  additive 123, 289
  antagonism 68
  biological 72
  definition 68
  higher order 317
  individual decision-making 72
  multiplicative 71, 123, 289
  public health 72, 123
  statistical 71
  synergy 68

Kuru 327

Law of death 171
Law of large numbers 180
Law of mortality 153, 154, 197
Least squares regression 180
Leeches 37
Leukaemia 24, 264, 266, 271
Life insurance 149
Life table 153, 155, 156, 181, 184, 191, 197, 218, 225, 280
Lip cancer 300
Liver cancer 274
Logic 105
Longitudinal study 250
Lung cancer 58-62, 64, 76, 87, 102, 118, 120, 121, 220, 246, 248, 251, 253, 262, 268, 270, 276, 279, 283, 284, 289, 304, 306, 310, 315, 318, 342
Lymphomas 343

Malaria 209
Matching 123, 322
Mathematics 90, 105, 207
Measles 110, 167
Medicine 159, 160, 203, 211, 221, 251, 275, 291, 309, 328, 337, 349
MEDLINE 292
Menu surveillance 202
Mesothelioma 287, 342
Methods 4
  definition 4
Miasma 145
Miasmatic 137, 147
Mining 277
Mortality 9
  definition 9
Mortality difference 70
Myocardial infarction 253

Nested case-control studies 123
  See case-control study
Nickel 262
Nosology 134
Number needed to treat 28

Obesity 342
Occupation 270, 275
Odds 8, 9, 25, 76, 83, 185
  definition 8, 9
  prevalence 25

Odds Ratio   64, 66, 76, 77, 79, 81, 82, 83, 120, 192, 271, 272, 299, 321, 324, 333, 348
  case-base   82
  incidence density   82
  traditional   82
Opsonic index   213
Outbreak   130, 199, 208
Outbreak investigations   130, 200
Oyster   202

Pellagra   49-52, 85, 251, 300
  niacin   52
Penile cancer   303
Period   268
  effect   267
Person-times   19, 20, 22, 80, 187, 188, 192, 193, 253, 261, 288
  man-years   253, 263
Person-years   19, 20, 22, 288
Phthisis   16, 159, 161, 170, 190, 297
Physics   90, 91, 105, 121, 328, 348
Physiology   130
Plague   11-13, 83, 157, 294
Plausibility   74
Pneumoconiosis   278
Pneumonia   38, 57, 161
Population thinking   5, 7
  definition   5
  predictions   7
Poverty   50
  pellagra   50
Precision   328

Prevalence   9, 23, 64, 113, 117, 235, 240
  definition   9
  incidence   24
Prevention   27, 32
  paradox   27
Preventive trials   251
Probability   99, 100, 160, 162, 173, 174, 178, 185
  two usages   100
Prognosis   159, 166
Proportion   12, 15, 30, 76, 77, 83, 160, 168, 185, 186, 247, 299
Proportional mortality ratio   283
Prospective study   78, 226, 233, 250, 253, 267
  See cohort
Puerperal fever   110, 339

Radiation   264, 267, 279, 281
Radon   281
Radiotherapy   266
Randomisation   220, 221, 318, 320, 329
  randomised trial   335
Rare disease assumption   82, 88, 123, 192
Rates   9, 13, 17, 18, 22, 30, 53, 70, 107, 116, 122, 153-155, 160-162, 164, 165, 169, 176, 178, 181, 183, 184, 187, 188, 191, 193, 226-228, 252, 253, 261, 288, 334
  adjusted   50
  age-specific   156
  cross-sectional   54
  definition   9
  standardised   50, 116

Ratio   8, 9, 12, 14, 63, 70, 81, 82, 114, 180, 184, 191, 258,
  definition   8, 9
  excess mortality   256
Reference group   35
Registries   88, 231, 233, 240
Relative incidence rates   79
Relative odds   299
Relative risk   51, 64, 71, 76, 77, 79, 82, 110, 111, 120, 122, 123, 132, 265, 274, 319
Retrospective   253
Retrospective study   59, 78, 86, 122, 292, 308
  See case-control
  synthetic   79
Risk difference   64
Risks   8, 9, 17, 19, 21, 29, 30, 39, 51, 107, 122, 183, 191, 193, 226, 250, 258, 324
  definition   8, 9

Scarlet fever   213
Screening   120, 335
Scurvy   33, 34, 36, 105
Serum treatment   57
Simpson's paradox   354
Smallpox   18, 130, 134, 146, 154, 157, 161, 163, 172, 181, 185, 190, 195, 212, 341
Smoking   59, 60, 62, 64, 76, 88, 102, 120, 191, 220, 251, 254, 258, 304, 310, 315, 342
Sociology   118

Subject index

Specificity 74, 103, 104, 281
Standard 156
  Healthy Districts 156
Standardised mortality ratio 263, 277, 282, 284, 285, 334
SMR 284, 285
Statistical test 74
Statistics 10, 121, 149, 180, 196, 200, 203, 208, 211, 212, 216, 218, 221,
  origin 10
Strength of association 29, 73, 103, 104
Survey 86, 236, 251
Synergy 71, 289, 355
  See interaction
Syphilis 130, 134, 169

Temporality 74, 103, 104
Textbook 86, 112, 120, 121, 191, 262, 294, 315, 323, 331, 352, 358, 361, 362
Tobacco 253
Toxic-shock syndrome 310
Trohoc 329, 365
Tuberculosis 16, 17, 53, 85, 201, 213, 220, 223, 244, 253, 261, 286, 297, 341, 344
Twins 58
Typhoid 86, 201, 202, 203, 216
Typhoid fever 144, 196, 293
Typhus 179, 206, 215, 293

Uranium 279

Vaccination 168, 341
Vaginal adenocarcinoma 310
Validity 331
Varicella 168
Vital statistics 129, 149, 152, 184, 195, 207, 252, 267, 295
Vitamin A 273
Vitamin B1 111
Vitamin C 36

Whooping cough 220

Yellow fever 294

Zymads 138
Zymotic 134, 155

405

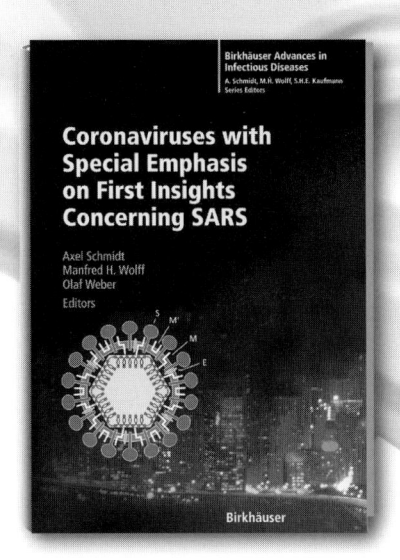

Where quality meets scientific research...

Birkhäuser

Schmidt, A. / Wolff, M. H. / Weber, O., all University Witten/Herdecke, Germany (Eds.)

Coronaviruses with Special Emphasis on First Insights Concerning SARS

2005. Approx. 300 pages. Hardcover
ISBN 3-7643-6462-9
BAID - Birkhäuser Advances in Infectious Diseases

The outbreak of SARS (Severe acute respiratory syndrome), an atypical pneumonia, has received much attention and coverage by the media and has consequently had a high impact on the public. The infectivity and route of transmission of the disease appear unusual, and it turned out to be a highly relevant threat for medical staff.

This monograph provides comprehensive information on the newest insights into the SARS epidemic and the responsible infectious agent. Background information on Coronaviridae (coronavirus/torovirus) and coronavirus/torovirus-associated infections in humans and animals is also given.

The volume will be a valuable source of information for researchers and clinicians in virology, epidemiology and biomedicine.

For orders originating from all over the world except USA and Canada:
Birkhäuser Verlag AG
c/o SAG GmbH & Co
Haberstrasse 7
D-69126 Heidelberg
Fax: +49 / 6221 / 345 4 229
e-mail: sales@birkhauser.ch
http://www.birkhauser.ch

For orders originating in the USA and Canada:
Birkhäuser
333 Meadowland Parkway
USA-Secaucus
NJ 07094-2491
Fax: +1 201 348 4505
e-mail: orders@birkhauser.com